The
HUMAN SKELETON
In
FORENSIC MEDICINE

The
HUMAN SKELETON
In
FORENSIC MEDICINE

Third Printing

By

WILTON MARION KROGMAN, Ph.D., LL.D. (h.c.)

Professor of Physical Anthropology
Graduate School of Medicine
University of Pennsylvania
Director, Philadelphia Center for
  Research in Child Growth
Philadelphia, Pennsylvania

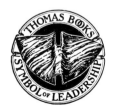

CHARLES C THOMAS · PUBLISHER

Springfield · Illinois · U.S.A.

Published and Distributed Throughout the World by
CHARLES C THOMAS • PUBLISHER
Bannerstone House
301-327 East Lawrence Avenue, Springfield, Illinois, U.S.A.

First Printing, 1962
Second Printing, 1973
Third Printing, 1978

With THOMAS BOOKS *careful attention is given to all details of
manufacturing and design. It is the Publisher's desire to present books that
are satisfactory as to their physical qualities and artistic possibilities and
appropriate for their particular use.* THOMAS BOOKS *will be true to those
laws of quality that assure a good name and good will.*

Printed in the United States of America

To

T. Wingate Todd

With Whom I Studied

and

From Whom I Learned

Preface

This book is the result of some thirty years of experience, not only with human skeletal material, per se, but with the identification of unknown bones. The theme of intrinsic variability and its range has been a major concern during all this time. As a result there is a constant emphasis in this book upon the *reliability* of the many different determinations to be made when solving, as it were, for "x, the unknown."

In 1958–59 I began unearthing and checking source material pertinent to a book such as this. With the aid of two of my graduate students, Mr. William Haviland and Mr. Wayne O. Wallace, Jr., I selected data from every major anatomical and anthropological journal from date of founding onward: American, English, German, French, Italian, Portuguese. The libraries of the University of Pennsylvania, including the University Museum, were opened to me. Mr. Elliott Morse, Librarian of the College of Physicians of Philadelphia, was very helpful, and the College Library was a veritable "Comstock Lode" of original references. Wherever I have cited an opinion, or used a Table or an illustration, I have given full and complete source credit.

The manuscript was typed by Mrs. Harry Jackson. It was proof-read with me by Mr. Francis E. Johnston. With their competent aid I am sure that all basic data are factually correct.

I have tried to make this book as broad and as complete in its application as I possibly could. The inclusion of data was terminated as of Dec. 31, 1960. If this book is generally useful then I have labored well. If it has any shortcomings I hope they may be called to my attention for I accept full and complete responsibility for form, style, and content of this book.

WILTON MARION KROGMAN

Contents

List of Illustrations

List of Tables

The
HUMAN SKELETON
In
FORENSIC MEDICINE

I.

Introduction

GENERAL STATEMENT OF SCOPE AND PROBLEMS

This book will deal with *bones* only. While I recognize the importance of *teeth* in forensic medicine I have decided that they are the subjects of a volume of their own. Hence, the dentition will be mentioned merely in passing. In dealing with bones I shall limit myself to the skeletal remains of deceased persons only. I shall, of course, discuss correlative evidence gained from studies of the living, but in the main medicolegal cases involving the bones of a living individual should in most cases be the concern of the orthopedist, the roentgenologist, and the pathologist.*

What, then, is the purpose, the aim, of this book?

First and foremost, it will not make the reader an "expert" in the field of the identification of human skeletal remains. It is my hope to acquaint the law enforcement agencies of the world with what the bones tell and how they tell it. This is to say, I hope to answer questions as to types of information gained from the bones; moreover, answer in terms of absolute and/or relative reliability, so far as this can be done. I do not flatter myself that this is a he-who-runs-and-reads-may-learn kind of book. It is a meaty, specialized, questioning, and evaluating exposition of our present

---

* I would make several exceptions here. I have been a consultant in several hundred adoption cases of unknown or suspect paternity, i.e., racial background. Here the problem is the possible presence or nonpresence of genes other than Caucasoid ("white"). A subsidiary problem may be skeletal age and evaluation of maturational status. I have also worked on immigration cases (non-Caucasoid) where chronological age is uncertain and skeletal age became of import in the assessment of whether the individual was under or over 21 years of age. These are special cases, not ordinarily within the scope of a book such as this, although Chapter II is certainly pertinent.

3

state of knowledge. It is not definitive, in whole or in part, for there are too many lacunae in our studies, our experiences, and our testings. It is a fact to be noted that much of the data we use for age, for sex, for race, in the bones were collected without medicolegal objectives firmly in view. For the most part, we must rely upon the studies of extensive dissecting-room populations, which are notoriously biased samples of the total population. Hence, we must always face the question, "How valid, to begin with, *are* our so-called norms for age, for sex, for race, for stature, . . .?" I hope to cope with this problem in terms of variability and reliability as we go from Chapter to Chapter.

In every sense, therefore, this book is a guide, a *vade mecum*, a reference book. (Hooton, '43, Snow, '48, Stewart, '51, and Brues, '58, have sketched this concept succinctly.) It will not have the elaborate, detailed precision of the Bertillon ('89) system (see also Wilder and Wentworth, '18, Morland, '50, Rhodes, '56). The bones simply do not lend themselves to Bertillon's quasi-shorthand system of cataloguing slight variations as for eyes, nose, lips, ears and so on.

While I am at it I may as well state certain other limitations. When bones are brought in for identification the first sorting-out should be human vs. non-human.* This book assumes that a comparison must be made, by the investigator, wherever there is a doubt. By this I mean that texts in comparative and human anatomy should be available as collateral references. In this book I offer Appendix I which is a brief over-view of the human skeleton and its parts.

From time to time I shall refer to certain dimensions or measurements of the skull or long bones of the human skeleton. In some parts of the book, notably with reference to the pelvis, I have cited measuring technique in some detail. In the main, however, I have taken the stand that this is not a book on bone-measuring. The investigator should have access to certain texts in physical anthropology (see References, Chapter VII). In Appendix II I offer definitions of the more common measurements referred to in this book.

* Stewart ('59) writes of the disconcerting similarities between the skeleton of bear-paws and human hands and feet. A useful general reference on non-human bones is that of Cornwall ('56).

The identification of human skeletal remains is a critical matter. A *fully qualified specialist* in this area must be extremely well grounded in comparative osteology, human osteology, craniometry and osteometry, and racial morphology. Moreover, he must have had extensive experience with the study of large series of human skeletal material. In this book I shall refer to the Todd Collection (Dept. Anatomy, Western Reserve University, Cleveland, Ohio) and The Terry Collection (Dept. Anatomy, Washington University, St. Louis, Mo.) as the best sources to study American white and American Negro skeletal material. Museums in Washington, D.C. (U.S. National Museum), New York (American Museum of Natural History), Boston (Peabody Museum, Harvard University) and Chicago (Chicago Natural History Museum) will round out the picture for the American Indian. This gives coverage for Caucasoid, Negroid, Mongoloid as represented in America. In addition, of course, there is in the Museums skeletal material (mostly skulls) representing the peoples of the world. Abroad there are excellent Museums in London, Paris, Berlin, Munich, and Rome, as major examples. I am sure that there are many others in the world (notably S. Africa, India, Japan) that I do not know from personal experience. I stress all these collections of human skeletons for one reason: they are extensive enough to convey important information concerning the *extreme variability* which is manifest in all aspects of identification: in size, shape, sex differences, age criteria, racial traits, and so on. To identify a single lot of bones one must be able to fit it accurately into a tremendous jigsaw puzzle within the total range of variation.*

All this training and background is to be found within the ranks of those who have qualified as Physical Anthropologists. This is not to say that all Physical Anthropologists are "bone-ologists," but merely to say that those who have specialized in skeletal studies are pretty apt to be qualified for identification consultation.

Up to this point I've been rather on the negative side of the picture. It is time, now, to turn to more positive considerations.

* Here again, I impose another limitation. I do not feel it my obligation to write about statistics. I have used the mean, the standard deviation, the standard error, the coefficient of correlation, assuming that the reader knows these or will go to an elementary text to define them. Where I've referred to elaborate statistics, as in variance, I've cited authorities in the *References*.

The whole theme of death-to-life reconstruction is presented in Chapters IX and X. The skull-to-head theme has been pretty well developed, employing osteology and osteometry plus soft tissue studies, and utilizing recently developed roentgenographic cephalometric techniques. As for miscellaneous criteria of individuality, they must be handled on a case-to-case basis as they turn up. I have, as an example, considered amputations in Chapter VIII.

It is obvious that all the mechanics of skeletal identification must focus upon an individual, a single human being. We measure in the mass; we identify an isolate, i.e., we have to pick out one from the total. We are not investigating in the usual case, 100 deaths, but one at a time! As we apply each set of criteria, each norm, as age, sex, race, stature, etc., the problem of reliability emerges, in terms of the relative variability of each set of data. We shall find that not only do these sets of criteria differ in reliability, but that, in addition, the same set may differ with respect to the completeness of the available skeletal material, the age factor, and so on.

In this book it will appear that too much information has been concentrated upon two major groups, American white and American Negro. This is not accidental, for it is a reflection that basic studies have been founded on these two peoples. We know they are mixed; the whites a blend of the many European races and nations that have come to the U. S., the Negroes a blend of their West African ancestry, plus white, plus American Indian admixture. I have studied the skeletal remains of all races at the Hunterian Museum at the Royal College of Surgeons, London, England, and the admirable von Luschan Collection of African material at the American Museum of Natural History. But all this does not preclude the fact that the norms I use are of the two groups above mentioned.

This leads me to another problem to which I now turn but which I certainly won't solve, viz., the problem of race-mixture as it may show up in the skeleton (see Todd, '29, Krogman, '36). Our knowledge is very uncertain, for we don't know enough of human genetics. Here is an outline of a case I worked on where white-Negro admixture suggested itself in the bones sent to me for study (female, young adult):

Skeletal trait	White	Negro	Uncertain
I. Skull			
1. Shape (breadth/length)	–	–	x
2. Height (height/length)	–	x	–
3. Total face proportions	–	x	–
4. Upper face proportions	–	x	–
5. Orbital shape	–	–	x
6. Interorbital width	x	–	–
7. Nasal aperture	–	–	x
8. Palate shape	x	–	–
9. Forehead contour	–	x	–
10. Roof or vault contour	–	–	x
11. Facial slope	–	–	x
12. Teeth: size, form	–	x	–
13. Upper front teeth	x	–	–
14. Lower jaw contour	x	–	–
Totals	4	5	5
II. Long bones, pelvis			
1. Shape of thigh bone	–	–	x
2. Shape of shin bone	x	–	–
3. Shape of sacrum	x	–	–
4. Proportions of pelvis	x	–	–
5. Form of pelvis	–	–	x
6. Forearm/upper arm ratio	–	–	x
7. Shin/thigh ratio	–	–	x
8. Arm/leg ratio	–	x	–
Totals	3	1	4
Over-all	7	6	9

In this tabulation "uncertain" may mean: (1) that the trait is nonracial, i.e., the same for all members of *H. sapiens,* or (2) that we just don't know. At all events in the skull the 14 traits ascribed to white or Negro are about 50-50, while in the eight traits of the long bones and pelvis white dominates in a 3:1 ratio in those definitely ascribed. I defined the bones as more white than Negro, possibly $^5/_8$–$^3/_8$. The identified woman was, as carefully as a family history could elucidate, $^1/_2$–$^1/_2$, white-Negro.

I want to turn, now, to the very practical consideration of *what to do* when bones are discovered. I envision two major classes of law enforcement units: (1) the more metropolitan areas where Medical Examiner's Offices and/or Coroner's Physicians are available, with their relatively complete pathological laboratories and radiographic set-ups; (2) more out-of-town agencies where the principal laboratory facilities and consultation services are apt to be in smaller and regional hospitals; and, in more isolated areas, the only readily available advice must come from the local general practitioner or the local biology teacher. What is written below is mainly for the second group, though the first group could well note procedures.

Most finds of bones occur accidentally. Only rarely is one led to the scene of burial by the suspect or the accused. Then it is relatively simple to "start from scratch." Let us assume that someone uncovers a bone or bones and calls the police. From this point on authority and responsibility devolve upon representatives of law enforcement. A bone or bones are involved; that is the beginning.

1. Is it *human*? It must be compared with a human skeleton. For this turn first to the local physician or dentist, either of whom may at least have a skull; or seek aid in the Biology Dept. of the local High School, or, possibly, local College or University; if none of these are of available help, turn to a text book in Anatomy. The local physician usually has one. Let us say it is human.

2. Now to the *site* where the bone or bones were found. It is to be hoped that the finder didn't paw around too much, before the police got there. If an archaeologist is in the neighborhood, either professional or amateur, he may be of aid. Usually such a person has dug "Indian mounds" and has some skill in exhumation; most important of all, he has some ability to recognize a "primary" or a "secondary" (intrusive) burial by observing a profile-section of the excavation. If such a profile does not show any "lensing," i.e., any break in soil continuity, then the burial is probably primary; moreover, it is then safe to say it is a relatively old interment, for the soil has achieved a degree of homogeneity. Many accidental skeletal finds in the U.S. are of prehistoric American Indians (Mongoloid; see Chapter VII). If they are Amerind then often artefacts (arrows, etc.) or potsherds are present. These should be looked for. Usually burials of aboriginal Amerinds are flexed (arms and legs folded against the trunk). It will be wise to note two precautions here: (1) take a sample, or samples, of the soil, putting such soil in labelled jars; (2) have available two screens, one with $1/4''$ mesh, the other with $1/8''$ mesh, as they may be required.

3. *Photograph* the site as at first encountered and then take step-by-step photographs until the exhumation is complete. This will

give a serial record of progressive exposure, including shots of the excavation itself and of the bones as they are uncovered.

4. Now to the *bones*. With the bone, or bones, initially found at hand try to fit them back into the hole, in possible context as first seen. This should give some idea of the orientation of the skeleton, whether at upper (skull), middle (shoulder, backbone, ribs, arm, pelvis), or lower ends (leg). I think it is best to start uncovering, carefully, at the skull end first, for this is better in identifying a bone-by-bone exposure. If no biologist (physician or teacher) is present, constant reference to an anatomical text book will be necessary. Each bone, especially the long bones, can be identified by text pictures.

5. If the body is completely skeletonized the foregoing holds as stated. If *soft parts* are still present (skin, muscles, hair, etc.) *all* such material should be preserved. The possibility of finger-prints must be considered, plus other pertinent information to be gained from careful study by a pathologist. If no soft parts, as such, are present, the bones should be carefully scanned to see if any sites of muscle attachment (ligaments) still show tissue remains. If none are present then signs of erosion (surface flaking, pitting, etc.) should be looked for. All these are factors in estimating dura-tion of interment.

6. If the bones are by now fairly well exposed, assuming that this is a relatively complete skeleton, the *age factor* should be reck-oned with. I am aware that most skeletal ageing problems, in identification work, have to do with adult material. But this may not always be the case. Hence, in Chapter II, I have dealt with the prenatal skeleton, and with bone-age in the first two decades of postnatal life. I suggest as a first age-check to go to the head of the humerus. If it is not united (if the head is separate from the shaft) then an individual below 20 years is represented; if it is united, then an adult skeleton is present. If the bones are im-mature then great care must be used to recover all bone-growth centers (epiphyses), especially from the ends of the long bones. If pelvic remains are present they should all be recovered, especially the pubic symphysis area. Here careful exhumation plus screen-ing the soil will yield very important age evidence. At the same time, if skull and mandible are present, all *teeth* should be recovered.

The anterior teeth, above and below (incisors, canines, and often premolars, see Krogman, '35), are apt to fall out of their sockets. They should be saved as evidence for age, sex, and race determination.

7.   At this stage the skeleton (skeletal parts) should be fully exposed, providing an over-all estimate of relative completeness and state of preservation.   This should be noted in descriptive writing (notes) and in photography *before any bones are taken from the earth.*   I advise strongly against taking up each bone as exposed; leave everything *in situ* until exposure is complete, compatible with remains present.   Now the bones may be carefully removed. The best thing is to put skull, mandible, and teeth in one container; each arm, ribs, vertebra, pelvis, each leg, in separate containers. They are then ready for removal to police headquarters or to a aboratory, as the case may be.*

At this point I'd like to present notes made available to me by Mr. Dean E. Clark, Lab. Supervisor, Mo. Basin Project, River Basin Surveys, Smithsonian Institution, Lincoln, Neb.   For work in the *field* the following applies:

No preservative is used except in case of extreme fragility.   Bones that are in fair to good condition and can readily be lifted receive no treatment other than *removal of excess dirt.*   Even a rather fragile bone may be lifted after being freed from surrounding dirt.   It is then carefully wrapped in soft tissue paper.   If bones are excavated while damp, they are immediately removed from direct sunlight and placed under shelter to *dry slowly.*

When treatment is required, the preservative used is $^3/_4$ lb. of gum arabic in one gallon of water plus a few drops of formaldehyde. This solution is brushed or dropped onto the first exposed portion of a bone.   When it has been absorbed, more of the bone is exposed and treated, etc., etc.   After being lifted, bones so treated are also dried under shelter.   The gum arabic may later be removed by sponging with water.

* Alvar solution thickens as the acetone evaporates and this loss must be replaced. Also, Alvar solution adhering to bone surfaces tends to whiten when relative humidity is high.   This tendency is greatly reduced by holding the cage of bones directly in a fan breeze immediately after dripping ceases.

In the *laboratory* the following applies:

> Brushes and wooden picks and scrapers are used to remove most
> of the remaining dirt from bones in better condition. They are
> then washed, without being immersed, by brushing with lukewarm
> water. They dry naturally on wire racks. Bones in poorer condi-
> tion are dry cleaned by gentle scraping and brushing. Light appli-
> cations of acetone help to remove tight dirt.
>
> When bones are clean and thoroughly dry, they are placed in a
> wire cage which is lowered into a tank containing a solution of
> one pound of Alvar 7/70 to three quarts of acetone.* Immersion
> is continued until bubbling ceases. The cage is then raised and
> excess solution drains back into the tank. When dripping ceases
> the bones are placed on wire drying racks. They are turned fre-
> quently to prevent sticking. The solution is brushed onto very
> fragile bones, repeated applications generally being necessary to
> seal cancellous exposures.

While the foregoing notes apply specifically to bones recovered
in archaeological "digs" they are nonetheless applicable to problems
of the uncovering, removal, and preservation of bones in medicolegal cases.

8. In Medical Examiner's labs, or in those of the Coroner's
Physician, all necessary equipment is usually available. Else-
where it may be necessary to send the bones to a local hospital or
a physician's office. The bones should be carefully x-rayed:
skull and jaws, pelvis, and long bones; for pelvis and long bones
one side (right or left) is enough, unless there is evidence to suggest
the need for symmetrical comparison. At the same time all age,
sex, race, etc., evidence should be assessed and interpreted according to techniques and information available in this book.

9. It is always possible, of course, to send the skeletal material,
carefully packed, labelled, and annotated, to the FBI, to the State
Crime Lab, to a nearby Medical Examiner or Coroner's Physician,
or to a specialist in skeletal identification at a University (usually
Dept. of Physical Anthropology or Dept. of Anthropology). A

---

* Remove earth from the bones prior to any form of transport. This is especially true
of the skull. Usually the inside of the skull is filled with earth. As the earth dries it
forms a hard ball which, in transit, becomes an effective battering-ram. Many a
skull, perfect at the site of exhumation, has reached the lab in fragments, pounded to
pieces by the endocranial ball of earth.

complete report can then be sent to the cooperating local law enforcement agency.   It should be added that these sources of referral will be glad to advise and aid at all stages of the investigation,
i.e., from the first finding of the bone or bones until completed
exhumation.   In last analysis, however, the success of the whole
identification problem hinges upon the "firing line" personnel
who do the actual spade-work, in the literal sense of exhumation,
and in the figurative sense of care of documentation.

ABBREVIATIONS USED IN ALL REFERENCES

Acta Anat. = Acta Anatomica
Acta Odont. Scand. = Acta Odontologica Scandinavica
Am. Anth. = American Anthropologist
Am. Assoc. Hist. Med. = American Association for the History of Medi-
cine
AJA = American Journal of Anatomy
Am. J. Dis. Children = American Journal of Diseases of Children
AJOG = American Journal of Obstetrics and Gynecology
Am. J. Orthod. = American Journal of Orthodontics
AJPA = American Journal of Physical Anthropology
Am. J. Roentgenol. (Rad. Ther.) (Nucl. Med.) = American Journal of
Roentgenology (Radium Therapy) (Nuclear Medicine)
Am. J. Surg. = American Journal of Surgery
Anat. Anz. = Anatomischer Anzeiger
Anat. Rec. = Anatomical Record
Ann. Surg. = Annals of Surgery
Anth. Anzeig = Anthropologischer Anzeiger
Arch. de Antropol. Crim. Psich. e Med. Legale = Archiv de Antropologia,
Criminal Psichologia e Medicíne Legale
Arch. f. Anth. = Archiv für Anthropologie
Arch. Int. Med. = Archives of Internal Medicine
Arch. Ital di Anat. e di Embriol. = Archiv Italiano di Anatomia e di
Embriologia
Arch. Path. = Archives of Pathology
Boston Med. and Surg. J. = Boston Medical and Surgical Journal
Bull. et Mem. de la Soc. d'Anth. Paris = Bulletins et Mémoires de la
Société d'Anthropologie de Paris.
Bull. Johns Hopkins Hosp. = Bulletin of the Johns Hopkins Hospital
Bull. Schweiz. Gesellsch. f. Anthropol. u. Ethnol. = Bulletin der schweiz-
eren Gesellschaft für Anthropologie und Ethnologie.

Child Dev. = Child Development
Clin. Pediat. = Clinical Pediatrics
Compt. Rend. Soc. Anat. = Comptes Rendu de l'Societie Anatomie
Contrib. paro o Estudo da Antropol. Portug. = Contribuçãoes paro o Estudo da Antropologia Portuguesa.
Eugen. News = Eugenical News
Finger Print. and Ident. Mag. = Finger Print and Identification Magazine
FBI Law Enforce. Bull. = FBI Law Enforcement Bulletin
Grad. Med. = Graduate Medicine
Hiroshima J. Med. Sci. = Hiroshima Journal of Medical Science
HB = Human Biology
Indian J. Med. Res. = Indian Journal of Medical Research
Indian J. Ped. = Indian Journal of Pediatrics
Indian Med. Rec. = Indian Medical Record
JA = Journal of Anatomy
JAMA = Journal of the American Medical Association
JAP = Journal of Anatomy and Physiology
J. Anth. Soc. Nippon = Journal of the Anthropological Society of Nippon
JBJS = Journal of Bone and Joint Surgery
J. Crim. Law, Criminol. and Police Sci. = Journal of Criminal Law, Criminology, and Police Science
J. Dent. Assoc. S. Africa = Journal of the Dental Association of South Africa
J. Forensic Med. = Journal of Forensic Medicine
J. Forensic Sci. = Journal of Forensic Sciences
J. Immunol. = Journal of Immunology
J. Malayan Branch Br. Med. Assn. = Journal of the Malayan Branch of the British Medical Association
J. Negro Educ. = Journal of Negro Education
JRAI = Journal of the Royal Anthropological Institute
L'Anth. = L'Anthropologie
MAGW = Mitteilungen der Anthropologischer Gesellschaft von Wien
Med. J. Austral. = Medical Journal of Australia
Medico-Legal and Criminol. Rev. = Medico-Legal and Criminology Review
Med. Radiog. and Photog. = Medical Radiography and Photography
Monatsch. f. Ohrenh. = Monatsschrift für Ohrenheilkunde
Phil. Trans. Roy. Soc. London = Philosophical Transactions of the Royal Society, London.
Police College Mag. = Police College Magazine

Publ. Fac. Sci. Univ. Masaryk = Publications of the Faculty of Science, Universitas Masaryk.

Rev. de la Assoc. Med. Argent. = Revue de la Association Medicale d'Argentina

Rev. Mem. de L'Ecole d'Anth. = Revue et Memoire de l'Ecole d'Anthropologie

S. Afr. J. Med. Sci. = South African Journal of Medical Sciences

Tab. Biol. = Tabulae Biologicae

Temple Law Quart. = Temple Law Quarterly

Trans. Roy. Soc. Trop. Med. and Hygiene = Transactions of the Royal Society of Tropical Medicine and Hygiene

Virginia Med. Monthly = Virginia Medical Monthly

Wenner-Gren Found. for Anth. Research. = Wenner-Gren Foundation for Anthropological Research, New York

ZE = Zeitschrift für Ethnologie

ZMA = Zeitschrift für Morphologie und Anthropologie

REFERENCES

BERTILLON, A.: Identification of the criminal classes by the anthropometrical method. Del. 11-22-85 at *Internat Penitentiary Cong., Rome.* Spottiswoode, London (transl. from Fr.), 1889.

BRUES, A. M.: Identification of skeletal remains. *J. Crim. Law, Criminol. and Police Sci., 48(5)*:551–563, 1958.

CORNWALL, I. W.: *Bones for the Archaeologist* London, Phoenix House. Macmillan, N.Y., 1956.

CORNWALL, I. W.: *Soils for the Archaeologist.* London, Phoenix House. Macmillan, N.Y., 1958.

DUTRA, F. R.: Identification of person and determination of cause of death from skeletal remains, *Arch. Path., 38*:339–349, 1944.

HOOTON, E. A.: Medico-legal aspects of physical anthropology. *Clinics, 1(6)*: 1612–1624, 1943.

KROGMAN, W. M.: Missing teeth in skulls and dental caries. *AJPA, 20(1)*:43–49, 1935.

KROGMAN, W. M.: The inheritance of non-pathologic physical traits in Man. *Eugen. News, 21(6)*:139–146, 1936.

KROGMAN, W. M.: The role of physical anthropology in forensic medicine: An historical survey. (mimeo) *Am. Assoc. Hist. Med.,* N. Y., 31st Ann. Meeting, 1958.

MORLAND, N.: *An Outline of Scientific Criminology.* Philos. Library, N.Y., 1950.

RHODES, H. T. F.: *Alphonse Bertillon: Father of Scientific Detection.* Abelard-Schuman, N.Y., 1956.

SNOW, C. E.: The identification of the unknown war dead. *AJPA n.s., 6(3)*:323–328, 1948.

STEWART, T. D., CORNWELL, W. S., DUGGINS, O. H., HOYME, L. E. and TROTTER, M.: Preliminary bibliography on human identification, VIII Wenner-Gren Summer Seminar in Phys. Anth. (Mimeo). Washington, D.C., 1955. See *Science, 122(3175)*:883–884. Nov. 4, 1955.

STEWART, T. D.: What the bones tell. *FBI Law Enforce Bull., 20(2)*:2–5; 19, 1951.

STEWART, T. D.: Bear paw remains closely resemble human remains. *FBI Law Enforce. Bull., 28(11)*:18–21, 1959.

TODD, T. W.: Entrenched Negro physical features. *HB, 1(1)*:57–69, 1929.

WILDER, H. H. and WENTWORTH, B.: *Personal Identification.* (ed. 1) Badger, Boston. 1918; ed. 2 by Wentworth and Wilder, T. G. Cooke Publ., Chicago. 1932.

II

Skeletal Age: Earlier Years

A. CRITERIA OF AGE IN THE HUMAN SKELETON: POSTNATAL APPEARANCE AND UNION OF CENTERS OF OSSIFICATION

1. General Considerations

The bones of the human skeleton (as is true of the mammalian skeleton generally) develop from a number of separate centers of ossification and growth.   This is true especially of the long bones (arm, leg; hand, foot), but the other bones share in this process also (vertebral column, thorax, shoulder and hip girdles).   In this Section we shall limit ourselves to the postnatal period of about the first three decades of life.   Some idea of the complexity of the overall ossification problem may be gleaned by the estimation that at the 11th prenatal week in humans there are some 806 centers of bone growth, at birth about 450, while the adult skeleton numbers only 206 bones.   From the 11th prenatal week to the time of final union some 600 centers of bone growth have "disappeared," i.e., they have coalesced or united with adjacent centers to give rise to the definitive adult bones as we know them.   This process of appearance and union has, in the normal human skeleton, a *sequence* and a *time* that makes of it a reliable age indicator.

With the exception of several bones in the skull, the bones of the skeleton are preformed in cartilage.   The cartilage takes on the characteristic shape of the bone-to-be and is, in very fact, the matrix within which ossification will occur.   A typical long bone, a tibia, for example, will have three centers or principal loci of growth: a mid-portion, the shaft, or *diaphysis;* and two end-portions, upper or proximal, and lower or distal, the *epiphysis*. These three, one diaphysis, two epiphyses, are the growth loci of the tibia. At either end, between diaphysis and epiphysis, is a plate of hyaline cartilage, which is the *diaphyseo-epiphyseal zone* (or *epiphyseal plane* or *line* or *disk*). It is here that growth actually occurs, and it is here that epiphyseal union occurs.

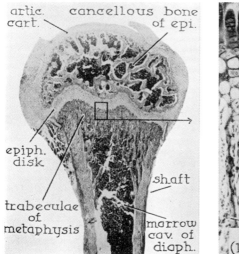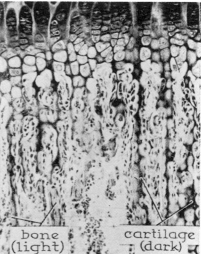

Fig. 1. Low-power photomicrograph (to left) of a longitudinal section through the upper end of a growing rat long bone to show diaphyseo-epiphyseal relationships. To the right is the boxed area under higher magnification.

In Figures 1–2 (from Ham, '57) the diaphyseo-epiphyseal relationship is shown. Figure 1 shows the epiphysis (epi.), epiphyseal disk (epiph. disk) and shaft or diaphysis (diaph.) of an immature bone. As seen the record is one of *appearance* of the epiphysis; with time the cartilaginous epiphyseal disk will be replaced by bone and ephiphyseal *union* (between epiphysis and diaphysis) will occur. Figure 2 shows diagrammatically how a long bone gains in length and is remodelled in form.

All long bone shafts are ossified at birth and many parts of the rest of the skeleton are also ossified (see Section on fetal ossification). At birth only six epiphyseal centers are present: head of humerus (proximal); condyle of femur (distal); condyle of tibia (proximal); talus, calcaneus, and cuboid (tarsal bones in foot). The first

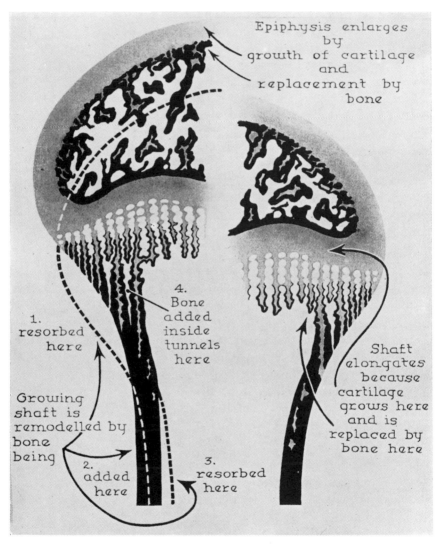

Fig. 2.   Schematic illustration of the growth and remodelling of a long bone.

three will unite with their respective shafts; the second three (as is true of all carpal bones of hand and tarsal bones of foot) will remain as discrete bones throughout life. As a rule ossification begins centrally in an epiphysis and spreads peripherally as it gets bigger. At first it is entirely amorphous; it is usually rounded, no bigger than a pin-head or a small lead shot. As it gets bigger it begins to take on more and more the osteological details of the bone part it will become, e.g., the condyle of the femur.

The foregoing brief notation of the appearance of ossification centers highlights the very important practical considerations outlined in Chapter I: in the exhumation of an obviously immature skeleton great care must be exercised to recover *all of the separate pieces of bone*. The earth must be carefully sifted, first with a sieve of $1/4''$ mesh, then with one with $1/8''$ mesh. Best of all, if it is possible, a specialist in skeletal identification should be called in when bones first show up. Usually the finding is accidental and is reported to the police. At this stage post a guard at the site and call for the help of the specialist. He knows what to look for and where (in progressive exhumation) to look for it. Every piece of bone tells its own story of its role in the individuality of its possessor, a story which, if properly unfolded, may result in an identification.

It is axiomatic in biology that stability is the exception, variability is the rule. That is to say, there really is no average; there is only a central tendency, with a normal range of variability clustering around it. It is within this predictable and measurable range that reliability lies. One does not say these bones are precisely so old, but, rather, these bones are approximately so old (or, to put it concretely, rarely can we say, "this skeleton is 35 years old"; instead we are more apt to say, "this skeleton is between 30–35 or 35–40 years old"). There is another axiom applicable here, i.e., that variability increases with age. As a general rule I'd say that ageing of bones is more precise with respect to *appearance* of centers of ossification than it is with respect to *union* of epiphyses.

2. The Appearance of Centers

In Figures 3–4 and Tables 1–3 (from Francis, Werle and Behm, '39, and Francis, '40) are presented basic data on the appearance

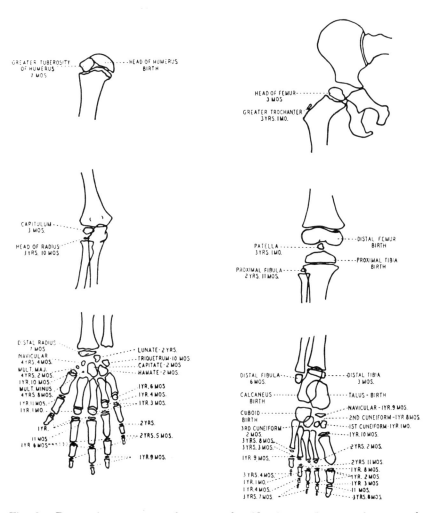

Fig. 3.   Dates of appearance of centers of ossification to 5 years of age—male whites.

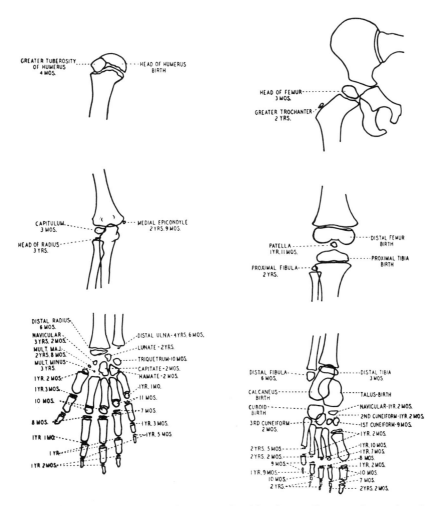

Fig 4.   Dates of appearance of centers of ossification to 5 years of age—female whites.

TABLE 1

AGE ORDER OF APPEARANCE OF OSSIFICATION CENTERS: SUPERIOR WHITE MALES*

Birth	**14 months**	**2 years, 2 months**
Calcaneus	4T-⎫1 phalanx	2 metatarsal
Talus	2T-⎭	**2 years, 5 months**
Femur, distal	3T-2 phalanx	2F-⎫3 phalanx
Tibia, proximal	**15 months**	5F-⎭
Cuboid	3 metacarpal	**2 years, 11 months**
Humerus, head	2T-2 phalanx	3 metatarsal
2 months	5F-1 phalanx	Fibula, proximal
Capitate	**16 months**	**3 years, 1 month**
Hamate	4T-2 phalanx	Femur, greater trochanter
Lateral cuneiform	4 metacarpal	Patella
3 months	**18 months**	**3 years, 3 months**
Femur, head	2F-⎫	4 metatarsal
Capitulum	3F-⎬2 phalanx	**3 years, 4 months**
Tibia, distal	4F-⎭	5T-3 phalanx
6 months	5 metacarpal	**3 years, 7 months**
Fibula, distal	**20 months**	3T-⎫3 phalanx
7 months	1T-1 phalanx	4T-⎭
Humerus, greater tuberosity	Middle cuneiform	**3 years, 8 months**
Radius, distal	**21 months**	5 metatarsal
10 months	3F-⎫3 phalanx	2T-3 phalanx
Triquetrum	4F-⎭	**3 years, 10 months**
11 months	Navicular of foot	Radius, proximal
3F-1 phalanx	5T-1 phalanx	**4 years, 2 months**
1T-2 phalanx	**22 months**	Multangulum majus
12 months	1 metacarpal	**4 years, 4 months**
2F-⎫1 phalanx	1 metatarsal	Navicular, hand
4F-⎭	**23 months**	**4 years, 8 months**
1F-2 phalanx	1F-1 phalanx	Multangulum minus
13 months	**2 years**	**5 years +**
3T-1 phalanx	5F-2 phalanx	Humerus, medial epicondyle
2 metacarpal	Lunate	Ulna, distal
Medial cuneiform		5T-2 phalanx

* From Francis, Werle, Behm, '39; cited as Table 1 in Krogman, '55.

TABLE 2
AGE ORDER OF APPEARANCE OF OSSIFICATION CENTERS: SUPERIOR WHITE FEMALES*

Birth	**10 months**	**21 months**
Calcaneus	2 metacarpal	5T-3 phalanx
Talus	2T-} 2 phalanx	**22 months**
Femur, distal	4T-}	3 metatarsal
Tibia, proximal	3 metacarpal	**23 months**
Cuboid	2T-1 phalanx	Patella
Humerus, head	Triquetrum	**2 years**
2 months	**11 months**	Lunate
Capitate	4 metacarpal	3T-} 3 phalanx
Hamate	5F-1 phalanx	4T-}
Lateral cuneiform	**12 months**	Fibula, proximal
3 months	4F-} 2 phalanx	Femur, greater trochanter
Femur, head	3F-}	**2 years, 2 months**
Capitulum	**13 months**	2T-3 phalanx
Tibia, distal	5 metacarpal	4 metatarsal
4 months	2F-2 phalanx	**2 years, 5 months**
Humerus, greater tuberosity	**14 months**	5 metatarsal
6 months	1 metacarpal	**2 years, 8 months**
Fibula, distal	1T-} 1 phalanx	Multangulum majus
Radius, distal	5F-}	**2 years, 9 months**
7 months	3F-} 3 phalanx	Humerus, medial epicondyle
1T-2 phalanx	4F-}	**3 years**
3F-} 1 phalanx	Navicular of foot	Radius, proximal
4F-}	Middle cuneiform	Multangulum minus
8 months	**15 months**	**3 years, 2 months**
2F-1 phalanx	1F-1 phalanx	Navicular, hand
1F-2 phalanx	5F-2 phalanx	**4 years, 6 months**
3T-1 phalanx	**17 months**	Ulna, distal
9 months	2F-} 3 phalanx	**5 years +**
3T-2 phalanx	5F-}	5T-2 phalanx
4T-1 phalanx	**19 months**	
Medial cuneiform	2 metatarsal	

* From Francis, Werle, Behm, '39; cited as Table 2 in Krogman, '55.

TABLE 3

AGE ORDER OF APPEARANCE OF CENTERS AFTER FIVE YEARS*

Center	White Male	White Female
Humerus, medial epicondyle	5:2	—
Ulna, distal	5:6	—
Calcaneal epiphysis (tuber)	6:2	—
Talar epiphysis	8:0	6:10
Humerus, trochlea	8:4	7:2
Olecranon	8:8	6:8
Femur, lesser trochanter	9:4	7:7
Pisiform	9:10	7:1
Sesamoid (flexor hallux brevis)	10:4	8:2
Humerus, lateral epicondyle	10:5	8:3
Tibial tubercle	10:10	9:0
Metatarsal V, proximal	11:0	8:7
Sesamoid (flexor pollex brevis)	11:8	9:4
Rib I, tubercle	13:3	10:0
Ilium, anterosuperior spine	13:4	9:3
Thoracic vertebra I, transverse process	13:4	11:4
Acromion	13:5	11:4
Iliac crest	13:5	12·0
Coracoid angle	13:10	11:3
Ischial tuberosity	15:0	13:2
Clavicle, medial	15:0+	14:6

* From Francis, '40; cited as Table 3 in Krogman, '55.

of major centers of ossification from birth to about 15 years or a bit older. The data are basically roentgenographic and are for white children only, of an upper ("superior") socio-economic bracket (the possibility of race differences will be noted later).*

In presenting the above data I must emphasize that the age-values given are single values only. I agree with Noback ('54) that adequate statistical data do not (with one or two exceptions) exist. I feel, however, that the data above presented by Francis and his associates are the most reliable. There are other tabulations on epiphyseal appearance available, to be sure,[†] but I find the ones presented the most useful and easiest to work with. In principle they represent optimum values, i.e., they give about the

* It is to be noted that Table 1 is for males, Table 2 is for females. The sex dichotomy is a real one, with the females advanced compared to males. Pryor ('23, '27/'28, '33) was among the first to establish this fact.

† See, for example, Davies and Parsons, '27/'28; Paterson, '29; Flecker, '32/'33, '42; Hodges, '33; Clark, '36; Girdany and Golden, '52, Drennan and Keen, '53. The studies by Flecker are by far the best to emphasize variability. These references will also be useful in the discussion of epiphyseal union. For detailed analysis of appearance of centers in the foot, only, with emphasis upon variability, the studies by Hasselwander ('02, '09/'10) and by Venning ('56a, '56b) are useful.

TABLE 4

AGES ASSIGNED BY VARIOUS AUTHORITIES FOR UNION OF EPIPHYSES*

Authority	Bryce ('11)	Dixon ('12)	Dwight ('11)	Gegenbaur ('92)	Henle ('71)	Krause ('09)	Lewis ('18)	Poirier ('11)	Terry ('21)	Testut ('21)	Thompson ('21)	Earliest	Latest	Difference
Epiphyses														
Humerus:														
Head	20–22	20–25	20	—	—	22	20	20–25	20	20–25	25	20	25	5 yrs.
Distal Ext.	17	17	15	18	15	16–17	17	16–17	17	16–18	16–17	15	18	3 "
Med. Epicond.	18	18	—	—	16	18	18	16–17	17	17–19	18–19	16	19	3 "
Radius:														
Proximal	17–19	18	16	17	16	16–17	17–18	16–19	17	16–20	18–20	16	20	4 "
Distal	18–20	21–25	19–20	20	19–20	20–21	20	20–25	20	20–25	20–25	18	25	7 "
Ulna:														
Proximal	17–19	17	16	17	15–16	16–17	16	20–21	16–17	16–20	16	15	21	6 "
Distal	18–20	20	18	20	20	20–21	20	22–24	18–20	20–25	20–23	18	25	7 "
Femur:														
Head	18–19	18–20	18	20–25	20	17–19	Puberty to 20	18–22	19	18	18–20	18	25	7 "
Lsr. Trochant.	18	18	19	20–25	—	17–19		18–22	17	18	18	17	25	8 "
Gtr. Trochant.	17	18	19	20–25	—	17–19		18–22	18	16–18	18–19	17	25	8 "
Distal Ext.	20	23–24	20	23	—	19–20		22–24	20	20–22	20–22	19	24	5 "
Tibia:														
Proximal	19–24	21	19–20	—	18–25	19	20	18–24	20–25	18–20	20–24	18	25	7 "
Distal	17–19	17–18	18	—	18–25	17–18	18	16–18	18	16–18	18	17	25	8 "
Fibula:														
Proximal	22–24	22–24	20	—	19–25	19	25	22–23	22	19–22	19	19	25	6 "
Distal	20–22	20	18–19	—	19–25	17–18	20	20–22	20	18–19	19	17	25	8 "
Scapula:														
Coracoid	Puberty	17	14–15	16–18	14–15	16–18	15	20–25	15	14–16	15–17	14	25	11 "
Acromion	22–25	22–25	18–19	—	16–17	19–21	—	20–25	20	17–18	25	16	25	9 "
Inf. Angle	25	22–24	20	—	20	21–22	25	—	25	22–25	20–25	20	25	5 "
Vert. Margin	25	22–24	20	—	21–22	21–22	25	25–28	25	20–24	20–25	20	28	8 "
Innominate:														
Primary Elements	Puberty	17–18	15	Puberty	Puberty	16–18	Puberty	15–20	18–20	15–16	16	15	20	5 "
Ischial Tuber.	18–25	18–20	20	24	22–24	17–24	20–25	18–20	20	15–20	20–25	15	25	10 "
Iliac Crest	18–25	18–20	20	24	22–24	17–24	20–25	20–25	20	24–25	22–25	17	25	8 "
Ramal Epiphysis	—	—	—	—	—	—	—	—	—	—	—	—	—	—
Clavicle	25	25	18	—	18	20–22	25	25	25	22–25	25	18	25	7 "

* From Stevenson, '24, Table 1.

80th percentile, or the age-values for the best-growing two in ten children.   This situation in itself offers one explanation for the wide age-differences so often noted in the literature.   Some authors cite age of *first* appearance, others of the *latest* appearance.   Some give an *average* age (50th percentile), others give an age of *total appearance* in the sample (100th percentile).   The 80th percentile is an acceptable "standard" or "norm" to use.

3. The Union of Centers

Without any doubt the study by Stevenson ('24) is an historical landmark in that it is the first study of epiphyseal union made on a sizeable sample (128 skeletons age 15–28 years) of *known* age, sex, and race.   It is important, also, because it is an osteological study, rather than a radiographic one.   It is a veritable landmark for it "cleared the air," so to speak, of the extreme variation found in earlier studies.*   An example of this is to be noted in Table 4.

The four stages recognized by Stevenson were: *no union; beginning union; recent union; complete union.*   The following quotation (pp. 58–59) is pertinent:

> Before beginning a specific investigation of the time and order of union of the various epiphyses, a preliminary study of the phenomenon as a whole was made in order to acquire a general appreciation of the progressive changes taking place at the epiphysodiaphyseal junction.   Through such a study it is possible to recognize four more or less distinct phases of epiphyseal union, each presenting characteristic and constant features.   (1) In the first, or stage of *no union*, the clearly evident hiatus between the epiphysis and diaphysis, as well as the characteristic saw-tooth-like external margins of the approximated diaphyseal and epiphyseal surfaces, present unmistakable evidence of the condition of nonunion.   In this stage the epiphysis has not infrequently become entirely separated from the diaphysis in the process of maceration, leaving a

---

* Lest I "over-sell" Stevenson I must point out that it has definite limitations: (1) "known age" is usually really "stated age," which is often rounded off to the nearest half-decade or decade;   (2) the number, 128, spread over 14 years and both sexes, becomes inadequate when broken down by age and sex;   (3) it is said that "dead material is defective material" and hence complete normality is not always achieved. But I still give Stevenson's work the palm as an historic "break-through" in the critical area of epiphyseal union.

billowy surface which is characteristic of this stage; a point to be noted in connection with the less frequent cases of epiphyses becoming forcibly separated at a later stage when partial union has taken place. (2) In the second, or stage of *beginning union*, a tendency is evident for the distinct superficial hiatus between epiphysis and diaphysis to be replaced by a line. The saw-tooth character of the approaching margins is gradually lost through the deposition of finely granular new bone in the depressions. Quite as characteristic of this stage is an occasional bridging over or knitting together of the two margins, an external manifestation of the process of obliteration of the space between the diaphysis and its epiphysis. This process of bridging over and progressive obliteration of the epiphyseal line becomes increasingly conspicuous from this stage on. Diaphyseal and epiphyseal surfaces resulting from the occasional complete separation of the epiphysis at this stage are not difficult to distinguish from those of the preceding stage when the filling in of the depressions by new bone deposition and the resultant smoothing out of the former rugged surface is noted. (3) The third, or stage of *recent union*, is the least definite of the four and offers at times some difficulty even to the most experienced observer. This stage is characterized chiefly by the retention of a fine line of demarcation, although the active process of bony union is plainly over. This line, which varies much in distinctness on different bones and in different skeletons, can be seen best in freshly macerated skeletons, when it usually, though not always, has a faintly reddish color. The line in question must be clearly distinguished from the "epiphyseal scar" which is occasionally met with in the fourth stage, and less frequently throughout life. (4) The fourth, or stage of *complete union*, represents the completion of the process of union and usually offers no difficulties in its recognition. In a certain small percentage of cases there may be a faint epiphyseal line persisting throughout life. Care must be taken in the case of such lines, however, especially in the case of the distal end of the femur and the proximal end of the tibia not to mistake a relatively conspicuous line of capsular attachment for the epiphyseal line itself.

In practice no union is scored in the Stevenson method as *O*, beginning as *B*, recent as *R*, complete as *C*. I have selected two bones, humerus and femur, to give an example of what has become

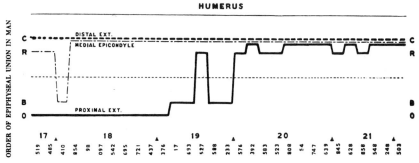

Fig. 5.   Age of union of epiphyses of humerus.

known as "Stevenson's epiphyseal keys."   In Figure 5 the humerus
is shown, in Figure 6 the femur.*

The sequence, for the age-period covered, is given by Stevenson
as follows (the order is variable, i.e., a given center may be before
or after another center, but in the main the sequence holds):

> Distal extremity of humerus
>   (Medial epicondyle of humerus)
> Coracoid process of scapula
> Three primary elements of innominate bone
> Head of radius
>   (Olecranon of ulna)
> Head of femur
>   (Lesser and greater trochanters of femur)
>   (Tuberosities of ribs)
> Distal extremities of tibia and fibula
> Proximal extremity of tibia
>   (Proximal extremity of fibula)
> Distal extremity of femur
> Tuberosity of ischium
> Distal extremities of radius and ulna
> Head of humerus
> Crest of ilium
> Heads of ribs
> Ramal epiphysis of pelvis
> Clavicle

In 1934, Stewart studied the sequence of epiphyseal union in two
Mongoloid samples: the American Indian (Pueblo of Southwest
U.S.), and the Eskimo.   He stated (p. 447) that "racial differences
in sequence of epiphyseal union are most apparent in connection
with earliest epiphyses" in Stevenson's list, i.e., the first six.   Stewart
also found greater variability than was implicit in Stevenson's
study, especially with reference to beginning union.

* In Figures 5–6 years 17–21 are shown.   The numbers in the line below the years are
the file numbers of the skeletons studied.   (Todd Collection.)

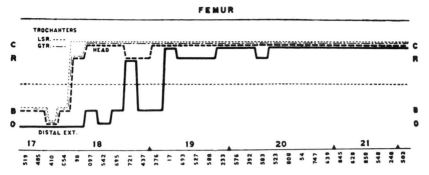

Fig. 6.   Age of union of epiphyses of femur.

Here is the sequence reported by Stewart for Eskimos and American Indians:

> Distal extremity of humerus
> ⌈Olecranon of ulna
> ⎢Primary elements of innominate
> ⌊Coracoid process of scapula
> Head of radius
> ⌈Medial epicondyle of humerus
> ⎢Calċaneus
> ⌊Anterior inferior spine of ilium
> ⌈Head of femur
> ⌊Lesser and greater trochanters
> Distal extremities of tibia and fibula
> Proximal extremity of tibia
> Proximal extremity of fibula
> Distal extremity of femur
> Acromion process of scapula
> Tuberosity of ischium (?)
> ⌈Distal extremity of radius and ulna
> ⌊Head of humerus
> Angle of scapula
> ⌈Ramal epiphysis of pelvis
> ⌊Vertebral border of scapula
> ⌈Crest of ilium
> ⌊Clavicle

The bracketted groups represent either union as a group or the presence of such great individual variation that precise order cannot be determined. This is also a difference pointed out by Stewart, viz., that apparently the sequence is not as clear-cut as Stevenson implies, for the epiphyses of the Eskimo, especially, cluster more.

There are two main factors to be considered here. The first is that Stevenson's series is admittedly numerically weak in the earlier age-ranges. The second is that Stevenson's population sample, American whites and mixed white-Negroes, was from a

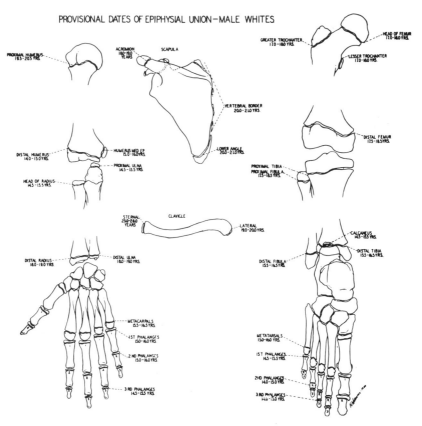

Fig. 7.   Dates of epiphyseal union—male whites.   Note that these are mean ages, only.   See text for discussion of variability.

dissecting room, representing, as Stewart says, "the dregs of a modern city population"; whereas the Pueblo and Eskimo are "pure subgroups of the yellow-brown race who lived in a natural environment." I am inclined to feel, therefore, that the difference between Stevenson and Stewart are more apparent than real. Sampling inadequacy (Stevenson) and vastly different socio-economic circumstances (Stewart) are probably the potent factors. It must be remembered, too, that sequence, not time (age) is at stake. Any time differences due to sequence shift are almost certainly within variable error. *Intra-racial variability is much more marked than inter-racial difference.*

The basic data on epiphyseal union from the Todd Collection may now be stated in terms of years (Todd, '30, Krogman, '39, '55). It is summarized in Table 5 and in Figure 7.

In supplement to this it will be well to note the data of Vandervael ('52, cited by Stewart, '54), for U.S. males, ages 18–38 years (225 skeletons of American soldiers killed in Europe), as shown in Table 6.

TABLE 5
POSTNATAL UNION OF CENTERS OF OSSIFICATION*

Scapula		Pelvis	
Acromion	18:0–19:0	Primary elements	13:0–15:0
Vertebral margin	20:0–21:0	Crest	18:0–19:0
Inferior angle	20:0–21:0	Tuberosity	19:0–20:0
Clavicle		Femur	
Sternal end	25:0–28:0	Head	17:0–18:0
Acromial end	19:0–20:0	Greater trochanter	17:0–18:0
Humerus		Lesser trochanter	17:0–18:0
Head	19:6–20:6	Distal	17:6–18:6
Distal	14:0–15:0	Tibia	
Medial epicondyle	15:0–16:0	Proximal	17:6–18:6
Radius		Distal	15:6–16:6
Proximal	14:6–15:6	Fibula	
Distal	18:0–19:0	Proximal	17:6–18:6
Ulna		Distal	15:6–16:6
Proximal	14:6–15:6	Calcaneal epiphysis	14:6–15:6
Distal	18:0–19:0	Foot	
Hand		Metatarsals	15:0–16:0
Metacarpals	15:6–16:6	Phalanges I	14:6–15:6
Phalanges I	15:0–16:0	Phalanges II	14:0–15:0
Phalanges II	15:0–16:0	Phalanges III	14:0–15:0
Phalanges III	14:6–15:6		

* From Krogman '55, Table 4. After Todd.

At this point I'd like to bring up the problem of *variability*. In Tables 1–3 and 5, and in Figures 3–4 and 7, I have presented certain data on appearance and union of centers of ossification. These data seem pretty categorical, i.e., they give rather precise timing, with, at best, a suggested range of about only one year. This is only a *central tendency*. In 1955, I discussed this problem and I wish to borrow from that paper in the next few paragraphs.

There is no such thing as an "average" individual. There are only individuals who, we hope, are acceptably variable, i.e., non-pathologic or "normal." Human biology is simply not amenable to the precision of the pure or exact sciences. Or, again, our species, genetically speaking, is so hybridized that norms or standards based on samples are not much more than approximations.

TABLE 6

EPIPHYSEAL UNION, U.S. MALES, 18–38 YEARS*

Epiphyses of femur, tibia and fibula:
Separate from diaphysis.................................... under 18 years
Uniting with diaphysis..................................... 17–18 years
Completely united with diaphysis.......................... over 18 years
Distal epiphyses of radius and ulna:
Separate from diaphysis.................................... under 19 years
Partially united with diaphysis............................ 18–19 years
United with diaphysis, but joint visible.................... 19–20 years
Completely united with diaphysis.......................... 20 years or over
Head of humerus:
Separate from diaphysis.................................... under 20 years
Partially united with diaphysis............................ 19–20 years
United with joint visible................................... 20–21 years
Completely united with diaphysis.......................... 21 years or over
Iliac crest and epiphyseal vertebral plates:
Completely separate....................................... under 20 years
Partially united... 19–20 years
Completely united... 20 years or over
Ischiatic tuberosity:
Epiphyseal plates separate................................. under 19 years
Plates partially united.................................... 18–19 years
Plates completely united.................................. 20 years or over
Sacrum:
Spaces between all of the sacral vertebral bodies.............. under 20 years
Spaces between S1 and S2 only............................ under 27 years
Complete union of the vertebral bodies..................... over 25 years
Medial epiphysis of clavicle:
Completely separate from diaphysis........................ under 20 years
Small osseous nodule adhering to center................... 20–22 years
Bony nodule more developed, partially united............... 23–24 years
Union almost complete..................................... 25–26 years
Union complete.. 26 years or more

* From Stewart, '54, p. 433.

TABLE 7

THE AGE DISTRIBUTION OF COMPLETE UNION FOR THE LONG BONE EPIPHYSES OF GROUP I* (IN %)

| | | Upper Extremity | | | Lower Extremity | | | | |
| | | | | | | Femur: | | | |
Age	No.	Humerus: med. epicond.	Radius: prox.	Ulna: prox.	Head	Gtr. troch.	Lsr. troch.	Tibia: dist.	Fibula: dist.
17–18	55	86	93	90	88	88	88	89	89
19	52	96	100	100	96	98	98	98	94
20	45	100			100	100	100	100	100
Total	152								

* McKern and Stewart, '57, Table 20.

At the risk of being particulate in a general statement, I'd like to offer an illustration in the field of ageing the bones, citing one example of appearance, one of union, of bony elements.

1) The *appearance of the capitate* is given as follows:

> Harding, V. V.
> Boys: 4% at birth, 50% at 0:3, 100% at 1:0.
> Girls: 7% at birth, 68% at 0:3, 100% at 0:9.
> Flory, 0:9 ± 0:6, males and females (9th l.m.–3:6, from literature)
> Todd, 0:2 males and females
> Pyle and Sontag
> Boys: 2.4 ± 1.8 mos.
> Girls: 2.3 ± 2.1 mos.
> Flecker, "majority," males at 0:6, females at 0:4

2) The *union of the proximal radial epiphysis* is given as follows:

> Harding, V. V.
>   *Mid 50%*   *Mid 80%*
> Boys: 15:2–16:6 14:6–(not given)
> Girls: 12:9–14:3 12:3–14:10
> Todd, 14:6–15:6 males and females; (females 1:0–2:0 earlier)
> Stewart, females 14:0, males 16:0
> Flecker, females "earliest" 13:0, males "earliest" 14:0
> "majority": females 14:0, males 16:0
> females "latest" 19:10, males 20:5

The ranges are terrific, especially for *appearance* time; the mean values, too, evidence some sort of biological uncertainty. What would an "expert" say here? To begin with, of course, he'd not rely upon a single center; but he'd find all carpo-metacarpo-phalangeal centers equally variable. The best he can do is, on the basis of knowledge and experience, to come to some sort of an opinion as to an approximate and acceptable age, (over-all or mean).

The same holds true, in principle, for the *union time*, though range is relatively not so great. For boys, 14:6–16:0 seems to be OK, for girls 12:3–15:6, though Flecker seems to be unperturbed at going as high as 20:5 and 19:10, respectively. Here, again, the evaluation and opinion of the expert must guide between the Scylla of "retardation" and the Charybdis of "acceleration," *both quite normal* as far as growth biology is concerned.

In handling data such as these there is an apparent difference between the *fact* of a normal range and the *stated opinion* of the expert as to the probable mean (over-all) age. It is his job to observe and state the one, and to evaluate the other.

McKern and Stewart ('57) reported on the skeletons of 450

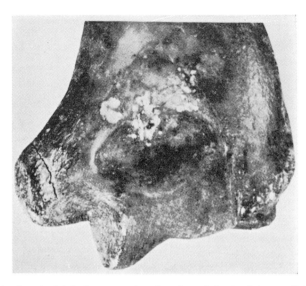

Fig. 8.   Distal end of right humerus showing the epiphysis of the medial epicondyle in stage 2 of union.   Note that union has begun inferiorly (#44, 18 yrs.).

American war-dead in the Korean conflict (age range 17–50 years). The authors have stressed the range of variation.   Here five stages were set up: 1 = non-union; 2 = $^{1}/_{4}$ united; 3 = $^{1}/_{2}$ united; 4 = $^{3}/_{4}$ united; 5 = complete union.   These are illustrated in Figures 8–11a.

The authors establish two main groups of epiphyseal union as follows:

Group I, early union
    Arm: *elbow* (distal humerus, medial epicondyle of humerus, proximal radius and ulna)
    Leg: *hip* (head and greater and lesser trochanters of femur); *ankle* (distal tibia and fibula)
Group II, late union
    Arm: *shoulder* (head of humerus); *wrist* (distal radius and ulna)
    Leg: *knee* (distal femur, proximal tibia and fibula).

These two Groups have complete union age-categories as follows:

Group		Age of complete union
I	ankle	20 years
	hip	20 "
	elbow	20 "
II		
	knee	23 years
	wrist	23 "
	shoulder	24 "

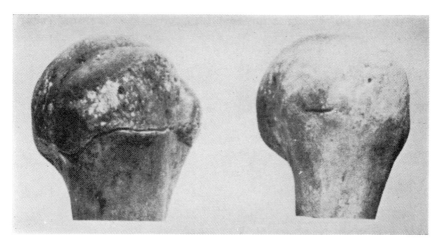

Fig. 9. Proximal end of right humeri, showing late stages of union: L, early stage 3 (#97, 20 yrs.); R, late stage 3 (#174, 20 yrs.).

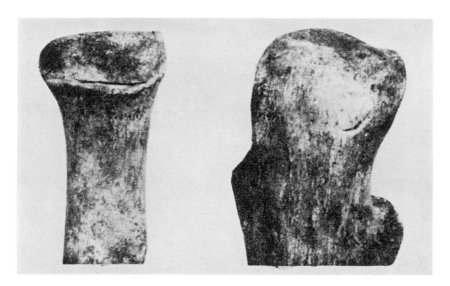

Fig. 10. Proximal end of right radius (L) and ulna (R) showing signs of recent union (#44).

TABLE 8

The Age Distribution for Stages of Union for the Long Bone Epiphyses of Group II*

| | | Upper Extremity | | | | | | | | | | | | | | | Lower Extremity | | | | | | | | | | | | | | | |
| | | Humerus (prox.) Stages | | | | | Radius (dist.) Stages | | | | | Ulna (dist.) Stages | | | | | Femur (dist.) Stages | | | | | Tibia (prox.) Stages | | | | | Fibula (prox.) Stages | | | | |
Age	No.	0	1	2	3	4	0	1	2	3	4	0	1	2	3	4	0	1	2	3	4	0	1	2	3	4	0	1	2	3	4
17–18	55	14	5	25	35	21	22	3	14	32	29	29	1	11	24	35	16	2	3	18	61	2	2	7	23	66	14		3	12	71
19	52	5	2	10	58	25	7	—	5	48	40	7	—	5	32	56	4	—	1	9	86	1	—	1	17	81	4		6	4	86
20	45	2	2	4	40	52	4	—	2	24	70	4	2	—	24	70			2	9	89				13	87			2	—	98
21	37			2	27	71				19	81				10	90				8	92				5	95				5	95
22	24				12	88				12	88				8	92					100				4	96					100
23	26				4	96					100					100										100					
24+	136					100																									

| Total | 375 |

* From McKern and Stewart, '57, Table 21.

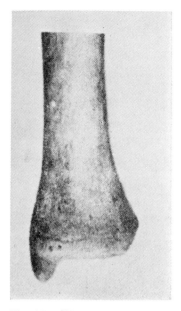
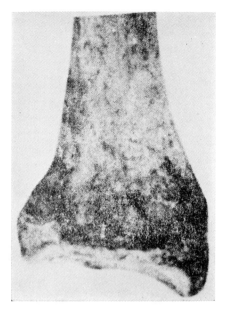

Fig. 11.   Distal end of L ulna (post. view, on L), showing stage 4 (#99, 17 yrs.).
Fig. 11a.   Distal end of L radius (ant. view, on R), also stage 4 (#250, 22 yrs.).

The above are based on the "100% principle." In Table 7 the epiphyses of Group I are shown in terms of % completely united at ages 17–18, 19, and 20 years.

In Table 8 the epiphyses of Group II are shown in % of each Stage, from years 17–18 to 24+ years.

Tables 7 and 8 point an important lesson in terms of the identification of an *individual* skeleton. Take the medial epicondyle of the humerus as an example (Table 7): 86% of 55 showed complete union at 17–18 years, 96% of 52 at 19 years, and 100% of 45 at 20 years (a spread of from 17–20 years). Or take proximal humerus as an example (Table 8): 21% of 55 showed Stage 4 (complete union) at 17–18 years; progressive increase of % until 100% of 136 at 24 years plus (a spread of from 17–24 years)+. Normal union may occur at any age within these total age-ranges.

McKern ('57) has tackled the problem of variability with respect to individuality by what he calls "combined maturational activity." He first sets up Groups I-V as follows:

Group   I.   Sampling of total maturation: 11 sutures (including vault, circum-
              meatal and accessory) and 38 postcranial epiphyses.
Group   II.   Sampling of 38 postcranial epiphyses.
Group III.   Sampling of 12 postcranial epiphyses:

Humerus, prox.	Clavicle, med. end
Humerus, med. epicondyle	Scapula, acromion
Radius, dist.	Vertebral centra
Femur head	Iliac crest
Femur, dist.	Ischial ramus
Tibia, prox.	Sacrum, lat. joints

Group IV.   Total number (15) of long bone epiphyses.
Group   V.   Nine postcranial epiphyses selected on the basis of the regularity of their
              overall pattern of maturation and on the distinctive nature of their
              observed stages of terminal union:

Humerus, prox.	Clavicle, med. end
Humerus, med. epicondyle	Iliac crest
Radius, dist.	Sacrum, lat. joints
Femur head	Sacrum, 3–4 joint
Femur, dist.	

Groups I, II, V, "proved to be the best predictors," but the author goes on to conclude (p. 408):

> The degree of relationship between combined maturational score and age has been tested for five groups of skeletal growth areas. The data indicate that an age estimation derived from the combined maturational activity of a small group of critical growth areas is as reliable as an estimation based on the total number of maturative events. To the identification specialist, this information means that instead of the usual practice of emphasizing complete skeletal coverage, dependable age estimations can be obtained from the combined maturational activity of a small number of critical areas. Also, because of the tested reliability of the symphyseal surface of the pubic bone, the use of other ageing criteria is necessary only where the pubic symphysis is damaged or missing (at least for age groups over 17 years).

In Figure 12, McKern demonstrates the foregoing graphically.

While Stevenson has four stages (O, B, R, C) and McKern and Stewart have five (0–4), the total process of epiphyseal maturation and union shows a quite detailed and integrated series of progressive changes. These can be seen grossly in the x-ray films of reasonably well preserved skeletal material. Todd ('30, p. 193) presents *nine roentgenographic stages* as follows:

> The *first* extends to the period when diaphysial and epiphysial bone approximate each other but as yet show no intimate relation, the adjacent surfaces being ill-defined and composed of cancellous tissue.

The *second* is the stage of obscuration of the adjacent bony surfaces by their transformation into thick hazy zones.

The *third* stage shows clearing of the haze with appearance of a fine delimiting surface of more condensed tissue shown on the roentgenogram as a fine white line.

The *fourth* stage exhibits billowing of adjacent surfaces.

In the *fifth* the adjacent surfaces show reciprocal outlines which are parallel to each other.

In the *sixth* the gap between adjacent surfaces is narrowed.

The *seventh* is the stage of commencing union when the fine white billowed outlines break up.

In the *eighth* stage union is complete though recent, and appears on the naked bone as a fine red line.

The *ninth* stage is that of perfected union with continuity of trabeculae ·from shaft to epiphysis.

The problem of evaluating and comparing epiphyseal union on the actual bone and on the x-ray film is a difficult one. At the risk of seeming arbitrary I'd place my bet for accuracy and reliability on the bone rather than on the x-ray film. I've done both and I know how misleading an x-ray film can be ("a confused medley of shadows" as Todd has called it). In the film the "scar" of recent union (the maintenance of radiographic opacity at the site of the piled-up calcification adjacent to the epiphyseo-diaphyseal plane) may persist several years *after* demonstrable complete union in the bone itself. Here I find myself in a fundamental disagreement with Keen ('50, cited by Drennan and Keen, '53). The statement is made that "the periods of fusion indicated by radiographs of the bony extremities are approximately three years earlier than the periods of fusion indicated by anatomical evidence and as given in anatomy textbooks, because epiphyseal lines can remain visible on the bone for a considerable time after the radiographs indicate that fusion has taken place." In Figures 13 and 14 I reproduce their Figures 8 and 9. In the illustration of the humerus I'd record the degree of union as *B* (Todd) or 1 (McKern and Stewart), *on the bone*. In the *x-ray film*, since union has begun centrally (which is normal) I'd certainly go no further than *B+* or 2, i.e., with the x-ray film depth is gained and hence some increase in progress toward union becomes obvious. The same reasoning

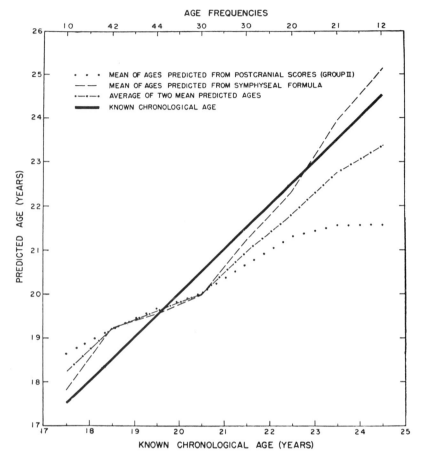

Fig. 12. Graph showing the relationships between mean predicted ages, the average mean predicted age, and known age.

applies to the illustration of the femur; certainly in the distal or condylar end I'd follow the bone rather than the film!

Actually the differences between bone and film (between, say Stages *B* or *B*+, or between Stages 1 or 2) is not too great: probably no more than ± six months or so. I cannot accept the "three years earlier" dictum in favor of the x-ray film. Nor can I accept a persistent "scar" as evidence of incomplete union or even of recent union. The problem of total duration from State *O* to *C*, or from Stage 0–4, has never been adequately tackled, but it is

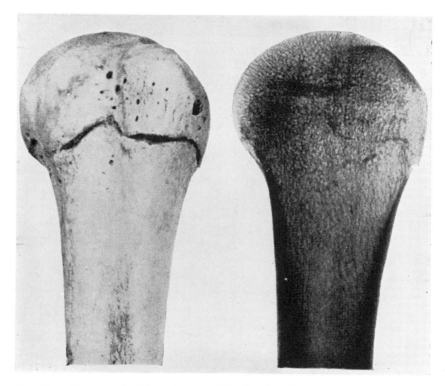

Fig. 13. Photograph (L) and x-ray (R) of a female humerus, age unknown. The epiphyseal "gap" is plainly seen on the bone, but some trabeculation across the gap has occurred.   The x-ray film suggests a higher degree of union, for it has begun in the depths, i.e., centrally.

probably of the order of 12–18 months, give or take a few months either way, i.e., in an individual bone, once union has begun.

With the foregoing discussion in mind I recommend Flecker's ('32/'33, pp. 158-159) over-view tabulation of appearance and union of centers of ossification as seen roentgenographically.   It is in pretty fair agreement with others similarly derived (see, for example, Clark, '36), and in his '42 article Flecker discusses the theme of variability; his '32/'33 data are as in Table 9.

If hand skeleton is reasonably complete (with at least several metacarpal and phalangeal epiphyses) and if knee is similarly present (distal femur with its epiphysis, proximal tibia with its epiphysis) then the x-ray films thereof may be compared with the

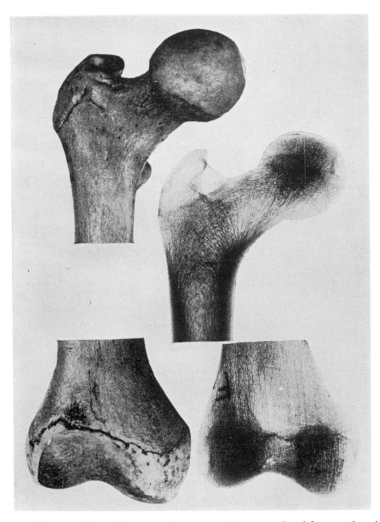

Fig. 14. Photographs and x-rays of upper and lower ends of femur of male of stated age at death of 23 years. In the upper end the head and trochanter have begun to unite (L side), while in the x-ray degree of union seems to suggest a "scar of recent union." In the lower end the photograph and the x-ray show a similar contrast.

TABLE 9

CHRONOLOGICAL ORDER OF APPEARANCE AND FUSION OF EPIPHYSES*

Before birth:		
Both sexes	Appearance	Head of humerus, distal femur, proximal tibia, calcaneum, talus
Female	"	Cuboid
During first year:		
Both sexes	Appearance	Hamate, capitate, head of femur, third cuneiform
Female	"	Capitulum, distal radius, distal tibia, distal fibula
Male	"	Cuboid
During second year:		
Both sexes	Appearance	Proximal phalanges of inner four fingers
Female	"	First metacarpal, distal phalanges of thumb, middle and ring fingers, tarsal navicular, first and second cuneiforms
Male	"	Capitulum, distal epiphysis of radius, distal fibula
At age of 2:		
Both sexes	Appearance	Inner four metacarpals, first metatarsal, proximal phalanges of toes, distal phalanx of hallux
Female	"	Proximal phalanx of thumb, middle row of phalanges of fingers
Male	"	First metacarpal, distal phalanx of thumb, and distal phalanx of index, first cuneiform
At age of 3:		
Female	Appearance	Patella, proximal fibula, second metatarsal, third metatarsal, middle phalanges of second, third and fourth toes, distal phalanges of third and fourth toes
Male	Appearance	Triquetrum, proximal phalanx of thumb, middle phalanges of middle and ring fingers, tarsal navicular, second cuneiform
At the age of 4:		
Both sexes	Appearance	Fourth metatarsal
Female	"	Head of radius, fifth metatarsal
	Fusion	Greater tubercle to head of humerus
Male	Appearance	Lunate, middle phalanges of index and little fingers, distal phalanges of middle and ring fingers, second metatarsal, third metatarsal, middle phalanx of second toe
At the age of 5:		
Both sexes	Appearance	Navicular (carpal), multangulum majus, greater trochanter, distal phalanx of second toe
Female	"	Medial epicondyle, distal ulna, lunate, triquetrum, multangulum minus, distal phalanx of index
Male	"	Head of radius, distal phalanx of little finger, patella, proximal fibula, fifth metatarsal, middle phalanges of third and fourth toes, distal phalanges of third and fourth toes
	Fusion	Greater tubercle to head of humerus
At the age of 6:		
Male	Appearance	Medial epicondyle, distal ulna, multangulum minus
At the age of 7:		
Female	Appearance	Distal phalanx of little finger
	Fusion	Rami of ischium and pubis

TABLE 9 (*Continued*)

CHRONOLOGICAL ORDER OF APPEARANCE AND FUSION OF EPIPHYSES

At the age of 8:		
Both sexes	Appearance	Apophysis of calcaneus
Female	"	Olecranon
At the age of 9:		
Female	Appearance	Trochlea, pisiform
Male	Fusion	Rami of ischium and pubis
At the age of 10:		
Male	Appearance	Trochlea, olecranon
At the age of 11:		
Female	Appearance	Lateral epicondyle
Male	"	Pisiform
At the age of 12:		
Male	Appearance	Lateral epicondyle
At the age of 13:		
Female	Appearance	Proximal sesamoid of thumb
	Fusion	Lower conjoint epiphysis of humerus, distal phalanx of thumb, bodies ilium, ischium and pubis
Male	"	Capitulum to trochlea and lateral epicondyle
At the age of 14:		
Female	Appearance	Acromion, iliac crest, lesser trochanter
	Fusion	Olecranon, upper radius, proximal phalanx of ring finger, distal phalanx of thumb, head of femur, greater trochanter, distal tibia and fibula, apophysis calcaneus, first metatarsal, proximal phalanges of toes
Male	Appearance	Proximal sesamoid of thumb, base of fifth metatarsal
At the age of 15:		
Both sexes	Appearance	Sesamoid of little finger
	Fusion	Distal phalanges of second, third and fourth toes
Female	Appearance	Sesamoid of index and little fingers
	Fusion	Medial epicondyle, first metacarpal, proximal phalanx of thumb, distal phalanges of inner four fingers, proximal tibia, outer four metatarsals, middle phalanx of second toe, distal phalanges of inner four toes
Male	Appearance	Acromion
	Fusion	Ilium, ischium and pubis
At the age of 16:		
Female	Appearance	Distal sesamoid of thumb, tuber ischii
	Fusion	Inner four metacarpals, proximal phalanges of index, middle and little fingers, middle phalanges of fingers
Male	"	Lower conjoint epiphysis of humerus, medial epicondyle, olecranon, head of radius, distal phalanx of middle finger, apophysis of calcaneus
At the age of 17:		
Both sexes	Fusion	Acromion
Female	"	Upper conjoint epiphysis of humerus, distal ulna, distal femur, proximal fibula

Male	Appearance	Distal sesamoid of thumb
	Fusion	First metacarpal, proximal phalanges of thumb and ring finger, middle phalanges, index, middle and ring fingers, distal phalanges of thumb, index, ring and little fingers, head of femur, greater trochanter, distal tibia and fibula, metatarsals, proximal phalanges of toes, middle phalanx of second toe, distal phalanx of hallux

At the age of 18:

Female	Fusion	Distal radius
Male	"	Inner four metacarpals, proximal phalanges of index, middle and little fingers, middle phalanges of little finger, proximal tibia

At the age of 19:

Male	Appearance	Sesamoid of index, tuber ischii
	Fusion	Upper conjoint epiphysis of humerus, distal radius and ulna, distal femur, proximal fibula

At the age of 20:

Both sexes	Fusion	Iliac crest
Male	"	Tuber ischii

At the age of 21.

Both sexes	Appearance	Clavicle
Female	Fusion	Tuber ischii

At the age of 22:

Both sexes	Fusion	Clavicle

* From Flecker, '32/'33.

norms of two excellent *Atlases*, the hand by Greulich and Pyle ('59) and the knee by Pyle and Hoerr ('55). Acheson ('54) has developed the "Oxford method" for assessing skeletal age via the x-ray film but it is of limited value for identification purposes unless the majority of epiphyses are recovered.

Earlier mention was made of the deplorable absence of adequate statistical studies in either appearance or union of centers. A notable exception is the work of Pyle and Sontag ('43) who report on time and order of onset of ossification in 61 centers in the hand and foot in boys and girls (Table 10). Greulich and Pyle ('59) give mean and standard deviation for hand centers.

Obviously, Table 10 is of direct value in identification only if hands and/or feet are reasonably complete. Conceptually, however, it is very important for it emphasizes a basic variability that must replace a precise age with an approximate age; emphasis is upon the *chance* that estimated age is correct, with recognizable tolerance or "error" of so-and-so many months (or possibly years in the case of union).

In the x-ray films of growing long bones there are often observed,

TABLE 10

TIME AND ORDER OF ONSET OF OSSIFICATION*

	Boys					Girls			
Order of Appearance	No. of Boys	Mean Age in Months	Standard Deviation (Months)	Coefficient Variability (Per Cent) $100 \times \frac{SD}{M}$	Order of Appearance	No. of Girls	Mean Age in Months	Standard Deviation (Months)	Coefficient Variability (Per Cent) $100 \times \frac{SD}{M}$
1. Distal femur	50	0	0.1		1. Distal femur	50	0		
2. Proximal tibia	50	0.1	0.3		2. Proximal tibia	50	0.1		
3. Cuboid	50	0.5	0.7		3. Cuboid	50	0.4		
4. Head of humerus	50	0.7	0.8		4. Head of humerus	50	0.9		
*5. Capitate	50	2.4	1.8	73.1	*5. Capitate	50	2.3	2.1	92.1
*6. Hamate	50	3.4	2.2	67.2	*6. Hamate	50	2.5	2.3	91.7
7. Distal tibia	50	3.9	1.5	37.5	7. Distal tibia	50	3.4	1.4	41.2
8. Head of femur	50	4.4	2.0	45.9	8. Head of femur	50	3.7	1.6	44.1
*9. Lateral cuneiform	50	4.4	4.3	97.5	*9. Lateral cuneiform	50	3.8	4.4	113.6
*10. Capitulum	50	6.3	4.3	68.3	*10. Capitulum	50	4.1	3.6	87.5
*11. Gt. tuber. humerus	50	11.4	7.2	63.3	11. Gt. tuber. humerus	50	6.6	3.3	49.4
12. Distal fibula	50	12.5	4.1	33.0	12. Distal fibula	50	9.3	2.6	28.5
13. Distal radius	50	13.0	4.7	36.2	13. Prox. 3rd finger	50	10.4	3.1	29.7
14. Prox. 3rd finger	50	16.2	5.3	33.0	14. Distal 1st toe	50	10.6	2.8	26.5
15. Distal 1st toe	50	16.8	5.6	33.5	*15. Distal radius	50	10.8	4.4	41.1
16. Prox. 2nd finger	50	17.3	5.0	28.9	16. Proximal 2nd finger	50	11.0	3.0	27.4
17. Prox. 4th finger	50	17.7	5.4	30.8	17. Proximal 4th finger	50	11.1	3.2	29.1
18. Metacarpal II	50	17.9	5.1	28.3	18. Proximal 3rd toe	50	12.2	3.8	30.8
19. Distal 1st finger	50	18.4	6.2	33.9	19. Distal 1st finger	50	12.8	5.0	38.9
20. Prox. 3rd toe	50	19.5	5.2	26.5	20. Metacarpal II	50	12.8	3.7	29.0
21. Prox. 4th toe	50	21.0	5.1	24.3	21. Proximal 4th toe	50	13.6	3.8	28.0
22. Metacarpal III	50	21.1	6.4	30.2	22. Proximal 2nd toe	50	14.1	3.8	27.2
*23. Medial cuneiform	50	21.9	9.9	45.1	23. Metacarpal III	50	14.2	4.0	28.4
24. Prox. 5th finger	50	22.2	5.6	25.4	24. Proximal 5th finger	50	15.2	4.2	27.5
25. Prox. 2nd toe	50	22.2	5.8	26.2	25. Middle 4th finger	50	15.8	4.8	30.2
26. Metacarpal IV	50	23.6	7.1	29.9	26. Middle 3rd finger	50	15.9	4.9	30.8
27. Middle 3rd finger	50	24.9	7.6	30.6	27. Metacarpal IV	50	16.0	4.1	25.9
28. Middle 4th finger	50	24.9	7.8	31.2	*28. Medial cuneiform	50	16.7	8.5	50.7

No.	Center					No.	Center				
29.	Metacarpal V	50	8.0	26.0	30.5	29.	Metacarpal V	50	17.2	4.7	27.4
30.	Middle 2nd finger	50	7.5	26.9	27.8	30.	Middle 2nd finger	50	17.3	5.2	30.0
*31.	Triquetral	50	15.9	27.3	58.4	31.	Distal 4th finger	50	19.9	5.9	29.8
32.	Metatarsal I	50	4.7	27.7	17.1	32.	Metatarsal I	50	20.1	3.3	16.6
33.	Distal 3rd finger	50	6.4	27.8	23.2	33.	Distal 3rd finger	50	20.2	3.9	19.4
34.	Distal 4th finger	50	7.0	28.3	24.7	34.	Metacarpal I	50	20.3	5.3	26.0
*35.	Middle cuneiform	50	11.2	28.4	39.4	35.	Proximal 1st toe	50	20.3	5.5	27.1
36.	Metacarpal I	50	7.3	29.8	24.4	*36.	Middle cuneiform	50	21.3	7.6	35.8
37.	Prox. 1st toe	50	5.8	29.9	19.3	37.	Proximal 5th toe	50	21.3	4.8	22.4
38.	Prox. 5th toe	50	5.9	32.0	18.4	38.	Proximal 1st finger	50	21.6	5.1	23.8
*39.	Navicular (foot)	50	13.5	33.4	40.3	*39.	Triquetral	50	23.6	13.7	57.9
40.	Metatarsal II	50	6.8	33.4	20.4	40.	Middle 5th finger	50	24.9	7.9	31.7
41.	Prox. 1st finger	50	7.9	34.8	22.6	41.	Distal 5th finger	50	25.5	7.0	27.6
42.	Distal 2nd finger	48	7.9	37.0	21.4	*42.	Navicular (foot)	50	25.8	11.1	43.3
43.	Distal 5th finger	48	7.4	37.4	19.7	43.	Metatarsal II	50	25.8	6.1	23.6
44.	Middle 5th finger	48	11.7	40.3	29.0	44.	Distal 2nd finger	50	25.8	6.9	26.9
45.	Metatarsal III	47	7.9	41.5	19.0	45.	Metatarsal III	50	29.1	6.4	21.9
46.	Gt. troch. femur	48	7.6	42.6	17.9	46.	Gt. troch. femur	50	29.8	6.4	21.5
*47.	Lunate	48	19.3	46.0	42.3	47.	Distal 4th toe	50	30.7	7.9	25.9
48.	Proximal fibula	46	11.8	47.0	25.2	48.	Proximal fibula	50	32.6	9.3	28.5
49.	Metatarsal IV	46	9.0	48.7	18.5	49.	Distal 3rd toe	50	32.8	7.7	23.6
50.	Distal 4th toe	44	10.1	51.2	19.8	50.	Metatarsal IV	50	34.0	7.2	21.2
51.	Patella	36	11.6	51.9	22.4	*51.	Lunate	50	34.6	14.2	41.1
52.	Distal 3rd toe	44	11.2	53.5	20.9	52.	Patella	43	34.8	8.5	24.6
53.	Metatarsal V	45	10.6	53.6	19.7	53.	Distal 2nd toe	50	35.5	7.3	20.5
54.	Distal 2nd toe	41	11.4	57.0	20.0	54.	Metatarsal V	50	38.6	8.4	21.7
55.	Navicular hand	38	14.1	60.1	23.4	55.	Med. ep. humerus	47	41.3	9.9	24.1
56.	Proximal radius	37	17.2	63.5	27.1	*56.	Greater multangular	46	47.0	14.8	31.5
*57.	Greater multangular	39	19.7	64.3	30.7	57.	Proximal radius	46	47.5	12.1	25.4
58.	Lesser multangular	36	15.2	64.4	23.6	58.	Navicular hand	45	47.8	12.3	25.7
59.	Med. ep. humerus	37	17.5	73.6	23.8	*59.	Lesser multangular	44	48.3	14.8	30.6
60.	Distal ulna	31	10.6	82.4	12.9	60.	Distal ulna	42	63.2	15.3	24.3
61.	Epiph. calcaneus	31	14.0	89.6	15.6	61.	Epiph. calcaneus	42	63.7	11.8	18.4

* Centers marked with an asterisk show "the tendency toward greater variability in onset of ossification of carpal and tarsal bone centers as contrasted with epiphyses of long bones." From Pyle and Sontag, '43, Table I–II.

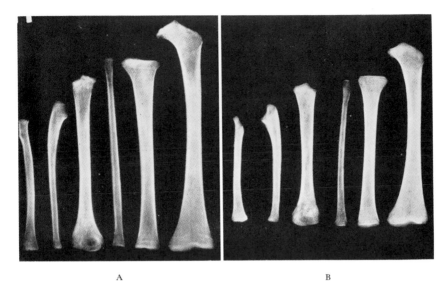

A   B

Fig. 15. X-ray films of long bones to show transverse striations at ends of shafts.
A, Skeleton A; B, Skeleton B.

at the diaphyseal ends, one or more transverse lines. These are
evidences of growth disturbance, and are called "scars of arrested
growth." They have been studied by Park and Howland ('21),
by Harris ('26) and by Todd ('33). I quote from Todd as follows:

> Certain of the deficiency diseases, notably scurvy and rickets,
> present very striking interferences with growth and development.
> Even when a child with scurvy is apparently well nourished there
> is an arrest of intercellular matrix formation at the growing ends
> of the bones which shows in the roentgenogram as a dense white
> line. Arrest of bony growth is the obvious consequence. Rickets
> does not affect the foundation substance so much as the actual
> texture of the bones. The secondary trabeculae, constituting the
> supply of mobile calcium, are absorbed . . .
>
> Associated with defects in appearance of ossific centers are the
> rings which are evident in all long bones after exanthemata. They
> mark pauses in bony growth. A crowded mass of these rings at
> the lower end of the tibia and less frequently at the lower end of
> the radius indicates a feeding problem or long continued low or
> intermittent fever . . .

In 1935, I examined two immature skeletons sent me from Harts-
burg, Mo. They were labelled A and B. The x-ray films of the

long bones (see Fig. 15, in which, from left to right, radius, ulna, humerus, fibula, tibia, femur, shafts only, are shown) showed transverse lines as follows (measurements in mm. are distances from ends of shaft):

Bone	Skeleton A	Skeleton B
Distal radius	2 scars: 7.2, 6.0	6 scars: 12.5, 7.0, 6.0, 4.3, 3.0, 1.0
Distal tibia	7 scars: 15.0, 12.5, 11.5, 9.8, 7.0, 5.2, 1.5	6 scars: 16.0, 10.1, 8.2, 6.0, 5.0, 3.3
Proximal tibia	3 scars: 9.8, 7.5, 6.2	4 scars, and cessation: 14.0, 7.5, 6.0, 3.0
Distal femur	4 scars: 16.0, 14.2, 12.0, 2.5	2 scars: 5.0, 2.5
Distal fibula	scar at end is indication of cessation of growth	5 scars and cessation: 12.0, 10.0, 6.0, 4.0, 2.5
Humerus	. . .	Cessation of growth, distal and proximal

The foregoing data led to the conclusion: In both individuals the scars of arrested development are evidence of either repeated illnesses or an intermittent illness of approximately $1^{1}/_{2}$ years duration. It is not without significance that in distal tibia of A and B there is a record of an illness at the same time: 15.0 and 16.0 mm., respectively. This virtual identity does not hold for the other bones, nor is there such complete uniformity thereafter. The fact remains, however, that the onset of illness was about the same for both, and that for $1^{1}/_{2}$ years prior to death both the children were very sickly.

In this case I felt that the two skeletons were those of siblings, i.e., brother and sister, brothers, or sisters.

4. Appearance and Union in Specific Bones Not Usually Given in Tabulated Data

Hands, feet, and long bones are the skeletal parts most frequently studied and discussed. There are, however, other bones that should be noted, and these will now be considered.

Clavicle (Todd and D'Errico, '28; McKern and Stewart, '57). Todd and D'Errico state that the medial (sternal) end begins to unite at 21–22 years, and is completely united by 25 years; the lateral (acromial) end "ossifies and unites in the twentieth year, barring anomalies." They point out that "the sternal epiphysis does not always completely ossify." No significant sex differences in union of either end was noted. McKern and Stewart conclude (p. 97):

As early as 18 years, but any time between 18–25 years, the epiphyseal cap begins to unite to the billowed surface of the medial end of the clavicle. Union begins at the approximate center of the face and spreads to the superior margin where it may progress either anteriorly or posteriorly. From 25–30 years the majority of cases are undergoing union. The last site of union is located, in the form of a fissure, along the inferior border. With the obliteration of these fissures (at age 31), the epiphysis is completely united.

Table 11, from McKern and Stewart, gives a good idea of age-range in Stages of union for the medial clavicular epiphysis.

Vertebrae (Todd and D'Errico, '26; Girdany and Golden, '52; McKern and Stewart, '57).

TABLE 11

Age Distribution of the Stages of Union for the Medial Clavicular Epiphysis (in %)*

Age	No.	Right Stage of Union					Left Stage of Union				
		0	1	2	3	4	0	1	2	3	4
17	10	—	—	—	—	—	—	—	—	—	—
18	45	90	10	—	—	—	86	12	2	—	—
19	52	79	13	8	—	—	73	21	4	—	—
20	45	69	28	11	2	—	56	35	7	2	—
21	37	36	43	13	8	—	47	32	13	8	—
22	24	4	27	39	30	—	1	33	37	29	—
23	26	—	11	43	40	6	—	8	43	40	9
24–25	27	—	3	10	52	37	—	3	10	52	37
26–27	25	—	—	—	36	64	—	—	—	36	64
28–29	18	—	—	—	31	69	—	—	—	31	69
30	11	—	—	—	9	91	—	—	—	9	91
31	54	—	—	—	—	100	—	—	—	—	100
Total	374										

* From McKern and Stewart, '57, Table 28.

Todd and D'Errico (pp. 28–29) studied the odontoid ossicle of C2 (second cervical vertebra): "A single center for the centrum appears about the third foetal month, twin centers for the base of the odontoid at the fourth or fifth month. These fuse with the body between the fourth and sixth years. The apical center appears about the second year and is united at about twelve years. This is the accepted description." They go on to say that "perhaps it would be safer to state that union occurs certainly before twelve years."

Girdany and Golden generalize that the vertebrae "ossify from three primary centers and nine secondary centers; any of these secondary centers, except for annular epiphyses, may fail to fuse." The primary centers, present at birth, are for the body and, bilaterally, for the neural arch; body and arch centers fuse in cervical vetebrae at three years, in lumbar at six years. Centers for spine, transverse processes, and superior and inferior articular processes, and for the mammillary processes of the lumbar vertebrae, appear at 16 years, unite at 25 years. Annular epiphyses (superiorly and inferiorly on the centrum or body) usually appear at or near puberty, but may do so as early as seven years. (Time of union is not stated). In first cervical vertebra (C1) an anterior center appears at birth (or within the first year) and unites at six years; the posterior tubercle fuses with the arch at three years. In the *sacrum* upper bodies fuse by 16 years, lower by 18 years, all by 30 years; lateral (auricular) epiphyses appear at 16–18 years, fuse by 25 years. Center for the first *coccygeal* vertebra (Co 1) appears at one year, for Co 2 at five to ten years, for Co 3 at 10–13 years, and for Co 4–5 at 15–18 years.

McKern and Stewart offer an overall evaluation for cervical, thoracic, and lumbar vertebrae as follows (p. 110) (only the two central epiphyses and that of the spinous process are noted):

> The presacral vertebral column is completely ossified by the 24th year. Noteworthy is the sequential pattern of ossification which shows the last signs of complete maturity occurring in the upper thoracic vertebrae (specifically, T-4 and T-5).
>
> Striations tend to disappear from the surface of the centra, starting at 23 years of age, but may persist in the lumbar region for many years. Other age changes, in the form of lipping of the anterior borders and the formation of spurs on the laminae of the dorsal arches, show a progressive increase in their occurrence and gross development. However, all are too variable to be of much assistance in age identification.

In Table 12 these authors give the Stages of the union of the superior and inferior epiphyseal rings (annular epiphyses).

For the *sacrum* McKern and Stewart conclude as follows (p. 154):

> The several elements comprising the sacrum begin to fuse from below upwards and along the sides. By 23 years ossification

is complete except often between the S 1–2 centra, where a gap may persist until the 32nd year. This gap seems to represent a sort of 'lapsed union' (see Todd and Lyon) which may be related to an extra wide intersegmental space.

The lateral joints of the sacrum also undergo changes but these are not very useful for ageing purposes.

Ribs (Girdany and Golden, '52; McKern and Stewart, '57). Girdany and Golden note centers for head and tubercles (no tubers cles in ribs 11–12) appearing at 14 years, fusing at 25 years.

McKern and Stewart conclude as follows (p. 160):

> No significant differences were noted due to right or left sides. The present data point to a probable age of 17 years for first appearance of complete union of the head epiphyses and a definite age of 24 years for the stage when all ribs are mature in all cases. However, ossification begins in the upper and lower ribs and slowly progresses toward the middle. Thus, the last ribs to become fully united are ribs 4 to 9.

Scapula (Cohn, '21; Girdany and Golden, '52; McKern and Stewart, '57). Cohn states that a center for the coracoid epiphysis may appear between birth and two years, but "is evident by three years." The center for the acromial process "is rarely evident before the middle of the 14th year," with "complete ossification" (union) about the mid-18th year. Girdany and Golden note the coracoid center at birth to one year, with union at 18 years; the epiphysis for the vertebral border appears at 15 years, unites at 20

TABLE 12

THE AGE DISTRIBUTION OF STAGES OF UNION FOR THE SUPERIOR AND INFERIOR EPIPHYSEAL RINGS OF THE PRESACRAL COLUMN AS A WHOLE (IN %)*

Age	No.	Superior Surface Stages					Inferior Surface Stages				
		0	1	2	3	4	0	1	2	3	4
17–18	54	5	22	37	23	13	2	24	37	23	13
19	50		10	30	36	24		8	32	48	14
20	43		7	14	33	46		7	14	37	42
21	35			20	27	63			20	36	44
22	24			4	8	88			4	8	88
23	26				7	93				11	89
24–25	27					100					100
Total	259										

* From McKern and Stewart, '57, Table 31.

years.   McKern and Stewart note that the scapula normally has six epiphyses: two for the coracoid process, and one each for the margin of the glenoid cavity, the acromion, the inferior angle, and the medial or vertebral border.   They report on only the last three epiphyses, plus "lipping" of the acromial facet and the glenoid fossa.   They conclude (p. 119):

> Though the epiphysis for the medial border lags in the early twenties, fusion for all three (acromion, inferior angle) is completed by 23rd year.
>
> The occurrence of lipping on the acromial facet and glenoid fossa cannot be used for other than supportive age evidence.

Later age-changes in the scapula have been studied by Graves ('22);   see also Todd ('39);   Cobb ('52);   Stewart ('54).   The following summary is taken from Stewart (p. 441):

> Age changes in the scapula due to ossification after maturity:
>
> Lipping of the circumferential margin of the glenoid fossa. Usually begins at the notch or depression located at the junction of the upper and middle thirds of the ventral margin (begins at 30–35 years).   The order of progression is usually ventral, inferior, dorsal and superior margins.
>
> Lipping of the clavicular facet.   Seldom uniform, but may involve entire margin (begins at 35–40 years).
>
> Appearance of a "plaque" or "facet" on the under side of the acromial process.   Often prolongs acromion tip from 2 to 8 mm. or more (begins at 35–40 or 40–45 years).
>
> Increasing demarcation of the triangular area at the base (vertebral margin) of the scapular spine.   Begins at 50 years or over.
>
> Appearance of cristae scapulae (50 years or over).   Although variable in number and development, they tend to become broader at their bases, more prominent and their apices more roughened or serrated with advancing years.

> Age changes in the scapula due to an atrophic process after maturity:
>
> Surface vascularity, seen as a number of fine delicate lines, like the marks on a dollar bill (below 25 years of age).   Diminish in visibility and finally disappear as age advances.   Vary also with fixation of bone.

Deep vascularity, seen as similar lines, but now by transillumination only (25–30 years). Tend to diminish with age but never
wholly disappear.

Atrophic spots—localized, discrete or coalescing areas of bone
atrophy—noted by transillumination, especially in the infraspinous fossa (begins at 45 years). Patchiness in vascularity
is probably a fore-runner of these spots.

Buckling and "pleating" of the infraspinous area (early 30's and
after), leading to actual distortion (40 years and over). These
phenomena appear to depend upon altered vascularity leading to irregular bone absorption (atrophy) especially of the
cancellous tissue.

B. CRITERIA OF AGE IN THE HUMAN SKELETON: PRENATAL OSSIFICATION

Fetal age is best stated in terms of lunar months (10 lunar
months of 28 days each = the human gestation period of 280 days),
although age in weeks is frequently given. Drennan and Keen
('53) give a useful tabulation of fetal age as follows, with particular
reference to the skeleton (Table 13).

Hill ('39) gives the following classification of fetal age by
crown-rump length:

Lunar month	C-R length (with range)
2	69 mm. (up to 80)
3	115 " (81–135)
4	157 " (136–175)
5	194 " (176–215)
6	233 " (216–255)
7 male	274 " ⎱ (256–285)
7 female	268 " ⎰
8 male	298 " ⎱ (286–315)
8 female	298 " ⎰
9 male	332 " ⎱ (316–340)
9 female	333 " ⎰
10 male	348 " ⎱ 341 plus
10 female	349 " ⎰

In a bit more detail Tchaperoff ('37) notes that no centers ossify
before the 7th week; by the 9th week all C and T vertebral bodies,
iliac wings, and femoral, tibial, fibular shafts have appeared;
between weeks 21–25 the calcaneus appears, and between weeks
24–28 the talus; by the 35th week the distal femoral epiphysis
has appeared, by the 37th week body of Co 1, and by the 39th
week the proximal tibial epiphysis.

The basic references in this Section are Flecker ('32), Hill ('39), and Noback and Robertson ('51). The first two are roentgenographic studies covering the entire prenatal period; the third is based on alizarine staining of the specimens and covers the first five prenatal months.

Flecker gives extensive data on *appearance* in terms of fetal length, basing his findings on 70 foeti, 30–334 mm. in length. In the *vertebral column* the cervical neural arches are present by 70 mm.; cervical bodies are present by 165 mm. +. Thoracic and lumbar vertebrae have all centers by 70 mm. In the sacrum bodies of S1-2

TABLE 13

THE MAIN POINTS BY WHICH THE AGE OF THE FETUS IS JUDGED BETWEEN THE THIRD MONTH OF INTRA-UTERINE LIFE AND THE TIME OF BIRTH*

Age of Fetus in Calendar Months	Crown-rump Length or Sitting Height	Other important Signs
End of third month	About 7 cm.	—
End of fourth month	About 13 cm.	—
End of fifth month	About 18 cm.	External genitalia sufficiently developed to enable the sex to be recognized. Primary centre of ossification of calcaneum has appeared.
End of sixth month	About 22 cm.	—
End of seventh month	About 26 cm.	Primary centre of ossification of talus has appeared. Fetus is viable.
End of eighth month	About 30 cm.	—
End of ninth month or just before birth	About 34 cm.	The testes have descended. The center of ossification in the lower epiphysis of the femur has appeared. The centre of ossification in the cuboid and sometimes one in the upper epiphysis of the tibia, has appeared.

* From Drennan and Keen, '53, Table 1.

are present by 70 mm., and by 90 mm. S1-5 bodies are all present (there is great variability here); sacral neural arches appear, for S1 at 109 mm., and for S1-5 by 171 mm. in males, 205 mm. in females; sacral lateral masses appear as three centers: first pair 180 mm. male, 220 mm. female; second pair 220 mm., both sexes; third pair 220 mm. male, 312 mm. female. In the coccyx Co 1 is present at 262 mm. female, 295 mm. male. In the *thorax* there are 11 pairs of ribs present by 70 mm., and the sternum has segments 1–3 for males at 180 mm., segments 1–4 for males at 218 mm., and all five segments at 283 mm. male, 285 mm. female. In the *upper extremity* the clavicle is present in males of 30 mm., the humerus is seen at 294 mm. female, 295 mm. male; no carpals were seen in Flecker's series; phalanges 2 of the hand were found at 109 mm. +. In the lower extremity the ilium is seen at 70 mm. +, the ischium at 109 mm. +, and the pubis at 165 mm. male, 205 mm. female; distal femur is seen at 262 mm. female, 263 mm. male; proximal tibia at 294 mm., both sexes; in the foot calcaneus is seen at 165 mm. male, 205 mm. female, talus at 180 mm. male, 205 mm. female, cuboid at 295 mm. male, 315 mm. female; phalanx 2 for toe II at 185 mm. male, 220 mm. female, for toe III at 171 mm. male, 220 mm. female, for toe IV at 275 mm. male, 233 mm. female, for toe V at 275 mm. male; phalanx 3 for toes II-V is seen at 109 mm. male, 150 mm. female. Hill ('39), who gives his data in lunar months 2–10, agrees substantially with Flecker.

Noback and Robertson state that there are three methods for observing prenatal ossification: (1) roentgenographic, as in Flecker, above; (2) serial sectioning; (3) clearing, then staining with alizarin red. Here, once more, the actual specimen takes precedence in reliability over the x-ray film thereof: "Data obtained from roentgenographs of embryos are of limited value, since the actual formation of a center precedes the time of its radiological recognition. An extreme example is the parietal bone, that is noted as appearing at 194 mm. CR radiologically (Hill, '39) at 31 to 45 mm. by the alizarin red method." The authors present their findings in very complete tabular form, including their own findings together with all previously recorded observations on human embryos based on (1) cleared, (2) cleared and stained with alizarin red, and (3) serially sectioned. Their conclusions are as follows (pp. 24–25):

> In the *skull*, the sequence is (1) facial and calvarial centers, (2) basicranial centers and (3) hyoid centers. In the *thorax*, the sequence is (1) costal centers, (2) thoracic vertebral centers and (3) sternal centers. In the *vertebral column*, the centers of the centra and neural arches appear concurrently, the neural arch centers appear cephalocaudally while the centrum centers, which first appear in the lower thoracic region, subsequently appear cephalically and caudally from their initial site of appearance.

In the *upper extremity*, the sequence is (1) humerus, (2) radius, (3) ulna, (4) distal phalanges, (5) metacarpals, (6) proximal phalanges and (7) middle phalanges. In the *lower extremity*, the sequence is (1) femur, (2) tibia, (3) fibula, (4) metatarsals, (5) distal phalanges, (6) proximal phalanges and (7) middle phalanges. The centers of the *pectoral girdle* appear before the *pelvic centers*. The sequence is (1) clavicle, (2) scapula, (3) ilium, (4) ischium and (5) pubis.

One pair of bilateral ossification centers may appear at a different time than the other center of the pair, but the degree of such asymmetry is usually slight.*

* The matter of sidedness or "handedness" may as well be settled once and for all: there is normally no difference, right and left sides (see Baer and Durkatz, '57; Dreizen, *et al.* '57).

A detailed radiographic study of the prenatal ossification of the *pelvis* is that of Francis ('51), as follows (compare with Flecker):

Element	*CR length*
Ilium	60 mm.
Ischium	130–140 mm.
Pubis	160 mm.
S1–S3	80–90 mm.
Centrum S4	160 mm.
Centrum S5	200 mm.
Trans. proc. S1–S5	soon after resp. central
First lat. sacral center	210 mm.
Second lat. sacral center	280 mm.
Third lat. sacral center	340 mm.
First Co center	Birth

The problem of ossification centers at *birth* is most ably handled by Adair and Scammon ('21) (see also Menees and Holly, '32) The conclusions of Adair and Scammon are as follows (pp. 57–59):

1. The inferior femoral epiphysis, judging from all available data, is present in about 1 case in 20 in the eighth fetal month, in 1 case in 3 in the ninth month, in 6 cases in 7 in the tenth month, and in about 19 cases in 20 at birth (full-term infants). If not present at birth, the center appears before the close of the first postnatal month. In our own series the center was present in 98 per cent of all newborn children.

2. The superior tibial epiphysis, judging from all available material, is almost never present before the ninth fetal month. It is found in 1 case in 17 in the ninth month, about 2 cases in 5 in the tenth month and in about seven-eighths of all full-term newborn children. It was present in 81 per cent of the cases in our series.

3. The cuboid, according to all available data, first appears at about the beginning of the ninth fetal month. It is present, on the average, in about 1 case in 25 in the ninth month, in about 1 case in 4 in the tenth month, and in about 3 cases in 5 in full-term newborn children. In our own series the center was present in a much smaller per cent of all cases than is reported by other investigators (38 per cent).

4. Two carpal ossification centers, those of the os capitatum (os magnum) and of the os hamatum (unciform), may be present in the newborn. In our series the os capitatum was present in 15 per cent and the os hamatum in 9 per cent of all cases.

5. There is a close relation between total body-length and frequency of ossification of the several centers discussed in this paper. A similar, but less close, correlation exists between frequency of ossification and the body-weight.

6. In our material the correlation of body-weight, total body-length and frequency of ossification with menstrual age was quite close for the middle members of the series ranging in menstrual age from 270 to 300 days. But the outlying cases (having a menstrual age of less than 270 or more than 300 days) show little relation between these measures of bodily development and age as determined from the menstrual history.

7. Our evidence points to the conclusion that ossification proceeds slightly more rapidly in females than in males during intrauterine life even though the weight and dimensions of the females are less than those of the males.

8. Our observations show no direct evidence of any relation between parity and the rate of ossification in intrauterine life.

9. Variations in the *number* of ossification centers present for individual bones were limited to the os capitatum and os cuboideum. The latter is formed from an extremely variable number of centers. When anomalies in the number of centers are present they are often asymmetrical.

10. Variations in the order of appearance of centers were decidedly unusual in our material, being confined to premature ossification of the os cuboideum (2 cases) and of the premature ossification of the os capitatum (2 cases).

11. The usual order of appearance of the centers under consideration is as follows: (a) Inferior femoral epiphysis; (b) Superior tibial epiphysis; (c) Cuboid; (d) Os capitatum; (e) Os hamatum.

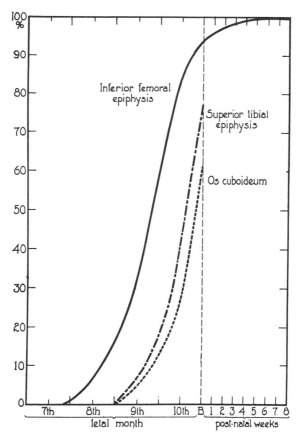

Fig. 16. Graphs showing the frequency of ossification in lower femur, upper tibia, and cuboid of the foot in later fetal life.

In Figure 16 the data by Adair and Scammon are graphically depicted for lower femur, upper tibia, and cuboid.

C. CRITERIA OF AGE IN THE HUMAN SKELETON: DIFFERENCES DUE TO RACE

This problem has not been systematically studied save for the possibility of differences in the first two decades of life, and even here studies have focussed mainly on evidence gained from hand and wrist, the so-called "carpal area" or "carpal age." There is a very serious limiting factor here; viz., there are norms or standards available only for an American white population. This raises the question of comparability: can we assess bone age in other racial samples via the American *Atlases* on the hand (Flory, Todd, Greulich and Pyle)? This question has been answered pragmatically, i.e., such *Atlases* have been used and the data available are based on the assumption that such use is valid.

For the *American Negro* Todd ('31), Kelly and Reynolds ('47), Christie ('49), and Kessler and Scott ('50) found Negro children to be a bit advanced during the first year of life. Platt ('56) found no difference between white and Negro children age 7–12 years (Negro samples from Florida and from Philadelphia). The Philadelphia findings were confirmed by Bass ('58) in a later study.

Data from *other racial* groups also suggest lack of racial differences genetically entrenched. For Japanese Sutow ('53) suggested a real difference to account for skeletal retardation of 6–24 months in Hiroshima boys 6–19 years of age and 9–24 months in Hiroshima girls 6–19 years of age. Greulich ('58) could find no such racial basis in his study of Japanese-Americans born in the U.S. For Guamanian children Greulich ('47) felt that exogenous factors were the cause of a measure of retardation. Much the same conclusion was reached by Cameron ('38) on Asian children generally, and by Webster and de Sarem ('52) on Ceylonese children. Abbie and Adey ('53) found no differences in Central Australian aboriginal children age three weeks to 19 years. Some general retardation was found in West African native children age 9–20 years by Weiner and Thambipillai ('52), in East African native children by Mackay ('52) and by Vincent ('54), and in South African native children by Beresowski and Lundie ('52), but again the difference between these samples and the white norms was ascribed to exogenous rather than endogenous factors. Borovansky and Hnevkovsky ('29) found no real differences in Czech children. Falkner *et al.*, ('58) studied age factors in the first two years of life in samples from London, Paris, Zurich, and Dakar, using Acheson's "Oxford method." The latter children were a bit advanced at birth, but by age two were somewhat retarded. Newman and Collazos ('57) found 200 boys from the Vicos Hacienda in the Peruvian Sierra to be nearly three years retarded (Greulich-Pyle *Atlas*), but dietary and intestinal parasitic factors are blamed. Basu ('38) tackled the problem of epiphyseal union, rather than that of appearance in Bengalese girls. He stated that "diaphyseo-epiphyseal union has a climatic and racial variability." He raised the question as to comparability of American (or European) standards, and expressed a doubt "whether there may be evolved one common standard for the whole of the heterogeneous population of India."

The most extensive tabulation for non-whites is that of Modi ('57) for East Indian children. I have adapted his data and present them in Table 14. It is a lengthy Table, but it highlights problems of sampling I have raised earlier in this Chapter. It also highlights the whole theme of applicability of "standards" and "group norms" to individual cases. Modi makes the following statement with which I find myself in general agreement.

> Owing to the variations in climatic, dietetic, hereditary and other factors affecting the people of the different Provinces of India it cannot be reasonably expected to formulate a uniform standard for the determination of the age of the union of epiphyses for the whole of India. However, from investigations carried out in certain Provinces it has been concluded that the age at which the union of epiphyses takes place in Indians is about 2 to 3 years in advance of the age incidence in Europeans and that the epiphysial union occurs in females somewhat earlier than in males.
>
> In ascertaining the age of young persons radiograms of any of the main joints of the upper or the lower extremity (of both sides of the body) should be taken, and an opinion should be given according to (Table 141) but it must be remembered that too much reliance should not be placed on this table as it merely indicates an average and is likely to vary in individual cases even of the same Province owing to the eccentricities of development.

For practical, working purposes we may assume that there are no racial differences in skeletal age that are truly genetic in origin. When working with populations other than white (American, European) factors of diet and health should be first carefully studied and evaluated.

In a sense the foregoing paragraph imposes a considerable limitation upon the use of available American or European ossification schedules. It may be argued that genetically they *do* apply, i.e., that the maturation process is characteristically the same for all

TABLE 14

AGE IN YEARS OF APPEARANCE AND FUSION OF EPIPHYSES IN EAST INDIANS*

	Galstaun (Bengalees)		Basu & Basu (Bengalees) Hindu Females	Hepworth (Punjabis)	Lall & Townsend (Females of United Provinces)	Lall & Nat (Males of United Provinces)	Pillai (Madrasis)
	Females	Males					
Clavicle (Sternal End):							
Appearance	14 to 16	15 to 19	—	—	—	—	—
Fusion	20	22	—	—	—	—	—
Base of Coracoid of Scapula:							
Appearance	2½ months	2½ months	—	—	—	—	—
Fusion	2½	2½	—	—	—	—	—
Coracoid Tip:							
Appearance	10 to 11	10 to 11	—	—	—	—	13
Fusion	16	16	—	—	—	—	14
Angle of Coracoid:							
Appearance	8 to 10	10 to 14	—	—	—	—	—
Fusion	16	17 to 18	—	—	—	—	—
Acromion:							
Appearance	12 to 14	14 to 17	—	—	—	—	13 to 14
Fusion	13 to 16	14 to 19	—	—	—	—	18
Humerus: Head							
Appearance	1	1	—	—	—	—	—
Fusion to shaft	14 to 16	14 to 18	16 to 17	17 to 18	—	—	14 to 17
Greater Tubercle:							
Appearance	2 to 4	2 to 4	—	—	—	—	—
Fusion to Head of Humerus	5 to 7	5 to 7	—	—	—	—	—
Fusion to lesser Tubercle	—	—	—	—	—	—	—
Humerus: Trochlea:							
Appearance	10	11	—	—	—	—	—
Fusion to Capitulum	9 to 13	11 to 15	12 to 13	—	—	—	—
Lateral Epicondyle							
Appearance	10	12	—	—	—	—	—
Fusion to Capitulum	10 to 12	11 to 16	12 to 13	14 to 15	—	—	13 to 14
Medial Epicondyle:							
Appearance	5	7	—	—	—	—	—
Fusion to shaft (Distal humeral epiphysis)	14	16	13 to 14	14½	14 to 15	15 to 17	14 to 17

Head of Radius:							
Appearance	6	8			16	17	14 to 17
Fusion	14	16	13 to 14	14 to 15	—	—	
Distal End of Radius:							
Appearance	1	1			—	—	
Fusion	16½	18	16 to 17	16 to 17	19	19	14 to 18
Olecranon:							
Appearance	9 to 12	11 to 13	13 to 14		15	16 or earlier	14 to 16
Fusion	15	17			—	—	
Distal End of Ulna:							
Appearance	8 to 10	10 to 11			—	—	
Fusion	17	18	16 to 17		19	19	14 to 18
Crest of Ilium:							
Appearance	14	17			—	—	
Fusion	17 to 19	19 to 20			—	—	14 to 18
Ischium and Pubis:							
Fusion	8½	8½			—	—	
Acetabulum:							
Disappearance of Triradiate Cartilage	14	15 to 16			—	—	11 to 14
Ischial Tuberosity:							
Appearance	14 to 16	16 to 18			—	—	
Fusion	20	20			—	—	
Head of Femur:							
Appearance	1	1			—	—	
Fusion	14 to 15	16 to 17	13 to 14	15½ to 17	—	—	14 to 15
Great Trochanter:							
Appearance	—	—			—	—	
Fusion	14	17	14	16 to 17	—	—	14 to 17
Lesser Trochanter:							
Appearance					—	—	
Fusion	15 to 17	15 to 17	13		—	—	14 to 17
Distal End of Femur:							
Appearance	Before birth	Before birth			—	—	
Fusion	14 to 17	14 to 17	16	16½ to 17½	—	—	14 to 17
Proximal End of Tibia:							
Appearance	Shortly before or after birth	Shortly before or after birth			—	—	
Fusion	14 to 15	15 to 17	15 to 16	16½ to 17½	—	—	14 to 17
Distal End of Tibia:							
Appearance	—	—			—	—	
Fusion	14.1 to 14.4	16	14 to 15	16 to 17½	—	—	14 to 17

TABLE 14 (*Continued*)

AGE IN YEARS OF APPEARANCE AND FUSION OF EPIPHYSES IN EAST INDIANS*

	Galstaun (Bengalees)		Basu & Basu (Bengalees) Hindu Females	Hepworth (Punjabis)	Lall & Townsend (Females of United Provinces)	Lall & Nat (Males of United Provinces)	Pillai (Madrasis)
	Females	*Males*					
Proximal End of Fibula:							
Appearance	—	—					
Fusion	14 to 16	14 to 16	16 to 17	16½ to 17½	—	—	14 to 17
Distal End of Fibula:							
Appearance	—	—					
Fusion	13 to 15	14 to 16	15	17 to 18	—	—	14 to 17
Patella:							
Appearance	4	3 to 7	—	—	—	—	—
Fusion	—	—	—	—	—	—	—
Carpal Bones:							
Capitate (Os magnum):							
Appearance	½	½	—	—	—	—	—
Hamate (Unciform):							
Appearance	8 to 14 months	8 to 14 months	—	—	—	—	—
Triquetrum (Cuneiform):							
Appearance	2 to 3	3 to 4	—	—	—	—	—
Lunate (Semilunar):							
Appearance	5	5	—	—	—	—	—
Multangulum Majus (Trapezium):							
Appearance	5 to 6	7	—	—	—	—	—
Multangulum Minus (Trapezoid):							
Appearance	5 to 6	4 to 7	—	—	—	—	—
Navicular (Scaphoid):							
Appearance	6	7 to 11	—	—	—	—	—
Pisiform:							
Appearance	9 to 12	12 to 17	—	—	—	—	10 to 12
First Metacarpal Bones:							
Appearance	3	4	—	—	—	—	—
Fusion	14 to 16	16 to 18	—	—	—	—	14 to 17

Second, third, fourth and fifth									
Metacarpal Bones:									
Appearance	2 to 3	3 to 4	—	—	—	—	—	—	—
Fusion	14 to 15	16 to 18	—	—	—	—	—	—	14 to 17
Phalanges of the Hand:									
Proximal Row:									
Appearance	1½	2 to 4	—	—	—	—	—	—	—
Fusion	14 to 15	17 to 18	—	—	—	—	—	—	14 to 17
Middle Row:									
Appearance	2 to 3	3	—	—	—	—	—	—	—
Fusion	14 to 16	16 to 18	—	—	—	—	—	—	14 to 17
Terminal Row:									
Appearance	3	3 to 5	—	—	—	—	—	—	—
Fusion	15	17 to 18	—	—	—	—	—	—	14 to 17
Tarsal Bones:									
Calcaneus (Os Calcis) and Talus (Astragalus):									
Appearance	At birth	At birth	—	—	—	—	—	—	—
Cuboid:									
Appearance	At birth	At birth	—	—	—	—	—	—	—
Internal Cuneiform:									
Appearance	1 to 3	1 to 4	—	—	—	—	—	—	—
Middle Cuneiform:									
Appearance	1 to 3	2 to 4	—	—	—	—	—	—	—
External Cuneiform:									
Appearance	1 to 3	1 to 4	—	—	—	—	—	—	—
Navicular:									
Appearance	1 to 3	2	—	—	—	—	—	—	—
Metatarsal Bones:									
Appearance	3	4 to 5	—	—	—	—	—	—	—
Fusion	14 to 15	16 to 18	—	—	—	—	—	—	14 to 17
Tarsal Phalanges:									
Proximal Row:									
Appearance	1 to 3	2 to 4	—	—	—	—	—	—	—
Fusion	14 to 15	16 to 18	—	—	—	—	—	—	14 to 17
Middle Row:									
Appearance	3 to 4	3 to 4	—	—	—	—	—	—	—
Fusion	14 to 15	16 to 18	—	—	—	—	—	—	14 to 17
Terminal Row:									
Appearance	4 to 6	4 to 6	—	—	—	—	—	—	—
Fusion	13 to 14	15 to 17	—	—	—	—	—	—	14 to 17

* From Modi, '57, pp. 32–35.

peoples. It may be argued, too, that environmentally they *do not* apply, i.e., that the maturation process is too labile, susceptible to the variable influences of diet, health, endocrine balance, etc. This two-horned dilemma is not amenable of precise solution at present. In the many cases of non-Caucasoid (many Negroid, fewer Mongoloid) that I have worked with I have used either the Todd or Greulich and Pyle standards (hand), or the Pyle and Hoerr standard (knee) as basic norms. In each individual case I have fitted the ossification picture into the norm-framework, allowing for all criteria and evidence of individuality that I scanned in the bones, either grossly or radiographically. The problem reduces itself to about the level of: either we use available standards or we don't. If we do use them we interpret and evaluate to the best of our ability.

Summarizing Statement

1. It has been my experience (and I am sure that this is rather general) that most cases of skeletal identification involve older (adult) material. But this does not deny the possibility that younger individuals may be involved; I have worked on a "baby farm" case where five skeletons were represented, two presumably prenatal (7–8 lunar months), two apparently at term, and one about six months old; I have worked on a baker's half-dozen of children's skeletons, ranging from about four years to 12 or so, plus several "teen-age" cases.

It is for this reason that I've included prenatal and postnatal *appearance* of centers, as well as the more frequently presented postnatal *union* of centers. In so doing two points of emphasis have emerged: (a) in fetal and immature postnatal skeletons (say, the first 20 years) great care of exhumation must be observed, not only care in the mechanics of recovery (sifting, sieving), but care in the knowledge of where to look for separate bony elements; it is true that an examination of a diaphyseal end will reveal union or non-union (see Figure 17), but it is equally true that presence of the epiphysis will yield a much more accurate and reliable estimation of age at time of death; (b) in immature postnatal skeletons (from about five years and on up to 18–19 or so) different age-tables should be used for males and females, in recognition of the

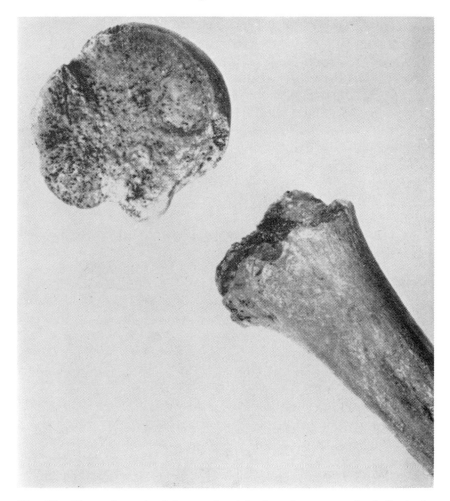

Fig. 17. View of proximal humeral epiphysis and upper end of diaphysis, showing characteristic appearance in non-union.

fact that the latter are advanced in maturation progress (a rough approximation is about one year between 5–10, about two years from 10–15, and about one year between 15–20).

2. The theme of *variability* has been discussed in the text of this Chapter, but it merits re-emphasis. The statement of skeletal age, based on bone development, is not absolute; it is relative. I have given many Tables the import of which is that of finality in

age determination, i.e., single absolute dates are given.   This is, of course, only a recognition of a central tendency, an "average." We know from our x-ray studies of well, healthy children that there are "early" and "late" maturers who are perfectly normal; for example, we might well have two boys both with chronological age of 10 years, yet the "bone age" of one might be 8:6, the other 11:6, a difference of 3:0; yet, there is nothing wrong with either of them.   In last analysis, an estimated skeletal age based on appearance and union must always be expressed in plus-and-minus terms, e.g. 10:0 ± 1:0 (10 years, plus or minus one year).   The studies of McKern and Stewart are basic contributions to the whole theme of variability.

Compounding an intrinsic, biological variability is the possibility of an extrinsic, physiological variability.   By this I mean that health, dietetic, and endocrinic factors (involving changed physiological states) may be superimposed upon the normal variability characteristic of all biological systems.   Here is an area where the specialist in bone identification approaches the frontier of pathology and in so doing joins forces with the pathologist.

3.   The evaluation of age on the bone and via the x-ray film (almost always centering on problems of *union*) is a moot problem. In the first place the duration from beginning union to complete union, in an individual case, is not well known.*   In the second place problems of the persistence of a "scar" of union (at the diaphyseo-epiphyseal plane) may provide a misleading radiographic picture.   Here is an area where longitudinal studies should throw light, i.e., the serial or follow-up x-ray study of a group of subjects through the years 17–21 or so.

4.   I see no valid reason to hold that there are any *racial* differences, in the sense that differences in sequence or time may be genetically entrenched and, hence, significant.   The available standards in this whole field of bone development are based on white

---

* Recently Noback, Moss and Lesczcynska ('60) have made available more precise information with respect to this problem.   They reported that from the beginning of *prefusion* (first radiographic sign of epiphyseal union) to *fusion* represented a time-elapse of 6.5–8.5 months.   The mean of the prefusion period was 6.5 ± 0.69 months, of the fusion period was 2.8 ± 0.3 months for a "fast" individual, 4.2 ± 0.4 months for a "slow" individual.   The mean of the fusion-process of a series of 15 hand epiphyses was 16 months (range of 4–28 months).

(American, European) material. I see no reason why these standards cannot apply to *all* peoples. To use Todd's term, such standards are "humanity-linked," not "stock-linked" or "race-linked." If there are differences, in an individual case, it is an intra-, not an inter-racial difference. In every individual case the bones must be carefully studied to see if they give any clue to an extrinsic modification. Then interpretation must take cognizance of both intrinsic and extrinsic variability: *not racial, but individual.*

5. Depending upon the completeness of recovered skeletal material in immature postnatal cases I feel that an accuracy of ± one year should be achieved. During this time, roughly the first two decades of postnatal life, the dentition may be used as a check. This statement emphasizes a point to be made over and over again: *in any case multiple criteria of skeletal age should be employed* wherever possible. Biological age in the skeleton is the sum of *all* skeletal age-changes, as shall be demonstrated in later Chapters.

REFERENCES

ABBIE, A. A. and ADEY, W. R.: Ossification in a Central Australian tribe. *HB,* *25(4)*:265–278, 1953.

ACHESON, R. M.: A method of assessing skeletal maturity from radiographs. *JA, 88*:498–508, 1954.

ADAIR, F. L. and SCAMMON, R. E.: A study of the ossification of the wrist, knee, and ankle at birth, with particular reference to the physical development and maturity of the newborn. *AJOG, 2*:37–60, 1921.

BACH, F. and MARTIN, R.: Grössen-und Massen-Verhältnisse beim Menschen. *Tab. Biol., 3*:617–719, 1926.

BAER, M. J. and DURKATZ, J.: Bilateral assymetry in skeletal maturation of the hand and wrist: A roentgenographic analysis. *AJPA n.s., 15(2)*:181–196, 1957.

BASS, W. M. III: A comparative study of the sequence and time of appearance of maturity indicators in the hand in white, Negro and Chinese children in the U.S. *Growth Center,* Phila., 1958. (Unpublished.)

BASU, S. K.: Medico-legal aspects of the determination of age of Bengalese girls. *Indian Med. Rec., 63(4)*:97–100, 1938a.

BASU, S. K. and BASU, S.: A contribution to the study of diaphyseo-epiphyseal relations at the elbow of the young Bengalese female. *Indian J. Ped.,* 5 (20); Oct. 1938b (4 pp., reprint).

BERESOWSKI, A. and LUNDIE, J. K.: Sequence in the time of ossification of the carpal bones of 705 African children from birth to 6 years of age. *S. Afr. J. Med. Sci., 17*:25–31, 1952.

BOROVANSKY, L. and HNEVKOVSKY, O.: The growth of the body and the process of ossification in Prague boys from 4 years to 19 years. *Anthropologie* (Prague), *7*:169–208, 1929.

BOYD, J. D. and TREVOR, J. C.: Race, sex, age, and stature from skeletal material, Chap. 7, Pt. 1, in Simpson, *op. cit.*, 1953.

CAMERON, J. A. P.: Estimation of age in Asiatic girls. *J. Malaya Branch Br. Med. Assn.*, *2(1)*:19–23, 1938.

CHRISTIE, A.: Prevalence and distribution of ossification centers in the newborn infant. *Am. J. Dis. Child.*, *77*:355–361, 1949.

CLARK, D. M.: The practical value of roentgenography of the epiphyses in the diagnosis of pre-adult endocrine disorders. *Am. J. Roentgenol.*, *35*:752–771, 1936.

COBB, W. M.: Skeleton. (pp. 791–856 in Lansing, *op. cit.* 1952).

COHN, I.: Observations on the normally developing shoulder. *Am. J. Roentgenol.*, *8*:721–729, 1921.

COWDRY, E. V. (ed.): *Problems of Ageing.* Williams and Wilkins, Baltimore, 1939.

DAVIES, D. A. and PARSONS, F. G.: The age order of the appearance and union of the normal epiphyses as seen in the X-ray. *JA*, *62*:58–71, 1927/28.

DREIZEN, S. *et al.*: Bilateral symmetry of skeletal maturation in the human hand and wrist. *Am. J. Dis. Children*, *93*:122–127, 1957.

DRENNAN, M. R. and KEEN, J. A.: Identity. (pp. 336–372 in Gordon, Turner, and Price, *op. cit.* 1953).

FALKNER, F., PERNOT-ROY, M. P., HABICH, H., SENECAL, J., and MASSÉ, G.: Some international comparisons of physical growth in the first two years of life. *Courrier*, Cent. Internat. de l'Enfance, Paris, *8*:1–11, 1958.

FLECKER, H.: Roentgenographic observations of the human skeleton prior to birth. *Med. J. Austral.*, *19*:640–643, 1932.

FLECKER, H.: Roentgenographic observations of the times of appearance of the epiphyses and their fusion with the diaphyses. *JA*, *67*:118–164, 1932/33.

FLECKER, H.: Time of appearance and fusion of ossification centers as observed by roentgenographic methods. *Am. J. Roentgenol. and Rad. Ther.*, *47(1)*:97–159, 1942.

FRANCIS, C. C.: The appearance of centers of ossification from 6–15 years. *AJPA*, *27(1)*:127–138, 1940.

FRANCIS, C. C.: Appearance of centers of ossification in human pelvis before birth. *Am. J. Roentgenol.*, *65*:778–783, 1951.

FRANCIS, C. C., WERLE, P. P. and BEHM, A.: The appearance of centers of ossification from birth to five years. *AJPA*, *24*:273–299, 1939.

GIRDANY, B. R. and GOLDEN, R.: Centers of ossification of the skeleton. *Am. J. Roentgenol.*, *68*:922–924, 1952.

GORDON, I., TURNER, R. and PRICE, T. W.: *Medical Jurisprudence*, (ed. 3), E. and S. Livingston, Edinburgh, 1953.

GRADWOHL, R. B. H. (ed.): *Legal Medicine.* Mosby, St. Louis, 1954.

GRAVES, W. W.: Observations on age changes in the scapula, *AJPA*, *5(1)*:21–33, 1922.

GREULICH, W. W.: The growth and development of Guamanian school children. *AJPA n.s., 9*:55–70, 1951.

GREULICH, W. W.: Growth of children of the same race under different environmental conditions. *Science, 127*:515–516, March 7, 1958.

GREULICH, W. W. and PYLE, S. I.: *Radiographic Atlas of Skeletal Development of the Hand and Wrist* (ed. 2), Stanford U. Press, 1959.

HAM, A. W.: *Histology.* (ed. 3), Lippincott, Phila., 1957.

HARRIS, H. A.: The growth of the long bones in childhood. *Arch. Int. Med., 38*: 785–806, 1926.

HASSELWANDER, A.: Untersuchungen über die Ossification des menschlichen Fussskeletts. *ZMA, 5*:438–508, 1902; *ZMA, 12*:1–140, 1909/10.

HILL, A. H.: Fetal age assessment by centers of ossification. *AJPA, 24(3)*:251–272, 1939.

HODGES, P. C.: An epiphyseal chart. *Am. J. Roentgenol., 30(6)*, Dec., 1933.

HRDLIČKA, A.: Practical anthropometry. Wistar Inst., Phila., 1939.

KELLY, H. J. and REYNOLDS, L.: Appearance and growth of ossification centers and increases in the body dimensions of white and Negro infants. *Am. J. Roentgenol., 57*:477–516, 1947.

KESSLER, A. and SCOTT, R.: Growth and development of Negro infants. II Relation of birth weight, body length, and epiphysial maturation. *Am. J. Dis. Child., 80*:370–378, 1950.

KROGMAN, W. M.: Life histories recorded in skeletons. *Am. Anth., 37(7)*:92–103, 1935.

KROGMAN, W. M.: A guide to the identification of human skeletal material. *FBI Law Enforce. Bull., 8(8)*:1–29, 1939.

KROGMAN, W. M.: The human skeleton in legal medicine: medical aspects. (pp. 1–92, in Levinson, *op. cit.* 1949).

KROGMAN, W. M.: The skeleton in forensic medicine. *Grad. Med.,* 17(2 and 3) Feb.-March, 1955.

KROGMAN, W. M.: Physical anthropologists as experts in human identification. (Paper given Sept. 7, 1955. Washington, D.C., at VIII Wenner-Gren Summer Seminar in Physical Anthropology; mimeo distribution only).

LANSING, A. I. (ed.): *Cowdry's Problems of Ageing.* (ed. 3) Williams and Wilkins, Baltimore. 1952.

LEVINSON, S. A. (ed.): *Symposium on Medicolegal Problems*, Series Two. Lippincott, Phila. 1949.

MACKAY, D. H.: Skeletal maturation in the hand: a study of development of East African children. *Trans. Roy. Soc. Trop. Med. and Hygiene, 46*:135–142, 1952.

McKERN, T. W.: Estimation of skeletal age from combined maturational activity. *AJPA n.s., 15(3)*:399–408, 1957.

McKERN, T. W. and STEWART, T. D.: Skeletal age changes in young American males, analyzed from the standpoint of identification. *Headqu. QM Res. and Dev. Command.,* Tech. Rep. EP-45, Natick, Mass., 1957.

MENEES, T. O. and HOLLY, E. L.: The ossification in the extremities of the new born. *Am. J. Roentgenol.*, *28(3)*:389–390, 1932.

MODI, J. P.: *Medical Jurisprudence and Toxicology* (ed. 12 by N. J. Modi), Tripathi Private, Ltd. Bombay, 1957.

NEWMAN, M. T. and COLLAZOS, C.: Growth and skeletal maturation in malnourished Indian boys from the Peruvian Sierra. *AJPA n.s.*, *15(3)*:431 (abst), 1957.

NOBACK, C. R.: The appearance of ossification centers and the fusion of bones. *AJPA n.s.*, *12(1)*:63–69, 1954.

NOBACK, C. R. and ROBERTSON, G. G.: Sequences of appearance of ossification centers in the human skeleton during the first five prenatal months. *AJA*, *89(1)*:1–28, 1951.

NOBACK, C. R., MOSS, M. L. and LESCZCYNSKA, E.: Digital epiphyseal fusion of the hand in adolescence: a longitudinal study. *AJPA n.s.* *18(1)*:13–18, 1960.

PARK, E. A. and HOWLAND, J.: The radiographic evidence of the influence of cod liver oil in rickets. *Bull. Johns Hopkins Hosp.*, *32*:341–344, 1921.

PATERSON, R. S.: A radiological investigation of the epiphyses of the long bones. *JA*, *64(1)*:28–46, 1929.

PLATT, R. A.: The skeletal maturation of Negro school children. M.A. Thesis, U. of Pa., Phila., 1956.

PRYOR, J. W.: Differences in the time of development of centers of ossification in the male and female skeleton. *Anat. Rec.*, *25(5)*:257–273, 1923.

PRYOR, J. W.: Difference in the ossification of the male and female skeleton. *JA*, *62*:499–506, 1927/28.

PRYOR, J. W.: Roentgenographic investigation of the time element in ossification. *Am. J. Roentgenol.*, *28*:798–804, 1933.

PYLE, S. I. and SONTAG, L. W.: Variability in onset of ossification in epiphyses and short bones of the extremities. *Am. J. Roentgenol.*, *49*:795–798, 1943.

PYLE, S. I. and HOERR, N. L.: *Radiographic Atlas of Skeletal Development of the Knee.* Thomas, Springfield, 1955.

SIMPSON, K. (ed.): *Modern Trends in Forensic Medicine.* Butterworth, London, 1953.

SIMPSON, K.: *Forensic Medicine* (ed. 3). Arnold, London, 1958.

SPEIJER, B.: Betekenis En Bepaling Van De Skeletleeftijd. Uitgevers Mattschappij. N.V., Leiden, Holland, 1950.

STEVENSON, P. H.: Age order of epiphyseal union in man. *AJPA*, *7(1)*:53–93, 1924.

STEWART, T. D.: Sequence of epiphyseal union, third molar eruption, and suture closure in Eskimos and American Indians. *AJPA*, *19(3)*:433–452, 1934.

STEWART, T. D.: Evaluation of evidence from the skeleton (pp. 407–450 in Gradwohl, *op. cit.*, 1954).

STEWART, T. D. and TROTTER, M. (eds.): Basic readings on the identifications of human skeletons: estimations of age. *Wenner-Gren. Found. for Anthrop. Research*, New York, 1954.

SUTOW, W. W.: Skeletal maturation in healthy Japanese children, 6–19 years of age; comparison with skeletal maturation in American children. *Hiroshima J. Med. Sci.*, 2:181–191, 1953 (cited in Greulich, '58).

SUTOW, W. W. and OHWADA, K.: Skeletal standards of healthy Japanese children, 6–19 years of age. *Clin. Pediat.* (Japanese), vol. 6, no. 11, 1953, (cited in Greulich, '58).

TCHAPEROFF, I. C. C.: *A Manual of Radiological Diagnosis for Students and General Practitioners.* Wood, Baltimore, 1937.

TODD, T. W.: The anatomical features of epiphyseal union. *Child Dev., 1(3)*: 186–194, 1930.

TODD, T. W.: Differential skeletal maturation in relation to sex, race, variability, and disease. *Child. Dev., 2(1)*:49–65, 1931.

TODD, T. W.: Growth and development of the skeleton (pp. 26–130 in *Growth and Development of the Child*, Pt. II: Anatomy and Physiology). Century Co., N.Y. 1933.

TODD, T. W.: Skeleton, locomotor system, and teeth. (pp. 278–338, in Cowdry, *op. cit.* 1939).

TODD, T. W. and D'ERRICO, JR., J.: The odontoid ossicle of the second cervical vertebra. *Ann. Surg., 81(1)*:20–31, 1926.

TODD, T. W. and D'ERRICO, JR., J.: The clavicular epiphyses. *AJA, 41(1)*:25–50, 1928.

VANDERVAEL, F. Critéres d'estimation de l'age des squelettes entre 18 et 38 ans. *S.A.S. Boll. Comitato internaz., per l'Unific. dei metodi e per la sintesi in antropologia e biologia. 25/26*:67–82, Bologna, 1952.

VENNING, P.: Radiological studies of variations in the segmentation and ossification of the digits of the human foot. I. Variation in the number of phalanges and centers of ossification of the toes. *AJPA n.s., 14(1)*:1–34, 1956a.

VENNING, P.: Radiological studies in variation in the segmentation and ossification of the digits of the human foot. II. Variation in length of the digit segments correlated with difference of segmentation and ossification of the toes. *AJPA n.s., 14(2)*:129–151, 1956b.

VINCENT, M.: L'enfant au Ruanda-Urundi *Inst. Royal Colonial Belge.* Sec. Sci. Nat. et Med. Mem. Vol. 23, fasc. 6. Brussels ,1954.

WEBSTER, G. and DE SAREM, G. S. W.: Estimation of age from bone development. Study of 567 Ceylonese children 9–16 years and 307 Ceylonese children age 4–8 years. *J. Crim. Law. Criminol. and Police Sci., 45(1)*:96–101; *45(2)*:236–239, 1952.

WEINER, J. S. and THAMBIPILLAI, V.: Skeletal maturation of West African Negroes *AJPA n.s., 10(4)*:407–418, 1952.

III

Skeletal Age: Later Years

I.   Suture Closure

1. GENERAL CONSIDERATIONS AND HISTORIC NOTES

The bones of the skull are separated by sutures which, in a sense, are analogous to epiphyseo-diaphyseal planes in that both are loci of growth, and that both have a sequence and timing of union. In the present discussion we shall limit ourselves to cranial sutures only, i.e., those of the brain-box rather than those of the facial skeleton.   This is seen in Table 15 (from Cobb, '52) and in Figure 18 (from Stewart, '54).

Just as epiphyseo-diaphyseal union most frequently begins centrally and proceeds peripherally, so does suture closure begin endocranially and proceed ectocranially, i.e., it begins inside the skull and progresses to the outside.   There is this difference, however, viz., that epiphyseal union is always complete in normal cases (with the possible exception of the ramal epiphysis of the ischium), whereas suture closure may be incomplete (so-called "lapsed union," which will be discussed later) in perfectly normal, healthy individuals.

The sutures and their relation to age and to race have excited comment over a long period of time.   Pommerol quotes Celsus, first century A.D., that crania devoid of sutures (i.e., sutures closed) occur more readily in warmer climates (Todd and Lyon, '24). Perhaps the most extravagant statement of all is that of Gratiolet in 1865 (Todd and Lyon, '25, p. 69):

"Has the long persistence of the patent sutures in the White race any relation to the almost indefinable perfection of their intelli-

76

gence? Does not this continuance of an infantile condition seem to indicate that the brain may, in these perfect men, remain capable of slow growth? Perhaps it is this which makes the perpetual youthfulness of spirit in the greatest thinkers seem able to defy old age and death. But in idiots and in Brutish races the cranium closes itself on the brain like a prison. It is no longer a temple divine, to use Malpighi's expression, but a sort of helmet capable of resisting heavy blows."

In 1885, Ribbé (Todd and Lyon, '24; also Montagu, '38) studied 50 skulls, 40 of which were white. He found earliest closure at 21 years, latest at 50, with greatest frequency at 40–45 years. In ageing skulls suture closure could not come closer than 15–20

TABLE 15
CRANIAL SUTURES AND SUBDIVISIONS FOR WHICH CLOSURE IS RECORDED*

No.	Suture	Subdivisions	Units	
1	Sagittal	Bregmatica, Vault vertica, obelica, lambdica	4	
2	Coronal	Bregmatica, complicata, pterica	3	
3	Lambdoid	Lambdica, media, asterica	3	
				10
		Circum-meatal		
4	Spheno-temporal	Superior, inferior	2	
5	Squamous	Anterior, posterior	2	
6	Parieto-mastoid	Taken as a whole	1	
7	Masto-occipital	Superior, media, inferior	3	
				8
		Accessory		
8	Spheno-parietal	Taken as a whole	1	
9	Spheno-frontal	Orbital, temporal	2	
				3
Total	. . . .		21	

* From Cobb, '52, Table 2.

years. In 1888, Schmidt said the basilar suture (spheno-occipital) united between 18–21 years, but possibly between 21–23 years. Vault suture closure began between 25–40 years, and was complete between 40–60 years. In 1890, Dwight noted that suture closure began endocranially, and concluded that "the time of closure of any particular part of a suture, and the order in which the process advances, are very uncertain." In 1905, Frédéric studied vault suture closure and in 1909/10 he studied closure of the facial sutures. He introduced a rating scale of 0 = patent (not closed), 1 = less than one-half closed, 2 = half closed, 3 = more than one-half closed, and 4 = totally closed. He felt that suture closure occurred later in females. In 1905, Parsons and Box stated that closure "may occur in a healthy skull before 30, though it is rare"; over 30 years there is always a "fair amount" of endocranial closure in coronal and sagittal sutures; over 50 years, usually, and over

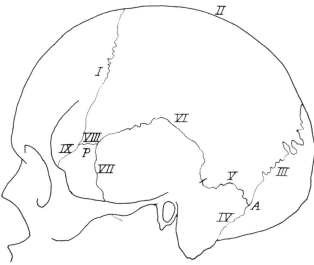

Fig. 18. Skull sutures: Vault group; coronal (I), sagittal (II), lambdoid (III); Circum-meatal group, masto-occipital (IV), parieto-mastoid (V), squamous (VI), spheno-temporal (VII); Accessory group, spheno-parietal (VIII), spheno-frontal (IX). P = Pterion, A = Asterion.

60 years, always, all endocranial sutures are "obliterated." The extreme variability and unreliability of ectocranial closure was emphasized. The later closure in females was suggested; it was further suggested that "simple sutures" (less serrated or denticulated) closed earlier. No differences, right and left, were noted. In 1917, von Lenhóssek quoted both Schwalbe and Frédéric on later closure in the female.

2. MODERN STUDIES IN SUTURE CLOSURE

In 1924–25, Todd and Lyon put the study of suture closure on a more adequate numerical basis. In a series of four papers ectocranial and endocranial closure was reported on for adult white and

Negro American males. To begin with a series of 307 male white skulls and 120 male Negro skulls was selected for study. However, 40 white skulls (13.3%) and 41 Negro skulls (34.2%) were excluded as "anomalous," i.e., irregularities in closure were noted. It was held that anomalous closure of one suture correlates with anomalous closure of all sutures in a given skull.* This business of rejecting skulls that did not "fit the picture," so to speak, has led to much criticism. At the very least elimination of extremes has given the data a spurious homogeneity as far as variability (range of variation) is concerned. On the other hand, assuming that extremes are more or less evenly removed at either end of the range, there is no valid reason to believe that the central tendency has been unduly influenced. The following, taken from Todd and Lyon ('24) suggests that this is true (Table 16):

TABLE 16
ESTIMATION OF AGE BY ENDOCRANIAL CLOSURE*

Skull	Suture Age Circa.	Actual Age	Dev.	Skull	Suture Age Circa.	Actual Age	Dev.
94	25	28	−3	618	30	30	
156	40	45	−5	649	27	22	+5
185	40	40		654	65	42	+23
267	25	25		671	35	33	+2
301	35	34	+1	678	40	38	+2
328	55	38	+17	708	45	32	+13
354	65	48	+17	711	43	47	−4
396	41	60	−19	772	37	40	−3
429	35	40	−5	786	43	45	−2
431	45	40	+5	794	33	32	+1
445	30	36	−6	799	35	36	−1
499	43	55	−12	823	30	33	−3
504	35	37	−2	828	58	68	−10
507	35	49	−14	876	43	ca 40	+3
617	37	32	+5	896	55	53	+2

Average of thirty. Suture age 40.2 years. Actual age 39.9 years. Dev. 6.2

* From Todd and Lyon, '24, Table III.

The ultimate result of this is to reduce the value of suture closure as an age criterion in individual cases. This was recognized by Todd and Lyon ('24, p. 379): ". . . it cannot be denied that so

* It should be noted that in eliminating a skull from the series the *whole skeleton* was first studied for further anomalies. Originally there were 58 female white skulls, 29 female Negro skulls, but the numbers were so reduced by the rejection of anomalous skulls that the female series was dropped.

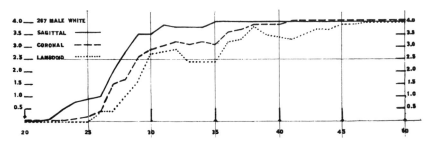

Fig. 19.   Endocranial suture closure in the vault, male white. Note great
activity at 26–30 yrs.

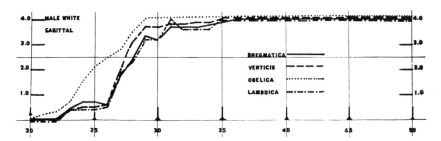

Fig. 20.   Endocranial suture closure in the sagittal suture, male white.   The
pars obelica follows a separate course.

far our work does not justify the uncontrolled use of suture closure
in estimation of age."

It is important to note that Todd and Lyon followed Frédéric
in the use of a rating scale of 0 to 4.   This may be seen in Figure
19, endocranial vault closure, and in Figure 20, endocranial closure
of the sagittal suture, both in male whites (Todd and Lyon, '24).
The use of this rating scale permits the creation of a "closure
formula" for a given skull, as for example, S2233, C211 right,
C211 left, L112 right, L112 left (S = sagittal, with its four parts,
C = coronal, with its three parts, L = lambdoid, with its three
parts).

The work of Todd and Lyon on vault and circum-meatal sutures
has been so ably summarized by Cobb ('52) that I reproduce his
Table 3 here (see Table 17):

It remains but to say that Todd and Lyon found no onset-timing

TABLE 17

AGES OF CRANIAL SUTURE CLOSURE*

	Endocranial						Ectocranial					
	Male White			Male Negro			Male White			Male Negro		
Suture	C**	T**	Remarks	C	T	Remarks	C	T	Remarks	C	T	Remarks
1. Sagittal	22	35	Slows at 31 at 3.9. Slow to 26	22	31	Slow to 26 complete	20	29	3.9 in obelica 2.4 alone; 2.9 in general Slow to 26	20	32	Slowly to 24. 2.9–3.6 in gen, 4.0 in obelica alone
2. Spheno-frontal orbital	22	64	Slows at 30 at 3.0. Final burst of act.	20	44	Slow to 26 complete	28	46	2.3 at 31, 3.8 at 46	21	35	3.5 at 35, may reach 4.0 at 43
3. Spheno-frontal temporal	22	65	Same	23	44	Slow to 26 complete	28	38	2.1 at 38, may reach 4.0 in old age	25	46	1.9 at 35
4. Coronal 1 and 2	24	38	Slows at 29 at 3.4	24	38	Slows at 32 at 3.6	26	29	Bregmatica at 2.3, complicata at 0.9	23	32	Breg. at 2.4, comp. at 1.7
5. Coronal 3	26	41	Slows at 29 at 2.1 rapid to ca. 30	25	44	Slows at 31 at 2.3	28	50	50 at 3.7, spurious rise at 21	25	35	35 at 2.8, spur. rise at 21
6. Lambdoid 1 and 2	26	42	Slows at 31 at 3.4	23	46	Slows at 30 at 2.5. Slow to 46	26	30	Spurious rise at 21. Lambdica 2.3, media 1.9	23	31	Lamb 2.4, media 2.0
7. Lambdoid 3	26	47	Slows at 30 at 2.2. Slow	27	46	Slows at 31 at 2.7. No further progress thereafter	26	?31	Not more than 1.0	22	?31	Not more than 1.0
8. Masto-occipital 3	26	72	32–48 at 3.2. Slow progress thereafter	17	30	30 at 3.3. No further progress thereafter	26	33	1.4 at 33, may reach 4.0 in old age	26	31	Spurious rise at 21 sec. act. at 50
9. Spheno-parietal	29	65	29–46 at 3.0	23	49	Slows at 30 at 2.7	28	38	2.0 at 38, 3.5 at 31, continues to old age	28	46	1.4 at 31
10. Spheno-temporal 2	30	67	Slow at once, 67 at 3.9, grad. progress	40	51	51 at 3.3. Oscillations thereafter	36	50?	Prob. never closes	50?	0	Prob. never closes
11. Spheno-temporal 1	31	64	31–62 at 2.5, 64 at 2.4. Burst of act. at 63	40	41	41 at 1.2, then oscil.	37	50?	Prob. never closes	50?	0	Prob. never closes
12. Masto-occipital	30	81	32–45 at 1.25, act. bet. 46 & 64, final burst	25	46	46 at 3.5, then oscil.	28	32	32 at 0.8–1.0, may reach 3.5 in old age	27	31	31 at 2.7, spur. rise ca. 18, sec. act. 50
13. Parieto-mastoid	37	81	Almost inact. till 50, slow thereafter	33	51	51 at 3.6, then oscil.	39	50?	Prob. never closes	50?	0	Prob. never closes
14. Squamous posterior	37	81	Bursts at 63 & 79, almost inact. till 62	40	49	49 at 1.7, then oscil.	38	50?	Prob. never closes	50?	0	Prob. never closes
15. Squamous anterior	37	81	Same	40	49	Same	38	50?	Prob. never closes	50?	0	Prob. never closes

* Compiled from data of Todd and Lyon. ** C = Commencement. T = Termination. (From Cobb, '52, Table 3.)

differences betweeen endocranial and ectocranial closure, but found the former a more reliable age-indicator since the latter so frequently showed lapsed union; they found no race differences (cf. Pittard and Kaufmann, '36); and no differences between right and left sides of the skull.

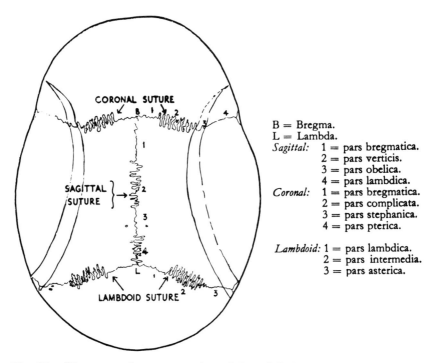

B = Bregma.
L = Lambda.
Sagittal: 1 = pars bregmatica.
    2 = pars verticis.
    3 = pars obelica.
    4 = pars lambdica.
Coronal: 1 = pars bregmatica.
    2 = pars complicata.
    3 = pars stephanica.
    4 = pars pterica.

Lambdoid: 1 = pars lambdica.
    2 = pars intermedia.
    3 = pars asterica.

Fig. 21. Diagrammatic representation of the subdivisions of the cranial vault sutures.

There have been several studies that have critically tested the reliability of suture closure as an age estimate. Of these that of McKern and Stewart ('57) is the most thorough and the most objective. They follow Singer in assigning four parts to the coronal, four to the sagittal, and three to the lambdoid (see Figure 21), but follow Todd and Lyon in a five-stage rating scale (0–1–2–3–4, though 2–3 are combined). The material upon which McKern and Stewart base their findings is the same as that used in the ossification studies.

TABLE 18

A SIMPLIFIED PRESENTATION OF THE STAGES OF SUTURE CLOSRUE TO SHOW ITS VARIABILITY: VAULT SUTURES (IN %)*

Age	No.	Sagittal Closures**				Lambdoid Closures**				Coronal Closures**			
		0	1	2,3	4	0	1	2,3	4	0	1	2,3	4
17–18	55	75	4	12	9	92	—	5	3	99	—	—	1
19	52	66	4	10	19	83	5	5	7	84	7	5	4
20	45	54	10	13	23	82	11	3	4	77	17	2	4
21	37	56	9	10	25	72	10	10	8	86	7	2	5
22	24	54	17	5	24	75	17	4	4	72	20	4	4
23	26	42	11	15	32	65	6	23	6	49	34	11	6
24–25	27	34	7	11	48	53	11	18	18	67	12	14	7
26–27	25	12	8	40	40	32	28	16	24	28	16	24	32
28–30	29	18	12	19	51	27	17	35	21	26	25	25	24
31–40	43	10	4	14	72	24	17	20	39	20	20	35	25
41–50	6	2	16	66	16	1	66	—	33	50	33	—	16
Total	369												

* From McKern and Stewart, '57, Table 8.
** 0: No closure anywhere. 1: No more than stage 1 anywhere. 2,3: No more than stages 2 or 3. 4: Stage 4 in some part.

Table 18 shows the extreme variability of vault suture closure. It should be compared with Figure 19 of this Section, taken from Todd and Lyons:

There is, obviously, a certain age-progression, i.e., from 17–18 years the % of Stage 0 decreases uniformly, as the % of Stage 4 increases, though not quite so uniformly: this is more true of sagittal than of lambdoid, and of lambdoid than coronal.

Now look at Tables 19 and 20, both concerned with vault suture closure. Here comparison should be made with Figure 20, this Section, from Todd and Lyon, dealing specifically with the sagittal suture. These two tables record site of beginning closure and site of final closure-stage, respectively. About all one can say is that closure *tends* to begin in 1st and 4th parts of sagittal, 1st part of lambdoid, and 1st and 4th parts of the coronal; final stage of closure *tends* to be registered in 1st and 2nd parts of sagittal, 1st or 2nd part of lambdoid, and 1st part of coronal.

There is an observation which must now be made: McKern and Stewart based their results on *ectocranial* suture closure only. On this score Todd and Lyon ('25, Pt II) have this to say: "Lapsed union . . . is characteristic of all ectocranial sutures. In consequence ectocranial sutures tend to remain in a state of incomplete

TABLE 19

LOCATIONS OF BEGINNING CLOSURE IN VAULT SUTURES* (IN %)

Age	No.	Sagittal				Lambdoid			Coronal			
		Pars breg.	Pars vert.	Pars obel.	Pars lamb.	Pars lamb.	Pars inter.	Pars aster.	Pars breg.	Pars comp.	Pars steph.	Pars pter.
17–18	55	—	4	8	—	4	1	2	4	2	—	2
19	52	11	15	11	6	6	4	4	8	6	4	1
20	45	9	22	15	24	9	11	7	2	13	9	2
21	37	10	16	5	19	16	10	8	2	8	2	2
22	24	20	20	16	25	12	20	4	20	16	8	8
23	26	7	19	11	23	11	11	7	19	19	23	34
24–25	27	26	19	30	26	26	26	26	15	14	19	22
26–27	25	23	1	1	23	3	1	2	3	3	1	37
28–30	29	9	12	9	25	12	29	9	16	29	12	16
31–40	43	11	18	13	17	28	11	18	28	28	18	17
41–50	6	16	16	16	33	50	50	16	33	33	—	16
Total	369											

* From McKern and Stewart, '57, Table 9.

union, some in a very high degree."* What is "lapsed union?" As the term implies it is incomplete union in the sense that a process once begun has not gone on to completion. Why this is so is not clear. The vault bones have a very specialized structure: they have two layers, an inner (tabula interna), and an outer (tabula externa), separated by a vascular spongy-bone space (the diploë). The impetus to closure seems to be from inner table to outer, i.e.,

TABLE 20
LOCATIONS OF FINAL STAGE OF CLOSURE IN VAULT SUTURES* (IN %)

Age	No.	Sagittal Parts compl. closed:				Lambdoid Parts compl. closed:			Coronal Parts compl. closed:			
		1	2	3	4	1	2	3	1	2	3	4
17–18	55	5	—	4	1	—	2	—	—	—	1	—
19	52	7	3	7	2	—	7	—	3	1	—	—
20	45	11	2	4	6	2	2	—	2	—	2	—
21	37	8	2	10	5	—	8	—	5	—	—	—
22	24	8	8	4	4	—	4	—	—	—	4	—
23	26	3	11	7	11	3	—	3	3	—	—	3
23–25	27	15	34	7	16	15	5	5	7	—	—	—
26–27	25	4	8	4	1	8	16	4	12	8	—	8
28–30	29	22	—	9	16	6	16	—	22	—	—	3
31–40	43	26	13	11	26	13	17	2	17	11	—	7
41–50	6	16	16	—	—	33	—	—	33	—	—	—
Total	369											

* From McKern and Stewart, '57, Table 10.

endocranial to ectocranial. Let us assume that the biological age is achieved so that closure is naturally in order; it begins inwardly and it spreads outwardly (inner to outer table). In many cases it will go on to completion and the suture is "closed" to the point where, on the outer bone, it is difficult to discern. Often, however, the closure force or process seems to lose energy, to dissipate itself, to halt short of completion. In these cases the closure has "lapsed"; the ectocranial suture is incompletely united. This, of itself, is often a recognizable feature, for the bone on either side of the outer suture is piled-up or, as Todd put it, "clawed" and turned in like the margins of the eyelids in cases of trachoma.

The point to be made is that ectocranial suture closure is so basically variable that it should not be the final arbiter of saying

* As early as 1910 Jones observed that "the external closure of the sutures may, however, be but very little evident when within the skull the obliteration of the sutures is complete."

sutures are "good" or "bad" age indicators. *Every effort should be made to ascertain endocranial closure.**

3. THE RELIABILITY OF SUTURES AS AGE CRITERIA

We have already noted that, historically, many writers have taken a very cautious view of the accuracy of age determination via suture closure, a view shared, in principle, by Todd and Lyons themselves. What of more recent views?

TABLE 21

AVERAGE DEVIATIONS IN YEARS OF VARIATIONS OF STATED FROM SKELETAL AGE*

Age	MW	FW	TW	MN	FN	TN	Total
10–19	5.0	—	5.0	3.4	2.5	2.9	3.6
20–29	6.6	4.2	5.4	4.3	4.2	4.2	4.8
30–39	9.3	6.8	8.0	8.5	9.7	9.1	8.6
40–49	6.1	11.7	8.8	11.5	5.5	8.5	8.7
50–59	12.0	—	12.0	9.4	10.0	9.7	10.8
60–69	9.8	7.0	8.4	15.0	—	15.0	10.6
70–79	13.0	16.0	14.5	26.0	17.0	21.0	18.0
80–89	10.0	—	10.0	25.0	—	25.0	17.5
Total	9.0	9.1	9.0	12.9	8.1	11.9	9.9

* From Cobb, '52, Table 6. (M = male, F = female, T = total, W = white, N = Negro.)

Hrdlička ('39), on ectocranial suture closure, said on the basis of this criterion alone "one could hardly be relied upon in age determination to within a closer limit than 10 years on either side of reality." In 1937, Cattaneo reported on 100 miscellaneous Argentine skulls and ruled that suture closure was only "a suggestive indicator" of age. In 1953, Singer concluded that estimation of "precise age at death of any individual, gauged only on the degree of closure of the vault sutures is a hazardous and unreliable process." In 1952 Cobb, using the Todd and Lyon schedules of suture closure, stated that age-assessment "can probably approximate the true age of an individual within plus or minus nine years" (p. 840). His supporting data are presented in Table 21.

An interesting historic note is not amiss here. Dobson ('52) studied the skull of John Thurtell, "The College Criminal," hanged at the age of 30 years on 1-9-1824. The remains went to the Royal College of Surgeons (London). It was noted that the

* I recommend either removal of the calvarium or a sagittal section of the skull in order to view the endocranial aspect of the skull.

vault sutures were "remarkably advanced for a subject of 30. Without they are completely closed and obliteration (*sic*) is advanced at pars obelionica and pars bregmatica of the sagittal suture." (In 1890 Dwight, and in 1905 Parsons, both said that union may be complete by 30 years of age.)

The work of McKern and Stewart ('57) is of great value here. They conclude that progress of suture closure "has only a very general relationship with age. So erratic is the onset and progress of closure that an adequate series will provide just about any pattern at any age level. Thus, as a guide for age determination, such a trend is of little use. In other words, suture closure, as either a direct or supportive evidence for skeletal age identification, is generally unreliable." In last analysis, "if other ageing areas of the skeleton are absent, then crude estimates can be made in terms of decades only."* Genovese and Messmacher ('59a, '59b) come to much the same conclusion, basing their findings on 101 male Mexican skulls of all ages and of known identity: for 47 "indigenas" and 54 "mestizos" the age difference between estimation via sutures, and actual age, was twelve years, eleven months for the former, nine years, five months for the latter (eleven years, one month over-all).

There is a residual problem to be mentioned, viz., that of the absolutely premature closure of one or more sutures. Terminology here is as follows: *precocious* closure is before age seven (the age at which cranial growth is about 95% complete); *premature* closure is after the age of seven, but considerably before the usual or "normal" age of closure. The following tabulation (Bolk, '15) gives an idea of observed frequency in a series of European white skulls of both sexes.

The *metopic suture*, present at birth between right and left halves of the frontal bone, usually closes at about two years of age. In a certain number of skulls it is persistant well into adult life. Meto-

---

* A very interesting example of the fallacy and/or danger of relying upon a *single* age-criterion (in the skull) is cited by Genovese ('60) and by Moss ('60). They examined a prehistoric skull (about 8,000–10,000 years old) excavated at Tepexpan, Mexico. In a first report M. T. Newman (pp. 97–98 in DeTerra, Romero, and Stewart '49) had, mainly on the basis of suture closure, assigned an age at time of death of 55–65 years. When the skull was restudied on a comparative basis, and when radiographic studies of the teeth were added, an age no greater than 25–30 years could be assigned.

ABSOLUTE FREQUENCY OF PREMATURE OBLITERATION IN 1820 SKULLS

	Times
Sut. masto-occipitalis	272
Sut. sagittalis	71
Sut. squamosa	17
Sut. parieto-mastoidea	16
Sut. coronalis	12
Sut. parieto-sphenoidalis	5
Sut. fronto-sphenoidalis	5
Sut. lambdoidea	5

pism is more frequent among whites and Mongoloids (about 10%) than among Negroids (about 2%) (Woo, '49; see also Montagu, '38).

4. OTHER AGE CRITERIA IN THE SKULL

Both Todd ('39) and Cobb ('52) note a series of changes which are in part rather subjective. Certainly they have not been standardized either by definition or by statistical analysis. The *texture* of a young adult skull is smooth and ivorine on both inner and outer surfaces; at about 40 years (± 5) the surface begins to assume a "matted," granular, rough-feeling, appearance. Certain *markings* appear with age: from age 25 years and on muscular markings (lines of attachment) become increasingly evident, especially on the side of the skull (temporal line), on the occiput (nuchal lines), and on the lateral side of the jawbone (masseteric attachment); on the inside of the skull, on either side of the sagittal suture, certain pits or depressions (called Pacchionian depressions) become more marked with age, both in depth and in frequency; also on the inside of the skull, laterally, the grooves for the middle meningeal artery become deeper. After about 50 years of age the *diploë* become less vascularly channeled (venous sinuses) and there is an increasing replacement by bone. There is no consistent age-change in the *thickness* of the vault bones. Todd summarizes all this as follows:

> "No obvious age changes are to be found in the markings of venous sinuses or in Pacchionian depressions although deepening of channels and sharpening of margins do occur in the grooves for meningeal veins with advancing years. Changes due to age alone in thickness of cranium and in diploë are not sufficient to emerge on statistical analysis. The cause of obliteration of sutures in childhood must be sought in phylogeny and is not an age character. Granularity of surface of cranium, thickening or thinning of vault,

multiple vascular pitting of parietal bones and gross changes in texture, often quite striking in the adult, are all features the cause for which must be sought in chronic nutritional defect or other constitutional infirmity. Halisteresis of cranial and facial bones, like halisteresis in the skeleton, does set in after fifty years. This however is indistinguishable from the osteoporosis consequent upon constitutional defect and may indeed be a sign of supervening infirmity."

Summarizing Statement

1. The sutures of the cranial vault and of the circum-meatal area are the best documented as far as age-changes are concerned. In our present state of knowledge it may be stated that there are no significant race, sex, or side (right/left) differences.

2. Due to the phenomenon of "lapsed union" ectocranially, the state of endocranial closure must take precedence in any evaluation of suture-age.

3. Estimation of age of the skull via suture closure is not reliable. I'd venture to place a skull in a decade, for example in the 20's or 30's or 40's, or at a decade mid-point, as 25–35, 35–45, and so on. If the skull is the only part present then this sort of age evaluation is the best one can do, and the statement is then diagnostic. If other bones are present, then suture age may become, at best, partially corroborative.

4. Other estimates of age in the skull, as texture, lineae, depressions, etc., are too subjective to be generally employed. A person with extensive experience may hazard an age approximation, but that is all.

REFERENCES

Bolk, L.: On the premature obliteration of sutures in the human skull. *AJA*, *17*:495–523, 1915.

Brooks, S. T.: 1955, (see *Refs.* Chap. IV).

Cattaneo, L.: Las suturas cranean en la determinacion de la edad. Examen de 100 craneos. *Rev. de la Assoc. Med. Argent.*, *50*:387–397, 1937.

Cobb, W. M.: 1952, (see *Refs.*, Chap. II).

DeTerra, H., Romero, J., and Stewart, T. D.: Tepexpan Man. *Viking Fund Publ. in Anthropol.*, No. 10, N.Y., 1949.

Dobson, J.: The College Criminal—John Thurtell. *J. Dent. Assoc. S., Afr.*, *7(7)*: 265–268, 1952.

Dwight, T.: The closure of the sutures as a sign of age. *Boston Med. and Surg. J.*, *122*:389–392, 1890.

Frédéric, J.: Untersuchungen über die normale obliteration der Schädelnähte. *ZMA*, *9*:373–456, 1905.

Frédéric, J.: Die Obliteration der Nähte des Gesichtsschädels. *ZMA*, *12*:371–440, 1909/10.

Genovese, S. T.: Revaluation of age, stature and sex of the Tepexpan remains Mexico. *AJPA n.s.*, *18(3)*:205–217, 1960.

Genovese, S. T. and Messmacher, M.: Valor de los patrones tradicionales para la determinacion de la edad por medio de/las suturas en craneos Mexicanos (Indigenas y Mestizos). *Cuadernos de Instituto de Historia.* Serie Antropol. No. 7, Mexico City, 1959.

Hrdlička, A.: 1939, (see *Refs.*, Chap. II).

Jones, F. Wood: Anatomical variations, and the determination of the age and sex of skeletons; pp. 221–262, in the Archaeological Survey of Nubia, Vol. II— Report on the Human Remains. Cairo: Natl. Printing Dept., 1910.

Lenhossék, M. von: Über Nahtverknocherung im Kindesalter. *Arch. für Anth. N.F.*, *15*:164–180, 1917.

McKern, T. W. and Stewart, T. D.: 1957, (see *Refs.*, Chap. II).

Montagu, M. F. A.: Ageing of the skull. *AJPA*, *23*:355–375, 1938.

Moss, M. L.: A reevaluation of the dental status and chronological age of the Tepexpan remains. *AJPA n.s.*, *18(1)*:71–72, 1960.

Parsons, F. G. and Box, C. R.: The relation of the cranial sutures to age. *JRAI*, *35*:30–38, 1905.

Pittard, E. and Kaufmann, H.: A propos de l'obliteration des sutures craniennes et de leur ordre d' apparition. Recherches sur les crânes de Boschimans, Hottentots, et Griquas. *L'Anth.*, *46*:351–358, 1936.

Schmidt, E.: Anthropologische Methoden: Anleitung zum Beobachten und Sammeln für Laboritorium und Reise. Veit Co., Leipzig, 1888.

Singer, R.: Estimation of age from cranial suture closure. *J. Forensic Med.*, *1(1)*:52–59, 1953.

Stewart, T. D.: 1954, (see *Refs.*, Chap. II).

Todd, T. W.: 1939, (see *Refs.*, Chap. II).

Todd, T. W. and Lyon, Jr., D. W.: Endocranial suture closure, its progress and age relationship Part I. Adult males of white stock. *AJPA*, *7(3)*:325–384, 1924.

Todd, T. W. and Lyon, Jr., D. W.: Cranial suture closure, its progress and age relationship. Part II. Ectocranial closure in adult males of white stock. *AJPA*, *8(1)*:23–45, 1925a.

Todd, T. W. and Lyon, Jr., D. W.: Cranial suture closure: its progress and age relationship. Part III. Endocranial closure in adult males of Negro stock. *AJPA*, *8(1)*:47–71, 1925b.

Todd, T. W. and Lyon, Jr., D. W.: Cranial suture closure: its progress and age relationship. Part IV. Ectocranial closure in adult males of Negro stock. *AJPA*, *8(2)*:149–168, 1925c.

Woo, Ju-Kang: Racial and sexual differences in the frontal curvature and its relation to metopism. *AJPA n.s.*, *7(2)*:215–26, 1949.

IV

Skeletal Age: Later Years

II   The Pelvis

1. THE PUBIC SYMPHYSIS

The right and left hip-bones (ossa innominata) meet in the mid-line in front to form the pubic symphysis.   The right and left pubic bones do not actually articulate: they are separated throughout life by the symphyseal cartilage.   Each pubic bone presents a symphyseal surface or face, which Todd ('20) stated to be "a modified diaphyso-epiphyseal plane and, as such, may be expected to show a metamorphosis, if not actual growth, as an age feature."

In evaluating the role of the pubic symphysis as an age indicator three major contributions are available: Todd (Studies I–VIII, '20–'30); Brooks ('55); McKern and Stewart ('57).   Todd's is the early and significant contribution, so we shall discuss it first.   In principle he considered each pubic symphysis to possess a more or less oval outline, with long axis supero-inferior; this oval had five main features: a surface; a ventral (outer) border or "rampart"; a dorsal (inner) border or "rampart"; a superior extremity; an inferior extremity; subsidiary features, found mainly on the surface were: "ridging" and "billowing," and "ossific nodules."   These are all descriptive osteological features.

Varying and progressive combinations of these features resulted in the establishment of 10 Phases of pubic symphysis age, ranging in age from 18–19 years to 50+ years.   These Phases were defined by Todd (I, '20) as follows (see also Fig. 22 and Table 22):

> I. *First Post-adolescent:*   18–19 years.   Symphysial surface
> rugged, traversed by horizontal ridges separated by well

marked grooves; no ossific nodules fusing with the surface; no definite delimiting margin; no definition of extremities (p. 301).

II. *Second Post-adolescent:* 20–21 years. Symphysial still rugged, traversed by horizontal ridges, the grooves between which are, however, becoming filled near the dorsal limit with a new formation of finely textured bone. This formation begins to obscure the hinder extremities of the horizontal ridges. Ossific nodules fusing with the upper symphysial face may occur; dorsal limiting margin begins to develop, no delimitation of extremities; foreshadowing of ventral bevel (pp. 302–303).

III. *Third Post-adolescent:* 22–24 years. Symphysial face shows progressive commencing formation of the dorsal plateau; presence of fusing ossific nodules; dorsal margin gradually becoming more defined; beveling as a result of ventral rarefaction becoming rapidly more pronounced; no delimitation of extremities (p. 304).

IV. *25–26 Years.* Great increase of ventral beveled area; corresponding delimitation of lower extremity (p. 305).

V. *27–30 Years.* Little or no change in symphysial face and dorsal plateau except that sporadic and premature attempts at the formation of a ventral rampart occur; lower extremity, like the dorsal margin, is increasing in clearness of definition; commencing formation of upper extremity with or without the intervention of a bony (ossific) nodule (p. 306).

VI. *30–35 Years.* More difficult to appraise correctly; essential feature is completion of oval outline of symphysial face. More individual variation than at younger ages; and terminal phases affect relatively minor details. Also, tendency for terminal phase to be cut short. Increasing definition of extremities; development and practical completion of ventral rampart; retention of granular appearance of symphysial face and ventral aspect of pubis; absence of lipping of symphysial margin (p. 308).

VII. *35–39 Years.* Paramount feature: face and ventral aspect change from granular texture to fine-grained or dense bone. Changes in symphyseal face and ventral aspect of pubis consequent upon diminishing activity; commencing bony outgrowth into attachments of tendons and ligaments, espe-

cially the gracilis tendon and sacro-tuberous ligament
(p. 310).

VIII. *39–44 Years*. Symphysial face generally smooth and inactive; ventral surface of pubis also inactive; oval outline
complete or approximately complete; extremities clearly
defined; no distinct "rim" to symphysial face; no marked
lipping of either dorsal or ventral margin (p. 311).

IX. *45–50 Years*. Characterized by well-marked "rim." Symphysial face presents a more or less marked rim; dorsal
margin uniformly lipped; ventral margin irregularly lipped
(p. 312).

X. *50 Years +*. Rarefaction of face and irregular ossification.
Symphysial face eroded and showing erratic ossification;
ventral border more or less broken down; disfigurement
increases with age (p. 313).

Of these Phases Todd remarked that as a whole they were "a
much more reliable age indicator from 20 years to 40 than after

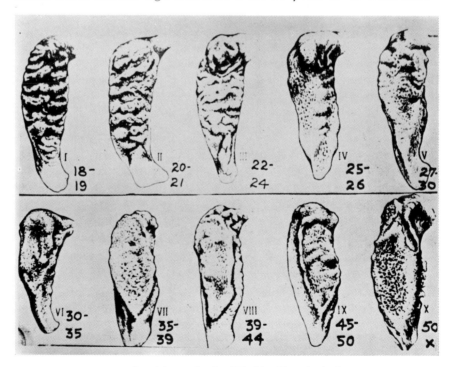

Fig. 22.   Modal standards of Todd's 10 typical phases.

TABLE 22

TEN PHASES IN POSTNATAL AGE-CHANGES IN THE PUBIC SYMPHYSIS*

Phase	Symphyseal Surface	Ossific Nodules	Ventral Margin	Dorsal Margin	Extremities
First 18–19	Rugged horiz. grooves, furrows and ridges	None	None	None	No definition
Second 20–21	Grooves filling dorsally and behind	May appear on sym. surf.	Ventral bevel begins	Begins	No definition
Third 22–24	Ridges and furrows progressively going	Present almost constantly	Beveling more pronounced	More definite dorsal plateau begins	No definition
Fourth 25–26	Rapidly going	Present	Beveling greatly increased	Complete dorsal plateau present	Lower commencing definition
Fifth 27–30	Little change	May be present	Sporadic attempt at ventral rampart	Completely defined	Lower clearer: upper extremity forming
Sixth 30–35	Granular appearance retained	May be present	Ventral rampart complete	Defined	Increasing def. upper and lower
Seventh 35–39	Texture finer; change due to diminishing activity	May be present	Complete	Defined	Carry on
Eighth 39–44	Smooth and inactive; no "rim"	May be present	No lipping	No lipping	Oval outline complete, extremities clearly outlined
Ninth 44–50	Rim present	May be present	Irregularly lipped	Uniformly lipped	Carry on
Tenth 50+	Erosion and erratic ossification			Broken down	

* From Krogman, '49, Table 3.

the latter age (p. 313). Further (p. 63, '21, Summary of Parts II–IV) he suggested that the Phases may be grouped into three periods: I–III, the post-adolescent stages; IV–VI, the various processes by which the symphysial outline is built up; VII–X, the period of gradual quiescence and secondary change. Todd found no race* or sex differences. Stewart ('57), however, feels that child-bearing may be a factor in causing certain symphyseal change ("pitting and irregularities in pubic symphyseal areas" were noted in female Eskimo pelves). He concluded that "assessment of age of females by the pubic symphysis cannot be as accurate as in the case of males."

In his 1923 study Todd uttered words of caution to the effect that ". . . unless it is absolutely unavoidable, the symphysis should never be used alone . . .Age prediction is at best an approximation: the most sanguine would not expect the prediction to be within less than two or three years if founded upon the entire skeleton, or to within less than five years if founded upon the pelvis alone" (p. 288).

In 1930, Todd (see also Burman *et al.*, '34) set up four Phases in the pubic symphysis discernible in the x-ray film, as follows (p. 283):

1. *25 Years.* Fine-texture body, undulating surface outline, no definition of extremities, no streak of compacta.
2. *26–39 Years.* Average-texture body, straight or faintly irregular surface outline, incompletely developed lower extremity, little or no grey streak of compacta.
3. *40–55 Years.* Average-texture body, a straight or irregular ventral outline, a well-developed lower extremity, and a fairly dense grey streak of compacta.
4. *55+ Years.* Open-texture body, an angular lower extremity, and a dense grey streak of compacta broken into patches marking the ventral margin.

Thus a real undulating outline with no definition of extremities and no grey streak of compacta, with a finely textured body, cannot occur later than twenty-five years. A straight or faintly marked irregular outline with an incompletely developed lower extremity, little or no grey streak, and a fine or averaged textured bone, defines

---

* Hanihara ('52) on 135 male Japanese skeletons found Todd's Phases workable, though they tended to over-age some specimens.

the age as between twenty-five and thirty-nine years. A well-developed lower extremity with a straight or irregular outline of the ventral face, a fairly dense grey streak, and an average textured body suggests forty to fifty-five years. A dense grey streak of outline broken into patches with an angular lower extremity and an open textured body characterizes the age as fifty-five or more. Considerable experience will guide the observer to a still closer estimate of age.

In Figure 23 (Todd, '30) are shown symphyseal age-traits via the x-ray film: youth, middle age, and senility (male whites, only).

TABLE 23
AGE CHARACTERISTICS OF THE UCMA AND WRU SERIES*

| | WRU Series | | | | UCMA Series | |
| | Male | | Female | | Male | Female |
Observer→	TWT	STB	TWT	STB	STB	STB
Total number in series	100	103	26	82	194	177
Coefficients of correlation						
Pubic and known age	.91	.87	.67	.72	—	—
Endocranial and known age	.78	.74	.56	.41	—	—
Pubic and endo-cranial age	.80	.73	.58	.40	—	—
Cranial and known age	—	.71	—	.38	—	—
Cranial and pubic age	—	.65	—·	.33	.39	.38
Mean cranial age	—	—	—	—	31.8 ± .50	29.7 ± .49
Mean pubic age	—	—	—	—	33.3 ± .58	39.6 ± .80
Mean of individual deviation of cranial from pubic age	—	—	—	—	±6.5	±11.6
Mean of individual excess of pubic over cranial age					+1.6	+9.7

* From Brooks, '55, Table 1.

I have checked Todd's basic data, i.e., the actual specimens upon which his studies are based, and have used his ten Phases for 30 years. They work, but they do tend to over-age, especially in the later decades of life. But, since they are applicable only in lustra of five years the five-year spread is enough to cover any over-lap.

In 1955 Brooks checked Todd and Lyons suture closure schedules and Todd's pubic Phase schedules on 470 aboriginal American Indians (UCMA Series = U. of Cal. Mus. Anthropol.) and 103 male

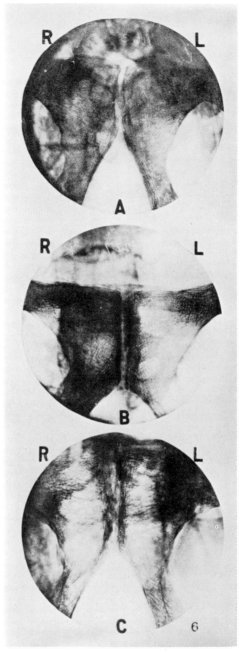

Fig. 23. Age-changes in the pubic symphysis as seen roentgenographically:
A, the fine texture of youth (male white, 26 yrs.) ; B, the average texture of middle
age (male white, 37 yrs.) ; C, open texture with streakiness of substance, characteristic of old age (male white, 81 yrs.).

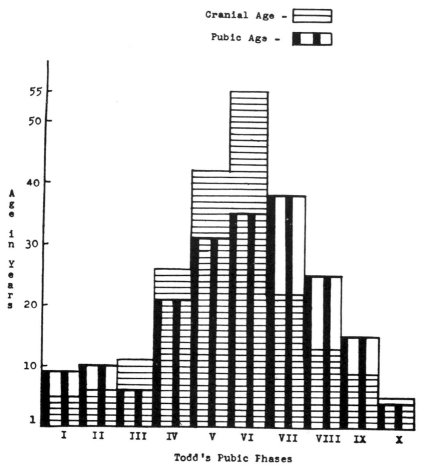

Fig. 24. Mortality curve, UCMA male.

skulls, 82 female skulls (WRU Series = Western Reserve Univ.). For the pubic symphysis Brooks found that estimates in males had a high correlation with known age; females were a bit lower. "Cranial age estimates, even endocranially determined, correlated poorly and should be used only with caution." These findings are presented in Table 23.

In Figures 24–25 the comparison between ageing via pubic Phases and via suture closure (cranial age) is shown for the UCMA Series,

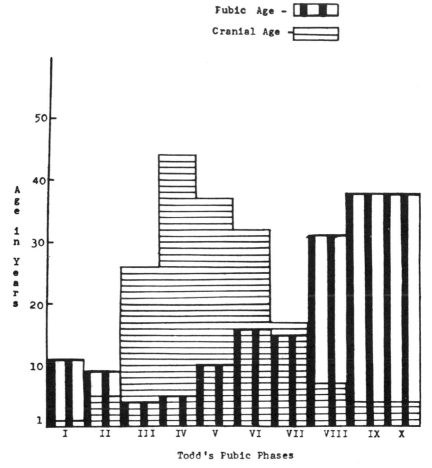

Fig. 25.   Mortality curve, UCMA female.

males and females, respectively.   The agreement is fair in males,
poor in females.

As a result of this study Brooks modified Todd's age limits for
the pubic symphysis by shifting Phases V–VIII about three years
downward (younger).   This is shown in Table 24, together with a
statement of prediction, both with reference to the pubic symphysis
and with reference to suture closure.

In 1957, McKern and Stewart made further and very useful

TABLE 24
LIMITS OF PUBIC PHASES, BASED ON WRU SERIES*

Pubic Phase	Age Limits According to TWT	Modified Limits	Overlapping Limits
I	17.5–19.5	17.5–19.5	17.0–20.0
II	19.5–21.5	19.5–21.5	19.0–22.0
III	21.5–24.5	21.5–24.0	20.0–25.0
IV	24.5–26.5	24.0–26.0	23.0–27.0
V	26.5–30.5	26.0–27.0	25.0–30.0
VI	30.5–35.5	27.0–33.5	27.0–35.0
VII	35.5–39.5	33.5–38.0	34.0–41.0
VIII	39.5–44.5	38.0–42.0	40.0–47.0
IX	44.5–50.5	42.0–50.5	45.0–50.0
X	50.5	50.5	48.0

Percentage of correct prediction

Sex	TWT Phase Limits	Modified Limits	Overlapping	Cranial Suture Closure
Male STB	30	61	72	45
Female STB	35	39	45	26
Male TWT	54	—	—	—
Female TWT	31	—	—	—

* From Brooks, '55, Table 2.

revisions. They started with Todd's nine morphological features of the pubic symphysis:

1. Ridges and furrows
2. Dorsal margin
3. Ventral bevelling
4. Lower extremity
5. Superior ossific nodule
6. Upper extremity
7. Ventral rampart
8. Dorsal plateau
9. Symphysial rim

It was noted by McKern and Stewart that feature 1 was divided by a longitudinal ridge or groove into dorsal and ventral halves; these were accordingly termed "dorsal demi-face" and "ventral demi-face." Obliteration of ridges and grooves was not considered a separate feature. It was then observed that features 4 and 2, 6 and 3, 5 and 7, were related (as paired) and that all six features might well be included in the description of the two demi-facets. Similarly feature 2 and 8, 3 and 7, were considered to be inter-related, and part of the demi-facet complex. This recombining leaves feature 9 as distinct.

As a result McKern and Stewart present *three components* of the pubic symphysis, each with *five developmental stages* as follows:

I. *Dorsal Plateau*
   0. Dorsal margin absent.
   1. A slight margin formation first appears in the middle third of the dorsal border.
   2. The dorsal margin extends along entire dorsal border.
   3. Filling in of grooves and resorption of ridges to form a beginning plateau in the middle third of the dorsal demi-face.
   4. The plateau still exhibiting vestiges of billowing extends over most of the dorsal demi-face.
   5. Billowing disappears completely and the surface of the entire demi-face becomes flat and slightly granulated.

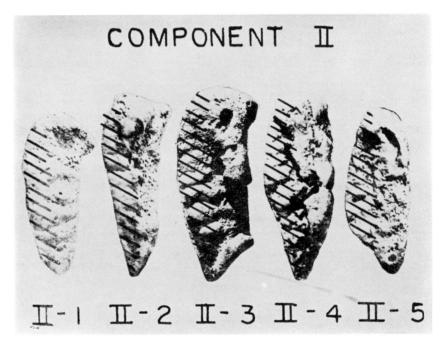

Fig. 26.   The five active stages of Component II.

II. *Ventral Rampart* (see Fig. 26)
   0. Ventral beveling is absent.
   1. Ventral beveling is present only at superior extremity of ventral border.
   2. Bevel extends inferiorly along ventral border.

3. The ventral rampart begins by means of bony extensions from either or both extremities.
4. The rampart is extensive but gaps are still evident along the earlier ventral border, most evident in the upper two-thirds.
5. The rampart is complete.

III. *Symphyseal Rim*

0. The symphysial rim is absent.
1. A partial dorsal rim is present, usually at the superior end of the dorsal margin, it is round and smooth in texture and elevated above the symphysial surface.
2. The dorsal rim is complete and the ventral rim is beginning to form. There is no particular beginning site.
3. The symphysial rim is complete. The enclosed symphysial surface is finely grained in texture and irregular or undulating in appearance.
4. The rim begins to break down. The face becomes smooth and flat and the rim is no longer round but sharply defined. There is some evidence of lipping on the ventral edge.
5. Further breakdown of the rim (especially along superior, ventral edge) and rarefaction of the symphysial face. There is also disintegration and erratic ossification along the ventral rim.

In Table 25 the authors present an age-range and distribution of Components and their stages:

A steady, uniform age-progression is obvious for all three Components.

In Table 26 the age limits of Components and stages are given:

With three variables taken 5 times the number of possible combinations is $5^3 = 125$. Actually, however, the authors found only 21 different formulae, as follows:

000	320	431	543
100	330	441	552
200	410	442	553
210	420	541	554
300	430	542	555
310			

The Components and their stages may be used to give a total score, which could, of course, range from 0 to 15. If all three

TABLE 25

THE AGE DISTRIBUTION OF COMPONENT STAGES IN THE PUBIC SYMPHYSIS*

Age**	No.	Component I Stages						Component II Stages						Component III Stages					
		0	1	2	3	4	5	0	1	2	3	4	5	0	1	2	3	4	5
17	5	5	8					5						5					
18	23	2	5	11	2			23						23					
19	57		5	35	16	1		51	5	1				57					
20	52		2	16	26	8		34	16	2				52					
21	33		1	4	20	8		8	13	5				31	2				
22	21				7	14		1	7	5	7	3		16	5				
23	29				6	20	3		5	4	5	3	1	15	14				
24	16				1	8	7			1	12	8	1	3	8	2	3		
25	8					3	5				7	7	2		3	3	2		
26	13					9	4				3	3	0		5	7	1		
27	12					7	5				3	10	3		4	3	5		
28	13					6	7				4	5	3		2	7	4		
29–30	15					1	14				2	7	4			9	4	2	
31–39	45						45					11	39			5	12	26	2
40–50	7						7					6	7					5	2
Total	349																		

* From McKern and Stewart, '57, Table 25.

** Represents age to the nearest year, for example, 17 = 16.5 to 17.4.

TABLE 26

AGE LIMITS OF THE COMPONENT STAGES IN THE PUBIC SYMPHYSIS*

Stage	Age Range	Mode
	Component I	
0	17.0–18.0	17.0
1	18.0–21.0	18.0
2	18.0–21.0	19.0
3	18.0–24.0	20.0
4	19.0–29.0	23.0
5	23.0+	31.0
	Component II	
0	17.0–22.0	19.0
1	19.0–23.0	20.0
2	19.0–24.0	22.0
3	21.0–28.0	23.0
4	22.0–33.0	26.0
5	24.0+	32.0
	Component III	
0	17.0–24.0	19.0
1	21.0–28.0	23.0
2	24.0–32.0	27.0
3	24.0–39.0	28.0
4	29.0+	35.0
5	38.0+	

* From McKern and Stewart, '57, Table 26.

Components are stage 0, the score is 0; if Component I is in stage 2, Component II in stage 2, and Component III in stage 3, the score is 7; and so on. Table 27 gives the age-range, mean age, and standard deviation for the total scores:

With the basic work of Todd and the refinements introduced by Brooks and by McKern and Stewart, the pubic symphysis takes its place as the most reliable indicator of age in the human skeleton.

2. THE PRIMARY ELEMENTS AND THE EPIPHYSES OF THE PELVIS

While the ossification of the pelvis has already been noted in another Chapter, it will be useful to amplify the theme at this point. The right and left pelvic bones (the innomonate bones) are made up of three separate bones: the pubic bone (pubis), anteriorly; the iliac bone (ilium), laterally; the ischial bone (ischium), postero-inferiorly. These are the *primary elements* of the pelvis, and they have a common point of meeting in the hip-socket (acetabulum).

It is generally accepted that "the union of the primary elements" refers mainly to their union at or near their common meeting

place in the hip socket. This occurs in the pubertal growing
period, at about 13 years in girls, 14 years in boys. McKern and
Stewart ('57) extend the concept of primary element union in both
time and locale. They report on final union of ischium and
pubis (at the postero-superior angle of the obturator foramen),
and of ilium and ischium (in the sciatic notch): "17 years represents the final age for union of the primary elements of the innominate (see Fig. 27).

TABLE 27

CALCULATED MEAN AGE, STANDARD DEVIATION AND AGE RANGES FOR THE TOTAL
SCORES OF THE SYMPHYSEAL FORMULAE*

Total Score	No.	Age Range for the Scores	Mean Age	Standard Deviation
0	7	–17	17.29	.49
1–2	76	17–20	19.04	.79
3	43	18–21	19.79	.85
4–5	51	18–23	20.84	1.13
6–7	26	20–24	22.42	.99
8–9	36	22–28	24.14	1.93
10	19	23–28	26.05	1.87
11–12–13	56	23–39	29.18	3.33
14	31	29+	35.84	3.89
15	4	36+	41.00	6.22
Total	349			

* From McKern and Stewart, '57, Table 27.

On the outer, upper free border of the ilium there is found the
iliac epiphysis. This center appears at around 12 years in girls,
13 years in boys (about a year before the union of the acetabular
junction of the three separate bones). Its union begins at or near
17 years and is completed at 23 years. McKern and Stewart
('57) recognize four stages of union as follows:

Stage I   Union begins internally near the ant. sup. spine (see
           Fig. 28).
Stage II
    Internally: Fused in anterior $1/2$; occasionally at the post. end.
    Externally: Fused at ant. sup. spine and in middle $1/3$ (some-
        times also at post. end, both externally and internally.
Stage III
    Internally: Ununited only at a point just above the junction of
        the iliac fossa and articular area.
    Externally: Ununited only at point of greatest ant. thickness

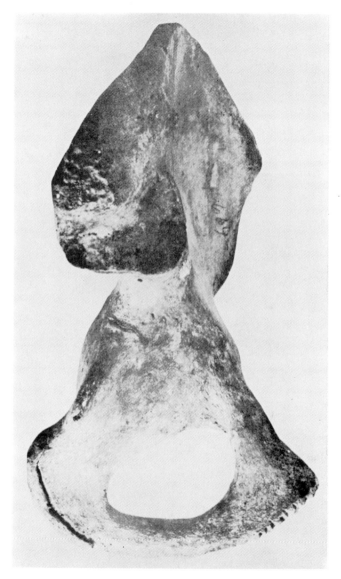

Fig. 27. Left hip bone showing stage 4 of union of primary elements (#425, 17 yrs.) (Note fissure in the sciatic notch marking line of union between ilium and ischium.

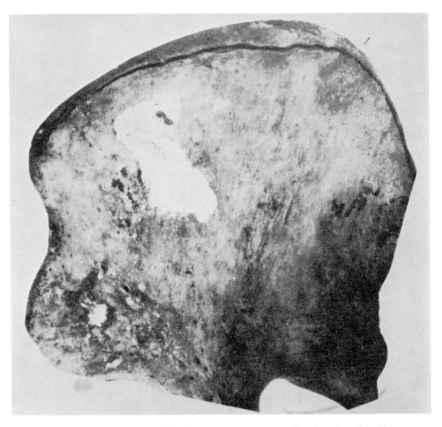

Fig. 28. External surface of R ilium, showing stage 1 of union for iliac crest.
(#319, 19 yrs.)   Note beginning union at anterior superior spine.

Stage IV (see Fig. 29).
    Completed union. (The fissures of stage III often persist as
    shallow grooves.)

Table 28 presents the age-variability of the union of the iliac
epiphysis.

Epiphyses are also found on the *ischial tuberosity* and on the *ischial
ramus*.   They usually represent a continuum, and appear at about
15 years in boys, 13 years in girls.   Union is completed by 23
years, with the external side of the ramus the last part to unite.*

---

* In Stevenson ('24) the ramal portion of the epiphysis is said to be unique in
that it is occasionally never fully united.

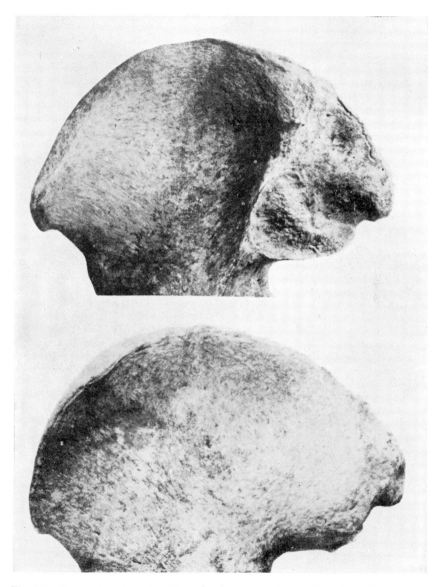

Fig. 29. Internal surface of R ilium (top) showing stage 4 for union of iliac crest; external surface of L ilium (bottom) showing stage 4 for union of iliac crest (#324, 19 yrs.).

TABLE 28

Epiphysis on Iliac Crest: Age Distribution of Stages of Union* (in %)

		Stages of Union				
Age	No.	0	1	2	3	4
17	10	40	10	10	40	—
18	45	18	16	26	20	20
19	52	5	4	27	28	36
20	45	2	6	4	24	64
21	37	—	5	8	13	74
22	24	—	—	4	4	92
23	26	—	—	—	—	100
Total	239					

* From McKern and Stewart, '57, Table 22.

TABLE 29

Epiphysis on Ischium: Age Distribution of Stages of Union: (in %)

		Stages of Union				
Age	No.	0	1	2	3	4
17	10	50	10	20	10	10
18	45	52	13	12	12	11
19	52	14	24	13	17	32
20	45	11	13	9	23	44
21	37	10	6	3	25	56
22	24	4	—	—	4	92
23	26	—	—	4	4	92
24–25	27	—	—	—	—	100
Total	266					

* From McKern and Stewart, '57, Table 24.

Table 29 presents the age-variability of the union of the ischial epiphysis.

The pelvic bone in its entirety is a focal area of age identification: 1) the appearance of iliac and ischial centers is correlated with puberty and early adolescence; 2) the union of the centers is correlated with young adulthood; 3) the pubic symphysis is correlated with the full vigor of the third, fourth, and fifth decades of life. In turn each of these three periods is correlated with other skeletal areas: (1) is timed with elbow and, possibly, basilar suture; (2) is correlated with wrist, shoulder, knee, and sternal end of clavicle; (3) is correlated (though less so) with union of sutures.

Summarizing Statement

1. The pubic symphysis is probably the best single criterion of the registration of age in the skeleton. Its age-range extends thru

the second, third, fourth and fifth decades, during which time it is reliably correlated with age-changes in long bones and in skull.

2. By itself the pubic symphysis should register age in lustra of five years. In correlation with other parts of the skeleton, when available, it should facilitate ageing within the five-year spans, especially in the third and fourth decades of life. In these decades, using pubic symphysis plus other skeletal criteria, I'd venture an accuracy of plus or minus two years.

REFERENCES

BROOKS, S. T.: Skeletal age at death: reliability of cranial and pubic age indicators. *AJPA, n.s., 13(4)*:567–597, 1955.

BURMAN, M., WEINKLE, I. N. and LANGSAM, M. J.: Adolescent osteochondritis of the symphysis pubis: with a consideration of the normal roentgenographic changes in the symphysis pubis. *JBJS, o.s. 32, n.s., 16*:649–657, 1934.

HANIHARA, K.: Age change in the male Japanese pubic bone. *J. Anth. Soc. Nippon, 62(698)*:245–260, 1952.

KROGMAN, W. M.: 1949, (see *Refs.*, Chap. II).

McKERN, T. W. and STEWART, T. D.: 1957, (see *Refs.*, Chap. II).

STEVENSON, P. H.: 1924, (see *Refs.*, Chap. II).

STEWART, T. D.: Distortion of the pubic symphyseal surface in females and its effect on age determination. *AJPA n.s., 15(1)*:9–18, 1957.

TODD, T. W.: Age changes in the pubic bone: I the male white pubis. *AJPA, 3(3)*:285–334, 1920.

TODD, T. W.: Age changes in the pubic bone: II the pubis of the male Negro-white hybrid; III the pubis of the white female; IV the pubis of the female Negro-white hybrid. *AJPA, 4(1)*:1–70, 1921.

TODD, T. W.: Age changes in the pubic bone: V Mammalian pubic metamorphosis. *AJPA, 4(4)*:333–406, 1921.

TODD, T. W.: Age changes in the pubic bone: VI the interpretation of variations in the symphysial area. *AJPA, 4(4)*:407–424, 1921.

TODD, T. W.: Age changes in the pubic symphysis: VII The anthropoid strain in human pubic symphyses of the third decade. *JA, 57(3)*:274–294, 1923.

TODD, T. W.: Age changes in the pubic bone: VIII Roentgenographic differentiation. *AJPA, 14(2)*:255–271, 1930.

V

Sexing Skeletal Remains

1. GENERAL CONSIDERATIONS, AND THE AGE FACTOR

There are a number of factors which inveigh against a high degree of accuracy in the sexing of unknown material. Among them are: (1) the often fragmentary or isolated nature of the remains available for study; (2) the evident age (at time of death) of the remains; (3) intrinsic variability and the absence of any real standards. Here is the problem of subjectivity vs. objectivity, of description vs. measurements, of "experience" vs. statistical "standardization." Most of the older studies of sex differences in the skeleton (skull and pelvis mainly) centered on morphological traits in a descriptive manner. The newer studies focus on morphometry in a largely quantitative and statistical sense.

How accurate can one be?

Years ago when I was at Western Reserve University I sexed a sample of 750 adult skeletons (white and Negro, male and female) from the Todd Collection. Lots of 50 were done at a time. This was a dissecting-room population and records of age, sex, and race were available. In the 15 lots of 50 each I scored as follows: entire skeleton 100%; pelvis alone 95%; skull alone 92%; pelvis plus skull 98%; long bones alone 80%; long bones plus pelvis 98%. Now, these are biased results. In a medical school the ratio of male to female cadavera is about 15:1. Hence, in any case in which I was in doubt, I had a 15:1 chance of being correct if I said male. Therefore, it is quite likely that all estimates should be lowered 5–10%, depending on the relative completeness of the material to be sexed.

Stewart ('48, '51) feels that for the entire adult skeleton, or for

112

the adult pelvis, or for one adult hip bone, he can sex correctly in 90–95% of cases; for adult skull alone about 80%; for adult major long bones alone "size alone determines the answer" ('51). Stewart ('48) said that Hrdlička on the adult skull alone hit 80%, but if mandible were present he hit 90%. In a series of 100 adult American Negro skeletons sexed by inspection (skeleton complete) Stewart scored 94%; but in this same series, using skull plus mandible, he scored only 77%.

TABLE 30
ASCERTAINMENTS OF SEX IN CHILDREN AT 2, 5 AND 8 YEARS OF AGE*

Sex	Age	N	Sex Correct	Sex Ambiguous	Sex Incorrect	% Correct
Boys	2	17	13	1	3	76
	5	17	15	1	1	88
	8	14	11	1	2	79
Girls	2	16	11	0	5	69
	5	16	10	0	6	63
	8	13	11	1	1	85
Both sexes combined	2	33	24	1	8	73
	5	33	25	1	7	76
	8	27	22	2	3	81

* From Hunt and Gleiser, '55, Table 1.

The foregoing discussion refers to adult material. When is "adult?" As a general rule definitive sexual traits in the skeleton are not manifest until after the full achievement of the secondary sex traits that appear during puberty. The dividing line between immaturity and maturity is somewhere around 15–18 years. Up to about this age sexing has been pretty much of a 50–50 guess proposition.*

Recently Hunt and Gleiser ('55) have scored dental development (Hurme, '48) and skeletal maturation (Greulich and Pyle, '58) in terms of sex differentiation. For dental age the formula $y = 0.95x$, and for skeletal age the formula $y = 0.80x$, were derived (y = age of girls, x = age of boys). In samples of children aged two, five, and eight years "hits" and "misses" are reported as follows (Table 30):

In evaluating their approach to immature remains Hunt and Gleiser conclude as follows:

* For an exception to this generalization see Sec. 3, dealing with sex differences in the pelvis.

On the basis of these equations, concurrent estimates of bone and
dental age by male standards should agree closely if the remains are
those of a boy, but should be more divergent if female standards
are applied.   The opposite is usually true if the remains belong to
a girl.   If bone and dental ages are assessed for the remains by the
standards of both sexes, the sex for which the standards agree best
is considered to be the correct one.

It is often stated that dimensionally the adult male:female ratio
is about 100:92, i.e., female measurements are about 92% of male
measurements.   This does not precisely hold for the entire living
body.   In 1901 Pfitzner stated as follows (female in % of male):*

Stature	93.5%	Head breadth	96.0%
Sitting height	94.5%	Head length	95.5%
Arm length	91.5%	Head height	96.0%
Leg length	93%	Face breadth	94.0%
Head circumference	96%	Face height	90.0%

These data, while referring to *body* measurements, may be taken
over to an approximation of skeletal sexual proportionality.   (See
Sec. 4, on the sexing of long bones.)

2. SEX DIFFERENCES IN THE SKULL

Traditionally the skull is the single most studied bone in physical
anthropology.   Archaeologists have concentrated on excavating
and preserving skulls, and much of our knowledge of human evolution is based on cranial remains.   Equally traditional, the sexing
of skulls has been based on an anatomical (osteological) basis,
so that descriptive features (traits) have ruled, rather than dimensions (size, proportions).   (See, as examples, the studies of Weisbach, 1868, Pittard, '00, Mobius, '07, and Parsons, '20.)

In Table 31 a tabulation of morphological sex-traits in the skull
is presented:

In amplification of this Table I'd like to summarize as follows
(Krogman, '39):

In sexing a skull the initial impression often is the deciding
factor: a large skull is generally male, a small skull female.   The
cranial capacity in the female averages 200 cc. less than the male,
though in the female the index of cerebral value is relatively higher.

---

* In '39/'40 Hug published elaborate tables of sex differences in cranial dimensions;
his data are partially summarized in Sec. 2.

The female skull is usually rounder than the male, i.e., the cranial index is two or more points greater. The cranio-facial proportions are about the same, though in the female the facial skeleton may be relatively more gracile. The general impression may be verified by observation of mandible, nasal aperture, orbits, cheekbones, supraorbital ridges, glabella, forehead contour, mastoid processes, occipital region, palate and teeth and base of skull. Insofar as several of these criteria are age-phenomena, appearing or becom-

TABLE 31
TRAITS DIAGNOSTIC OF SEX IN THE SKULL*

Trait	*Male*	*Female*
General size	Large (endocranial volume 200 cc. more)	Small
Architecture	Rugged	Smooth
Supra-orbital ridges	Medium to large	Small to medium
Mastoid processes	Medium to large	Small to medium
Occipital area	Muscle lines and protuberance marked	Muscle lines and protuberance not marked
Frontal eminences	Small	Large
Parietal eminences	Small	Large
Orbits	Squared, lower, relatively smaller, with rounded margins	Rounded, higher, relatively larger, with sharp margins
Forehead	Steeper, less rounded	Rounded, full, infantile
Cheek bones	Heavier, more laterally arched	Lighter, more compressed
Mandible	Larger, higher symphysis, broader ascending ramus	Small, with less corpal and ramal dimensions
Palate	Larger, broader, tends more to U-shape	Small, tends more to parabola
Occipital condyles	Large	Small
Teeth	Large; lower M1 more often 5-cusped	Small; molars most often 4-cusped

* From Krogman, '55, Table 9.

ing pronounced at puberty, and many are affected by the changes of senility, the description of sex differences must be limited to the ages of approximately 20–55.

The *mandible* in the male is larger and thicker, with greater body height, especially at the symphysis, and with a broader ascending ramus; the angle formed by body and ramus is less obtuse (under 125°); the condyles are larger and the chin is "square."

The *nasal aperture* in the male is higher and narrower and its margins are sharp rather than rounded. The male nasal bones are larger and tend to meet in the mid-line at a sharper angle.

The *orbits* are higher, more rounded and relatively larger, com-

pared to upper facial skeleton, in the female.   The orbital margins
are sharper, less rounded, than in the male.

The *cheek-bones* in the male are heavier, in the female lighter.
In the male they are usually described as medium to massive, in the
female slender to medium.

The *supraorbital ridges* are almost invariably much more strongly
developed in males than in females.   The males range from moderate to excessive development, the females from a mere trace to
moderate.   "Heavy" supraorbital ridges are typically male,
while a "trace" or "slight" are typically female.

Glabella (the forehead eminence above the root of the nose)
appears to keep pace with the supraorbital ridges.   A large glabella
is male, a small glabella is female.   It must be pointed out, however, that the range of variation is greater for glabella than for
the ridges, i.e., there is greater convergence toward an intermediate
type.

The *forehead contour* in the female is higher, smoother, more vertical, and may be rounded to the point of forward protrusion;
in general the pattern is more on the infantile ground-plan.

The *mastoid processes* (just back of the ear-hole) are definitely
larger in the male, smaller in the female.   The males range in
size from medium to large, in females from small to medium.

The *occipital region* presents several transverse lines and the external
occipital protuberance which are the sites of attachments of the
neck muscles.   The transverse lines are much more evident and the
protuberance much larger in the male.   A relatively smooth occipital bone is invariably female.

The *palate* is usually larger and broader in the male.   The shape
of the male arch tends more toward a ∪, due to the relative length
of the cheek tooth-row;   in the female the relative shortness of the
cheek tooth-row conduces to a parabolic shape.

The *teeth* are a bit larger in the male, but the greater variability
of tooth dimensions in the female tends to prevent sex discrimination
on the basis of size.

The *base of the skull* shows larger condyles, a relatively longer
foramen magnum and larger foramina generally in the male.   The
basilar portion of the occiput and the body of the sphenoid are
longer in the male.

These characters in their entirety should give a pretty good idea of sex in adult skulls. It may be observed that with respect to the majority of the characters used as the basis of assessment the female skull is negative, the male skull positive. If ranked in order we note: general size, and architecture, supraorbital ridges, mastoid processes, occipital region, cheek-bones, orbits, mandible and palate.

In 1939–40, Hug put sex differences in cranial dimensions on a fairly sound basis (German crania). Following are some of the basic absolute dimensions classified by him (in mm., except cranial capacity which is cc.):

Dimension and Classification	Male	Female
Max. skull length		
(very short)	(X–169)	(X–159)
short	X–179	X–169
average	180–189	170–179
long	190–X	180–X
(very long)	(200–X)	(190–X)
Max. skull breadth		
(very narrow)	(X–129)	(X–124)
narrow	X–139	X–134
average	140–149	135–144
broad	150–X	145–X
(very broad)	(160–X)	(155–X)
Skull height (from base)		
(very low)	(X–121)	(X–115)
low	X–129	X–123
average	130–137	124–131
high	138–X	132–X
(very high)	(146–X)	(140–X)
Skull height (from earhole)		
(very low)	(X–106)	(X–102)
low	X–112	X–108
average	113–118	109–114
high	119–X	115–X
(very high)	(125–X)	(121–X)
Horiz. circumference		
(very small)	(X–502)	(X–482)
small	X–519	X–499
average	520–534	500–514
large	535–X	515–X
(very large)	(552–X)	(532–X)
Cranial capacity		
(very small)	(X–1150)	(X–1000)
small	X–1300	X–1150
average	1301–1450	1151–1300
large	1451–X	1301–X
(very large)	(1601–X)	(1451–X)
Face breadth		
(very narrow)	(X–121)	(X–113)
narrow	X–129	X–121
average	130–137	122–129
broad	138–X	130–X

Dimension and Classifications	Male	Female
(very broad)	(146–X)	(138–X)
Face height (total)		
(very low)	(X–105)	(X–97)
low	X–113	X–105
average	114–121	106–113
high	122–X	114–X
(very high)	(130–X)	(122–X)
Face height (upper)		
(very low)	(X–63)	(X–59)
low	X–68	X–64
average	69–73	65–69
high	74–X	70–X
(very high)	(79–X)	(75–X)

A scrutiny of these data will reveal considerable size overlap, as between male and female. Obviously, no single dimension is diagnostic, but if *all* dimensions are large, in a male direction, then it is pretty safe to diagnose the skull as "male."

In 1950, Keen attempted to set up a battery of cranial traits and dimensions for adult skulls (juvenile and senile skulls excluded) "which will sex skulls with 85% accuracy." He chose three basic anatomical features (the supraorbital ridges, the external auditory meatus, the muscle markings on the occipital bone) and four basic measurements (maximum cranial length, facial breadth, depth of the infratemporal fossa, length of the mastoid process). For these four he calculated the mean and standard deviation for each sex. This gave a "male range," "a female range," and a "neutral zone." An example of this procedure may be seen for maximum cranial length:

	Male	Female
Mean	185.6 mm.	178.6 mm.
S.D.	6.2 mm.	6.9 mm.
±1 S.D.	179.4–191.8 mm.	171.7–185.5 mm.

Total range of both sexes is 171.7–191.8 mm. Probably male = 185 mm. +; probably female = 178 mm. −. Doubtful zone = 178–185 mm.*

* What is sauce for the goose is not necessarily sauce for the gander! Total range is not the sauce for all series of skulls, hence "zones" of sex difference may shift with the sample studied. Stewart ('54, quoting Simmons, '42) gives ranges for 1179 white male skulls and 182 white female skulls:

	Male	Female
Max. skull lgth.	158–210 mm.	157–193 mm.
Max. skull breadth	123–164 "	123–154 "
Cranial capacity	1099–1782 cc.	1070–1749 cc.

Keen used 50 male skulls, 50 female skulls of the "Cape Coloured" population of S. Africa, which he accepts as a homogeneous population. His data are presented in Table 32. Significance of sex difference is tested by the *critical ratio*. A C.R. value of over 2.5 is deemed significant, i.e., it is due to factors other than random chance.

It is interesting to note that each of the anatomical features (Nos. 21–23) shows a significant sex difference. Dimensions No. 1, 2, 7, 8, 9, 10, 12, 17, 20, all show Critical Ratios of 5.0 or more and hence are significant.

In recent years elaborate and detailed statistical studies, involving discriminant analysis,* have been made of sex differences in skull and long bones. Hanihara ('59) reports on such a study on Japanese skulls. The following measurements were taken:

X_1 max. lgth. of skull
X_2 max. brdth. of skull
X_3 ht. (total) of skull
X_4 face brdth.
X_5 upper face ht.

X_6 mandib. brdth.
X_7 symph. ht. of mand.
X_8 cond. ht. of mand.
X_9 ramal brdth. of mand.

In Table 33 Hanihara presents his basic data (N = size of sample, $\bar{x}$ = mean value of dimension, S_x = sums of squares of deviations, and u^2 = mean squares).

In Table 34 is presented the discriminant functions for the cranial measurements taken:

The procedure is roughly as follows: (1) take the measurements, X_1, X_2, . . . ; (2) compute Y, the discriminant function, from these measurements; (3) compare Y with the discriminant value: if the former is larger than the latter the skull is male, if the reverse it is female. In the last column of Table 34 the likelihood of error is calculated (range is from 10.29% to 16.93%). In a "blind test" Hanihara sexed 35 skulls (all male) taken at random from a known series of 98 individuals, using only measurements X_{i-4}. He missed four of the 35 (11.4% error). He had most trouble in sexing skulls with relatively broad or low vaults, and concluded that the method was not as good for skulls as it was for long bones.

---

* For an excellent summary of methodology in this statistical procedure see Thieme and Schull ('57b). (See Chap. VII for additional references.)

TABLE 32

STATISTICAL COMPARISON OF MALE AND FEMALE SKULLS OF THE CAPE COLOURED POPULATION IN MEASUREMENTS, INDICES AND SPECIA[L] FEATURES

(Measurements in Millimeters Unless Stated Otherwise)*

	50 Male Skulls			50 Female Skulls			Critical** Ratio of Difference
	Range	Mean ± ϵ	S.D.	Range	Mean ± ϵ	S.D.	
1. Maximum length	168–198	185.6 ± .9	6.2	165–192	178.6 ± 1.0	6.9	5.4
2. Length of base	90–110	100.1 ± .6	4.1	82–106	94.8 ± .7	4.6	5.8
3. Length of foramen magnum	30–44	36.3 ± .4	2.9	30–40	34.8 ± .3	2.4	3.0
4. Maximum breadth	124–150	135.4 ± .7	4.9	120–146	133.0 ± .8	5.9	2.2
5. Median sagittal arc	338–410	372.7 ± 2.1	15.0	332–392	364.3 ± 2.3	15.8	2.7
6. Basion-bregma height	118–142	131.4 ± .8	5.3	115–139	127.1 ± .7	4.8	3.9
7. Horizontal circumference	479–542	516.2 ± 2.1	14.5	465–528	498.3 ± 2.2	15.6	6.0
8. Cranial capacity (cc³)	1000–1750	1355 ± 16.8	117.9	950–1500	1199 ± 18.1	126.6	6.3
Cranial index (4/1)	67.5–80.5	73.5 ± .4	2.9	68.5–79.5	74.5 ± .4	2.9	1.7
Height-length index (6/1)	64.5–76.5	70.9 ± .4	2.5	66.5–75.5	71.3 ± .4	2.5	.7
Base-maximum length index (2/1)	49.5–57.5	54.0 ± .3	2.1	46.5–58.5	53.1 ± .3	2.4	2.1
Base-median sagittal arc index (2/5)	24.1–29.7	26.9 ± .2	1.4	22.0–29.0	26.1 ± .2	1.6	2.8
9. Total face height	97–130	116.8 ± 1.0	7.7	90–120	108.7 ± 1.2	8.6	5.1
10. Maximum bizygomatic diameter	116–140	128.2 ± .7	4.7	104–128	119.5 ± .8	5.5	8.0
Total facial index (9/10)	75.5–105.5	91.0 ± .9	6.6	75.5–105.5	91.0 ± .9	6.2	0.0
11. Weight of mandible	40–120g	79.8 ± 2.6g	18.2	24–88g	60.6 ± 2.3g	16.4	5.5
12. Angle of mandible	110–140°	125.3 ± 1.2°	8.2	113–143°	128.0 ± .9°	6.1	1.8
13. Weight of cranium	390–840g	618.0 ± 15.2g	106.5	340–840g	572.0 ± 15.9g	111.8	2.1

	Range	Mean ± SE	SD	Range	Mean ± SE	SD	Critical ratio
14. Nasion to bregma	112–145	129.3 ± .9	6.6	112–142	126.0 ± 1.0	7.0	2.5
15. Bregma to lambda	112–136	126.5 ± .9	6.7	100–145	121.7 ± 1.3	9.1	3.0
Index, frontal: parietal length (14/15)	83.0–113.0	102.6 ± .9	6.2	86.0–122.0	103.8 ± 1.1	7.9	.9
16. Depth of infra-temporal fossa	19–30	24.3 ± .4	2.6	18–29	21.2 ± .3	2.1	6.2
17. Length of mastoid process	21–27	29.3 ± .5	3.6	19–33	26.5 ± .4	3.1	4.4
18. Porion to superior temporal line	75–108	91.9 ± 1.0	7.2	75–99	87.1 ± 1.0	7.0	3.0
19. Porion to vertex	139–163	152.9 ± .9	6.0	124–160	150.0 ± 1.1	7.7	2.2
Index of temporal muscle extent (18/19)	51.0–71.0	60.1 ± .6	4.5	49.0–69.0	57.8 ± .7	4.6	2.5
20. Profile angle at nasion	114–154°	135.3 ± 1.1°	7.9	112–162°	146.4 ± 1.0°	6.7	7.5
21. Supraorbital ridges, 3 categories							
(1) nil or trace	12%			42%			
(2) medium	64%			58%			
(3) marked	24%			0%			
mean score		2.12 ± .08	.59		1.58 ± .07	.49	5.0
22. Occipital crest and nuchal lines, 4 categories							
(1) nil or trace	0%			22%			
(2) medium	54%			66%			
(3) pronounced	36%			12%			
(4) excessive	10%			0%			
mean score		2.56 ± .10	.67		1.90 ± .08	.57	5.1
23. Ridge at upper rim of auditory meatus, 3 categories							
(1) nil or trace	6%			46%			
(2) medium	40%			44%			
(3) marked	54%			10%			
mean score		2.48 ± .09	.61		1.64 ± .09	.65	6.5

* From Keen, '50, Table 1.

** Critical ratio $= M_1 - M_2/f_1^2 + f_2^2$. ($M$ = mean, f = standard error of the mean.)

TABLE 33
MEASUREMENTS OF JAPANESE SKULLS*

Measure-ment	Male				Female			
	N	$\bar{x}$	S_x	u^2	N	$\bar{x}$	S_x	u^2
X_1	64	180.1	2009.60	31.90	41	170.6	1950.37	48.76
	60	180.2	1909.80	32.37	40	170.8	1890.40	48.47
X_2	64	139.8	1667.20	26.46	41	136.8	935.21	23.38
	60	139.9	1621.40	27.48	40	136.6	865.60	22.19
X_3	64	138.2	1289.44	20.52	41	130.9	570.72	14.27
	60	138.4	1172.40	19.87	40	130.9	566.60	14.53
X_4	64	132.0	1338.88	21.25	41	125.5	708.89	17.72
	60	132.4	1184.40	20.07	40	125.5	714.00	18.31
X_5	64	69.3	1083.52	17.20	41	65.5	397.70	9.94
X_6	60	96.4	2466.60	41.81	40	88.9	1406.80	36.07
X_7	60	34.2	477.60	8.09	40	30.6	225.60	5.78
X_8	60	60.9	1023.60	17.35	40	54.1	393.60	10.09
X_9	60	33.3	493.80	8.37	40	31.1	219.60	5.63

* From Hanihara, '59, Table 1.

TABLE 34
DISCRIMINANT FUNCTIONS FOR JAPANESE SKULLS*

Object of Diagnosis	Discriminant Functions	Discrim-inant Value	Proba-bility of Misclassi-fication
Cranium	$Y = X_1 + 2.6139X_3 + 0.9959X_4 + 2.3642X_7 + 2.0552X_8$	850.6571	0.1029
	$Y = X_1 + 2.5192X_3 + 0.5855X_4 + 0.6607X_6 + 2.7126X_8$	807.3989	0.1075
	$Y = X_1 + 0.7850X_4 + 0.4040X_6 + 1.9808X_8$	428.0524	0.1357
	$Y = X_1 + 2.5602X_3 + 1.0836X_4 + 2.6045X_8$	809.7200	0.1107
	$Y = X_1 + 2.2707X_3 + 1.3910X_4 + 2.7075X_7$	748.3422	0.1122
Calvarium	$Y = X_1 - 0.0620X_2 + 1.8654X_3 + 1.2566X_4$	579.9567	0.1358
	$Y = X_1 + 0.2207X_2 + 1.0950X_4 + 0.5043X_5$	380.8439	0.1693
Mandibula	$Y = X_6 + 2.2354X_7 + 2.9493X_8 + 1.6730X_9$	388.5323	0.1439

* From Hanihara, '59, Table 2.

3. SEX DIFFERENCES IN THE PELVIS

The entire pelvic structure, i.e., its constituent bones and its total configuration, has long been regarded as a critical factor in the sexing of the human skeleton.* It takes on added value by virtue of the fact that it apparently differs from other skeletal sexual criteria in that sex differences are present from foetal life and onward.

In the *fetus* (30 American white, 107 British white, 96 American Negro) Boucher ('55, '57) found "significant sex differences" in the subpubic angle of American white and Negro fetuses. The

* Hoyme ('57) and Genovese ('59) give excellent historical résumés of the evaluation of sex differences in the pelvis.

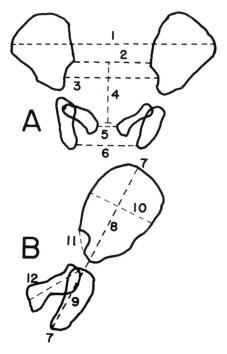

Fig. 30. The measurements, as taken from a pelvic tracing (A) and a hip tracing (B). In (A): 1, pelvis breadth; 2, inter-iliac breadth; 3, inlet breadth; 4, sagittal inlet, diameter; 5, inter-pubic breadth; 6, bi-ischial breadth. In (B): 7, pelvis height; 8, ilium length; 9, ischium length; 10, ilium breadth; 11, breadth of sciatic notch; 12, pubis length.

width and depth of the sciatic notch, and their increase with age, were also found to differ significantly between the sexes. "No sex differences have been found in the growth of the ischium or pubis with age, or of the ischium-pubis indices, either of the bony or cartilaginous pelves" ('57).

For the fetal sciatic notch ('55) the following index was derived:

$$\frac{\text{width of sciatic notch}}{\text{depth of sciatic notch}} \times 100$$

In females the index = 4.6–7.3 (central tendency 5.0–6.0).
In males the index = 3.9–5.0 (central tendency 4.0–5.0).

"The difference between the indices is sufficient to suggest that sex can be determined confidently from the ilium during fetal life" ('55). In American Negro and British white fetuses the index was found to be significantly higher in females than in males. No such sex difference was found in American white fetuses ('57).

Reynolds ('45) made roentgenometric studies of the bony pelvic girdle in *early infancy*. Studied were 46 boys, 49 girls, both American white, from birth to one year of age (serial x-ray films at birth, and at one, three, six, nine, 12 months).

The following measurements were taken on x-ray films, divided into two groups (see Figure 30) :*

Group A

Item	Description
Pelvis height	The maximum distance between the upper edge of the iliac crest and the lower margin of the ischium, taken on the left side. All ages.
Pelvis breadth	The maximum transverse distance between the outer borders of the iliac crests; corresponds to the bi-iliac. Birth and 1 month.
Inlet breadth	The maximum transverse diameter of the inlet. Birth and 1 month.
Inter-iliac breadth	The minimum distance between the ilia. Birth and 1 month.
Inter-pubic breadth	The minimum distance between the pubic bones. Traverses the area of the pubic symphysis. All ages.
Bi-ischial breadth	The minimum distance between the ischia. All ages.
Ilium length	The maximum length of the ilium, along its long axis. Left side; all ages. Intermediate in nature.
Pubis length	The maximum length of the pubis, along the shaft. Left side; all ages. Intermediate in nature.

Group B

Item	Description
Inlet, sagittal diameter	The anteroposterior distance between the centers of a line joining the posterior borders of the greater sciatic notch, and the center of a line defining the posterior surface of the pubic symphysis. Birth and 1 month.
Ilium breadth	The maximum breadth of the ilium, at right angles to the length. Left side; all ages.
Ischium length	The maximum length of the ischium along the shaft. Left side; all ages.
Breadth of greater sciatic notch	The breadth of the sacro-iliac notch, insofar as it is, at these age levels, contained entirely within the ilium. Left side; all ages.

From these dimensions the following indices and proportions were derived:

Item	Description
Pelvic index	Pelvis height/Pelvis breadth × 100. Birth and 1 month.
Inlet index	Inlet, sagittal diameter/Inlet breadth × 100. Birth and 1 month.
Iliac index	Ilium breadth/Ilium length × 100. All ages.

* Left side only, after tests at birth showed no differences between right and left sides.

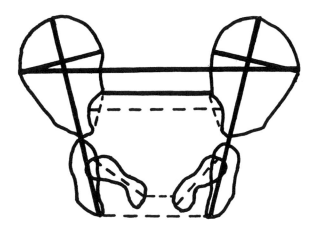

Fig. 31. Sex differences in pelvic measurements. Solid lines: boys tend to be larger; broken lines: girls tend to be larger.

Sacral index   Inter-iliac breadth/Pelvis breadth × 100. Birth and 1 month. This item is called "sacral index" because it represents approximately the relative breadth of the sacral region.

Relative inlet breadth   Inlet breadth/Pelvis breadth × 100. Birth and 1 month.

Anterior segment index   Inlet, sagittal diameter/Anterior segment × 100. Birth and 1 month. The anterior segment is that portion of the sagittal diameter of the inlet that lies in frcnt of the greatest transverse diameter of the inlet.

Reynold's conclusions on sex differences in the pelvis in the first postnatal year are as follows (see also Figure 31):

1. Boys show higher intercorrelations in measurements at birth than girls.

2. Significant sex differences in measurements and indices are found as follows: Boys lead in pelvis height, ilium breadth and ischio-iliac space. Girls lead in bi-ischial breadth, pubis length, breadth of greater sciatic notch, relative inlet breadth, and anterior segment index.

3. Suggestive, but not statistically significant sex differences, are found in pelvis breadth and iliac index (boys lead), and in inter-pubic breadth (girls lead).

4. Critical ratios of sex differences show a slight tendency to become smaller with age.

5. The possibility that pelvic tilt may be a causative factor in certain sex differences is discussed.

6. Measurements of girls tend to be more variable than measurements of boys.

7. The general pattern of sex differences in the pelvis, as shown by the present study, seems to favor the hypothesis that boys are larger in measurements relating to the outer structures of the pelvis, while girls are larger in measurements relating to the inner structures of the pelvis, including a relatively larger inlet.

In view of the studies of Hunt and Gleiser (see Sec. 1) on early sex differences in dental development and skeletal maturation, Reynold's observations on the first year are interesting. In boys, only, a positive correlation between pelvic size at 12 months and advanced ossification was found. "Larger pelves are associated with earlier appearance of ossification centers in boys." In both boys and girls a positive correlation between pelvic size at birth and age of appearance of first tooth was found. "Larger pelves are associated with earlier appearance of the first tooth." These conclusions are shown in Table 35.

TABLE 35

THE RELATION OF SIZE OF PELVIS TO SKELETAL AND TOOTH DEVELOPMENT*

	Boys			Girls		
Items Compared	*n*	*r*	*Signif-icant?*	*n*	*r*	*Signif-icant?*
Pelvis height (12 months) and skeletal age (Fels, 12 months)	29 + .50		Yes (1%)	29 + .19		No
Pelvis breadth (birth) and time of appearance of 1st tooth	39 + .33		Yes (5%)	43 + .22		No
Birth weight/Pelvis breadth and time of appearance of 1st tooth	38 + .23		No	43 + .30		Yes (5%)

* From Reynolds, '45, Table 18.

For the *prepuberal period* Reynolds ('47) studied the serial pelvic x-ray films of 92 American white boys, 91 American white girls, age two to nine years. The measurements and indices were as in the infant study, but three lengths and four angles were added (see Figure 32):

Inter-obturator breadth—The minimum transverse distance between the inner borders of the obturator foramina. (A)

Bi-trochanteric breadth—Maximum distance between the great trochanters. (A)

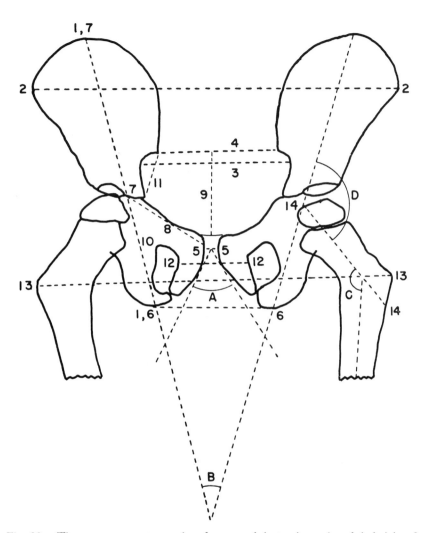

Fig. 32. The measurements as taken from a pelvic tracing: 1, pelvis height; 2, pelvis breadth; 3, inlet breadth; 4, inter-iliac breadth; 5, inter-pubic breadth; 6, inter-tuberal breadth; 7, ilium length; 8, pubis length; 9, inlet, sagittal diameter; 10, ischium length; 11, breadth of iliac notch; 12, interobturator breadth; 13, bitrochanteric breadth; 14, length of femoral neck; A, pubic angle; B, pelvic angle; C, femoral angle; D, femoral-pelvic angle.

Length of femoral neck—The distance, as measured in the mid-line of the femoral neck, from the upper edge of the proximal epiphysis to the outer margin of the shaft of the femur. Right, left, average. (A)

Pubic angle—The angle made by tangents to the inferior ramus of each pubis, converging at the point defining the center of the pubic symphysis.

Pelvic angle—The angle made by the convergence of lines defining the right and left pelvis heights.

Femoral angle—The angle made by the line defining the length of the femoral neck, at its junction with a line defining the mid-line of the shaft of the femur. Right, left, average.

Femoral-pelvic angle—The angle made by an extension of the line defining the length of the femoral neck, at its junction with the line defining pelvis height. Right, left, average.

Sex differences for this age period are summarized by Reynolds as follows:

1. Girls show higher intercorrelations in measurements at 34 months than boys. This finding is in contrast to the infant study, where the tendency toward higher intercorrelations was shown by the boys.

2. Significant sex differences at one or more age-levels are found as follows: Boys lead in pelvis height, pelvis breadth, inlet breadth, inter-iliac breadth, ilium length, ischium length, bi-trochanteric breadth, length of femoral neck and pelvic angle. Girls lead in inter-pubic breadth, intertuberal breadth, pubis length, breadth of iliac notch, inter-obturator breadth, pubic angle, femoral-pelvic angle and inlet index.

3. Critical ratios of sex differences are larger at 22 months than at any of the 6 succeeding age-levels. There appears to be a tendency for sex differences to become less pronounced with age.

4. Measurements of girls tend to be more variable than measurements of boys. This agrees with the results from the infant study.

5. The general pattern of sex differences in the prepuberal pelvis is in agreement with the results of the infant study. The suggestion is again made that, in prepuberal childhood as well as in infancy, boys are larger in measurements relating to the overall structure of the pelvis, while girls tend to be either absolutely or relatively larger in measurements relating to the inner structure of the pelvis, including the inlet.

TABLE 36

PRE-PUBERAL PELVIC MEASUREMENTS AND INDICES RANKED BY EFFECTIVENESS OF INTERCORRELATION*

Item	Rank	Rank When Related to Infant Study	Rank Shown in Infant Study
Bi-trochanteric breadth	1	—	—
Pelvis height	2	1	7
Pelvis breadth	3	2	3
Inlet breadth	4	3	1
Pubis length	5	4	8
Inter-tuberal breadth	6	5	11
Ischium length	7	6	9
Inter-obturator breadth	8	—	—
Inter-iliac breadth	9	7	4
Length of femoral neck	10	—	—
Ilium length	11	8	5
Inlet, sagittal diameter	12	9	2
Breadth of iliac notch	13	10	6
Inter-pubic breadth	14	11	10
Femoral-pelvic angle	15	—	—
Femoral angle	16	—	—
Pubic angle	17	—	—
Pelvic angle	18	—	—

* From Reynolds, '47, Table 6.

TABLE 37

SEX DIFFERENCES IN PELVIC MORPHOLOGY*

Trait	Male	Female
Pelvis as a whole	Massive, rugged, marked muscle sites	Less massive, gracile, smoother
Symphysis	Higher	Lower
Subpubic angle	V-shaped, sharp angle	U-shaped, rounded; broader divergent obtuse angle
Obturator foramen	Large, often ovoid	Small, triangular
Acetabulum	Large, tends to be directed laterally	Small, tends to be directed anterolaterally
Greater sciatic notch	Smaller, close, deep	Larger, wider, shallower
Ischiopubic rami	Slightly everted	Strongly everted
Sacro-iliac articulation	Large	Small, oblique
Preauricular sulcus	Not frequent	More frequent, better developed
Ilium	High, tends to be vertical	Lower, laterally divergent
Sacrum	Longer, narrower, with more evenly distributed curvature; often 5+ segments	Shorter, broader, with tendency to marked curve at S1-2 and S3-5; 5 segments the rule
Pelvic brim, or inlet	Heart-shaped	Circular, elliptical
True pelvis, or cavity	Relatively smaller	Oblique, shallow, spacious

* From Krogman, '55, Table 10; see also Stewart, '54, Table XV.

In Table 36 the measurements and angles are ranked in order of effective sexual differentiation in the pre-puberal pelves.

We may now turn to a consideration of sex differences in the *adult* pelvis. By far the most extensive and thorough reference here is Genovese ('59).

In the adult pelvis morphology, i.e., anatomical detail, looms large in problems of sexing. This is the "descriptive method." (sometimes called the "inspectional method"). Salient descriptive details are given in Table 37.

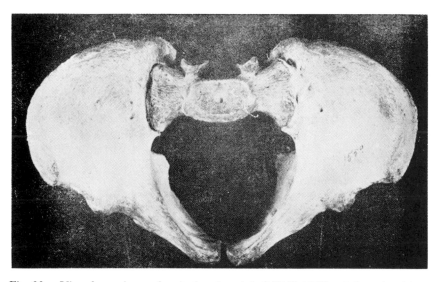

Fig. 33. View from above of typical male pelvis (WRU 1559), adult male white, to show narrowed pelvic inlet. Max. breadth across iliac crests is 287 mm; trans. breadth of inlet is 117 mm; index trans. brdth inlet/iliac brdth. = 40.8%.

Obviously a tabulation of this sort is based on almost a stereotype male and/or a stereotype female. The traits in the "male" and in the "female" columns are for ultra-masculine and ultra-feminine pelves (see Figs. 33–34). Furthermore there is the possibility that not *all* of the traits will be equally emphasized for masculinity or femininity, as the case may be. Also, there is no "weighting" of the traits: which one or two, or which cluster, tells more of sex difference than any of the others (singly or in groups). Finally, are these traits independent in the sense that any one will be modi-

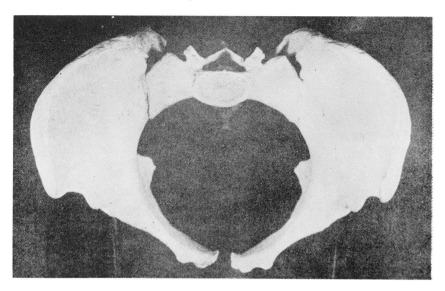

Fig. 34. View from above of typical female pelvis (WRU 781), adult female white, to show widened pelvic inlet. Max. breadth across iliac crests is 280 mm; trans. breadth of inlet is 141 mm; index = 50.4%.

fied in one direction or another as any other is similarly modified i.e., is there correlation between any two, or any group of, traits so that unit assessment is really counting the same tendency over and over?

A partial answer to these questions may be found in measurements of the pelvis, such as have been noted for the immature pelvis. One of the earliest metrical sex differences was claimed for Turner's *pelvic index:*

$$\frac{\text{a-p or conjugate diam.}}{\text{max. trans. diam.}} \times 100.*$$

The values assigned by Turner were:

Platypellic................ X–89.9 (trans. oval)
Mesatipellic.............. 90–94.9 (rounded)
Dolichopellic............. 95–X (long oval)

This has been modified by Greulich and Thoms ('38) as follows:

1. Dolichopellic—a-p or conj. diam. of inlet exceeds max. trans. diam.
2. Mesatipellic—max. trans. either equals conj. or exceeds it by no more than 1 cm.
3. Brachypellic—trans. diam. exceeds conj. by 1.1–2.9 cm.
4. Platypellic—trans. diam. exceeds conj. by 3 cm. +

* See Greulich and Thoms ('38, '39), Thoms and Greulich ('40), and Krukierek ('51).

They found the incidence of these pelvic types for samples of adult white females to be as follows (x-ray pelvimetry):

Type	*582* *Clinic women,* *per cent*	*104* *Student nurses,* *per cent*	*Total* *686 adult,* *per cent*
Dolichopellic	15.0	37.5	18.4
Mesatipellic	44.8	44.2	44.7
Brachypellic	34.3	18.2	31.8
Platypellic	5.6	. . .	4.7

These figures do not support the stereotype of the typically broad pelvic inlet of the female!*

A further sex comparison centers around groups of measurements made by Thoms and Greulich ('40) as follows (in cm.):

Pelvic inlet
  a-p diameter (A.P.)
  trans. diameter (Trans.)
  posterior sagittal diam. (P.S.)
Midpelvic plane
  a-p diameter (A.P.)
  trans. diameter (interspinous) (Trans.)
  post. sag. diam. (P.S.)
Pelvic outlet
  trans. diam. (Trans.)
  post. sag. diam. (bi-tuberous) (P.S.)

Average values, for pelvic types are as follows (in cm.):

200 WHITE FEMALES

Type	\begin{tabular}Inlet\end{tabular}			Midplane			Outlet	
	A.P.	Trans.	P.S.	A.P.	Trans.	P.S.	Trans.	P.S.
Dolichopellic	12.50	11.72	5.07	12.55	9.45	5.22	8.95	7.84
Mesatipellic	11.75	12.32	4.48	12.34	10.34	5.23	9.16	7.71
Brachypellic	11.06	12.67	4.15	12.01	10.32	5.23	8.92	8.05
Platypellic	9.0	12.67	2.75	11.67	10.45	4.71	9.12	7.58

69 WHITE MALES

Type	Inlet			Midplane			Outlet	
	A.P.	Trans.	P.S.	A.P.	Trans.	P.S.	Trans.	P.S.
Dolichopellic	12.30	11.60	4.89	12.43	8.54	4.47	10.65	7.68
Mesatipellic	11.46	11.87	4.01	12.07	8.66	4.22	10.75	7.49
Brachypellic	10.77	12.01	3.63	11.96	8.86	4.33	10.72	6.97

As regards pelvic types the male tends to be dolichopellic, the female mesati- to brachypellic. Platypellic pelves are rare in either

---

* In terms of Turner's pelvic index Greulich and Thoms ('39) found on 69 *males* that 5 (7.2%) were platypellic, 10 (14.5%) were mesatipellic, 54 (78.2%) were dolichopellic. The average index was 100.5, with a total range of 77.0–121.0. Caldwell and Moloy ('33) have suggested classification of female pelvic types from an obstetrical standpoint.

sex. As far as dimensions of pelvic inlet, midpelvic plane, and pelvic outlet are concerned, they vary more with pelvic type than they do with sex. The trans. diam. of inlet may be a bit larger in the female pelvis, the trans. diam. of outlet a bit larger in the male pelvis.

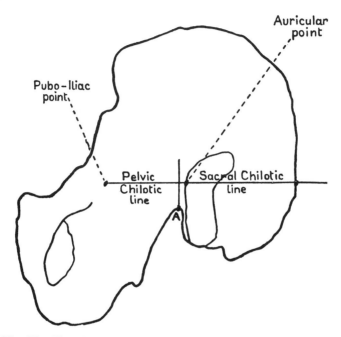

Fig. 35.   The determination of the "Chilotic Line" in the ilium.

In 1952, Sauter and Privat devised the "Cotylo-sciatic index." Two measurements were taken: a) distance from edge of acetabulum to adjacent border of sciatic notch; b) sciatic height, perpendicular to the same border, to the posterior iliac spine (where internal border of ilium joins the articular surface). If sciatic height is larger in females, and the acetabulo-sciatic distance is less, then the index a/b should show a sex difference. The authors used 50 male, 50 female, white pelves. The total average was 122.8 (73.8–185.3 range); the male average was 104.6 (73.8–128.9); the female average was 141.0 (92.5–185.3). The value 123 was set as an arbitrary male: female limit, since only six males (12%) were higher and 10 females (20%) were lower.

The acetabulum (hip-socket), as an entity, has been considered by several authors.   Shiiho ('14, '15) said that all acetabular dimensions are absolutely smaller in the female pelvis, and that the acetabulum "is more frontal in position."   Keil ('30) devised an index:

$$\frac{\text{surface area of acetabulum}}{\text{surface area of ilium}} \times 100.$$

The values derived were: male av. 13.57, S.D. 0.75, range 12.17–15.05; female av. 12.57, S.D. 0.79, range 10.42–14.01.

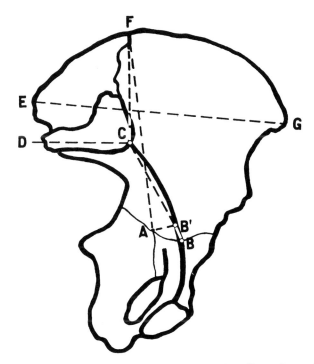

Fig. 36.   Left human os coxae, medial aspect, showing dimensions of the ilium.

The ilium, the laterally-placed flared-out part of the pelvis, has received considerable attention.   Derry ('09, '12, '23/'24) was an important early contributor.   He set up two end-points: (1) the *pubo-iliac*, on the ilio-pectineal line at the site of union of pubis and ilium; (2) the *auricular*, on the anterior margin of the auricular surface nearest the first point.   A line connecting points (1) and (2)

TABLE 38

RACE AND SEX DIFFERENCES IN THE ILIUM IN AMERICAN WHITES AND NEGROES*

| | White | | | | Negro | | | |
| | Male | | Female | | Male | | Female | |
Dimension	Av.	S.D.	Av.	S.D.	Av.	S.D.	Av.	S.D.
Lower iliac H	52.5	5.96	59.7	6.04	50.7	5.17	56.1	5.55
Upper iliac H	80.9	5.29	70.5	4.80	78.6	5.58	67.7	5.24
Direct iliac H	130.2	6.44	124.4	5.57	125.0	6.09	116.5	5.54
Iliac W	162.4	9.33	157.3	7.54	156.6	9.79	146.2	7.66
Subauric. angle	119.8°	8.44°	120.8°	9.73°	119.4°	5.42°	120.0°	7.74°
$\dfrac{\text{Upper iliac H}}{\text{Lower iliac H}}$	156.4%	—	119.2%	—	157.0%	—	121.9%	—
$\dfrac{\text{Iliac W}}{\text{Iliac H}}$	124.8%	—	126.4%	—	125.3%	—	125.6%	—

* From Straus, '27, Tables 3–7, 9–10.

is projected to the iliac crest and is termed the *chilotic line;* at point (2) it is divided into a pelvic and a sacral portion, giving rise to an index, sacral chilotic/pelvic chilotic (see Figure 35). The values derived are as follows: pelvic chilotic, male av. 54.5 mm., female av. 59.1 mm.; sacral chilotic, male av. 68.9 mm., female av. 60.8 mm.; total, male av. 123.4 mm., female av. 120.5 mm. The differences are not sufficient to be discriminative in individual instances (see Haeusermann, '25/'26).

The definitive study of the ilium is that of Straus ('27), based on the Todd Collection. (100 male whites, 50 male Negroes, 50 female whites, 44 female Negroes). Here both sex and race differences emerge for American whites and Negroes. Straus took four dimensions and one angle, as follows (see Figure 36):

1. Lower iliac height: distance along the ilio-pectineal line, from the auricular surface to the ilio-pubic junction (CB);

2. Upper iliac height: distance between the point where the ilio-pectineal line meets the auricular surface, and the iliac crest (at attachment of ilio-lumbar lig.) (CF);

3. Direct iliac height: distance between ilio-ischio-pubic tubercle and iliac crest (at attachment of ilio-lumbar lig.) (AF);

TABLE 39

LENGTH OF PUBIS AND ISCHIUM IN MM AND ISCHIUM-PUBIS INDEX*

	No.	Pubis Length				Ischium Length				Ischium-Pubis Index			
		Mean	Range	S.D.	C.V.	Mean	Range	S.D.	C.V.	Mean	Range	S.D.	C.V.
White male	100	73.8	65–83	4.1	5.6	88.4	(75–98)	4.3	4.9	83.6	(73–94)	4.0	4.8
White female	100	77.9	69–95	4.4	5.6	78.3	(69–93)	3.8	4.9	99.5	(91–115)	5.1	5.1
Negro male	50	69.2	60–88	4.7	6.8	86.6	(79–96)	3.6	4.1	79.9	(71–88)	4.0	5.0
Negro female	50	73.5	63–86	4.4	6.0	77.5	(67–86)	4.4	5.7	95.0	(84–106)	4.6	4.8

* From Washburn, '48, Table 1.

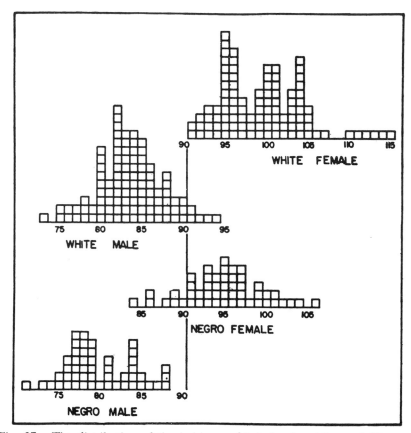

Fig. 37. The distribution of the ischium-pubis index in whites and Negroes.

4. Iliac width: maximum distance between anterior superior and posterior superior iliac spines (GE);

5. Subauricular angle: formed by lower border of the auricular surface and ilio-pectineal line projected from the auricular surface to the point where the ilio-pectineal line is crossed by a perpendicular from the ilio-ischio-pubic tubercle (Angle DCB').

Two indices are derived: (1) upper iliac height/lower iliac height; (2) iliac width/direct iliac height. In Table 38 is presented a summary of the means and standard deviations derived from Straus' study.

Male and female white pelves are larger than male and female Negro pelves. Male white and Negro pelves are larger than female white and Negro pelves in all absolute dimensions except lower iliac height. The upper iliac height/lower iliac height index is lower in females in both groups. There are no differences in the sub-auricular angle. The ilium in the Negro of both sexes is a bit less variable than in the white, but there is no sex difference in variability in either group.

General sex differences in both whites and Negroes, involving the ilium, are stated by Straus as follows: (1) the iliac crest has a steeper anterior and posterior slope in males; (2) the lower portion of the auricular surface ("the lower auricular arm") extends farther

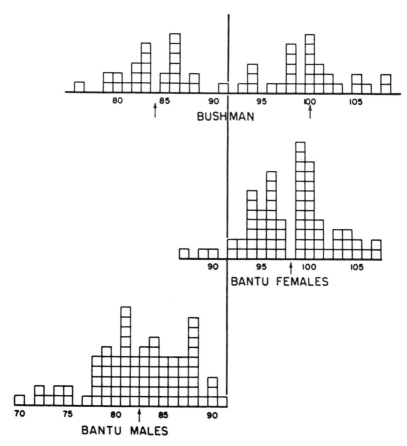

Fig. 38. The distribution of the ischium-pubis index in Bantu and Bushmen. Arrows point to the means.

backwards in males; (3) the sulcus preauricularis is absent to slight in males, but marked in females; (4) the greater sciatic notch is narrow and deep in males, broad and shallow in females.

After carefully evaluating his data Straus (p. 27) concluded as follows: "All of the characters studied, both quantitative and qualitative, vary so greatly and exhibit such marked sexual and stock-

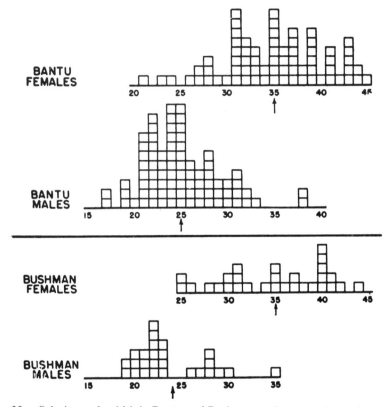

Fig. 39. Sciatic notch width in Bantu and Bushman. Arrows point to the mean.

linked hverlapping that they arc of limited value in sexing or determining racial affinities of pelves."

Genovese ('59) feels that one index, three dimensions, and four morphological traits are basic to sex differences in the pelvis. The index is:

$$\frac{\text{breadth of greater sciatic notch}}{\text{lowest point on gr. sci. notch to pyramidal proc.}}$$

TABLE 40

	"Female"				"Male"			
	Mean	Range	S.D.	C.V.	Mean	Range	S.D.	C.V.
Pubis Length, mm.	80.1	73–90	5.1	6.3	74.1	63–85	4.0	5.3
Ischium Length, mm.	81.0	72–89	5.0	6.1	88.4	79–98	4.0	4.5
Ischium-Pubis Index, %	98.8	91–109	3.8	3.8	83.9	73–92	3.7	4.4
Sciatic Notch Angle, degrees	74.4	61–93	7.1	9.5	50.4	26–65	8.4	16.6
Upper Iliac Height, mm.	64.2	50–76	5.4	8.4	72.4	61–85	5.2	7.2
Lower Iliac Height, mm.	61.8	54–77	6.9	11.1	54.5	42–67	5.4	9.9
Interiliac Index, %	104.5	73–140	14.1	13.4	133.6	100–177	15.9	11.9

* From Hanna and Washburn, '53, Table 1. Reprinted from *Human Biology* by permission of the Wayne State University Press.

The dimensions are: (1) minimum inferior breadth of the ilium; (2) height of acetabulum; (3) pubic height. The index and dimension (3) are greater in females, dimensions (1), (2), are greater in males. The four morphological traits are: (1) sulcus preauricularis; (2) subpubic angle; (3) the form of the greater sciatic notch; and (4) the pubic crest. Genovese concluded as follows:

> Agreement with the actual sex is arrived at in 94.5%, 94.2%, and 94.3% of cases by applying the respective metrical, morphological and combined criteria to the two known series. Corresponding values of 94.9%, 96.1%, and 97.7% are obtained for the large unidentified series, which had previously been sexed by anatomical appreciation. . . . A reliability of 95% can therefore be obtained from sex determination by means of the innominate bone, and more optimistic claims by other workers should be accepted with reserve.

Washburn ('48, '49) and Hanna and Washburn ('53) have focussed their attention on sex differences, dimensionally expressed in pubo-ischial relationships. Washburn ('48) points out the nonrelation of traits as a basic factor, e.g., "the sex difference in the sciatic notch belongs to a far different *system* (italics W.M.K.) from that in the pubic bone. . . . the sciatic notch is not correlated with the subpubic angle." He states that "the sex of over 75% of pelves can be determined by the notch alone, therefore theoretically

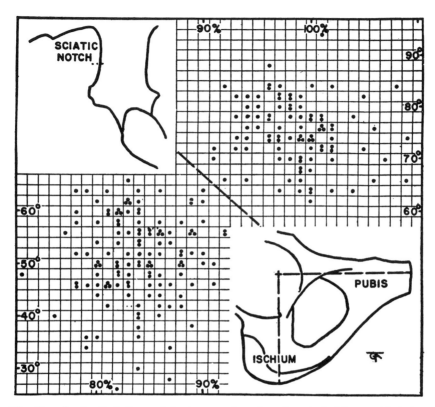

Fig. 40. Angle of sciatic notch in degrees plotted against the ischium-pubic index in %. Diagonal line separates "males" and "females."

well over 95% of skeletons can be sexed using the [ischium-pubic] index and an observation of the notch."

The dimensions taken by Washburn for his index are "length of ischium and pubis. . .from the point at which they meet in the acetabulum." * In Table 39 and in Figure 37 the results are given for male and female, Negro and white, pelves.

In 1949, Washburn tested his hypothesis on 152 skeletons of Bantu of known sex, and on 55 Bushman skeletons, mostly of unknown sex (i.e., excavated material). His findings are graphed

* Thieme and Schull ('57b) suggest the pubic dimension "from the nearest acetabulum border to the superior point of the pubic symphysis," and the ischial dimension "to the far border of the acetabulum." This method would include femoral head size. With this method 96.5% correctness in sexing was achieved.

in Figure 38. Comparatively the index may be tabulated as follows:

Group	Male	Female
American Negro	79.9	95.0
Bantu	82.5	98.1
American White	83.6	99.5
Bushman	83.7	100.0

In Figure 39 Washburn presents pertinent data on the width of the sciatic notch (in mm.) in Bantu and Bushman.

In these two series of pelves Washburn, using both the index and the notch, found that "the sex of over 98% of the skeletons could be determined."

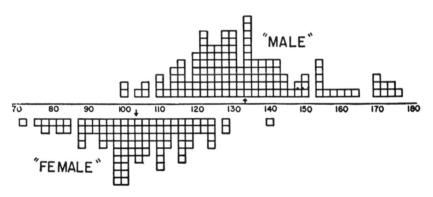

Fig. 41.   Distribution of interiliac index.

In 1953, Hanna and Washburn studied the pelves of 224 Alaskan Eskimos.   To the ischium-pubic index and the sciatic notch they added the "interiliac index."   The dimensional results are in Table 40.

Figures 40 and 41, both from Hanna and Washburn, relate sciatic notch and the index, and show sex differences in the interiliac index, respectively.   In this series the authors reported coefficients of correlation as follows:

	Male	Female
Ischium-pubis Index and Angle of Sciatic Notch	+.032	−.010
Ischium-pubis Index and Interiliac Index	−.008	+.001
Pubis length and Lower Iliac height	−.006	+.017
Ischium length and Upper Iliac height	+.040	+.037

4. SEX DIFFERENCES IN THE LONG BONES

One of the most obvious sex differences in the long bones is that typically male bones are longer and more "massive" than typically female bones.   Schultz ('37) observed that "the various human races differ but very little in the degree with which the males surpass the females in the length of the long bones."   Thieme and Schull ('57b) observe that "the expression of sexual dimorphism is relatively similar in pattern for all varieties of man."   The male: female ratio for long bone length hovers around 100:90.   Some years

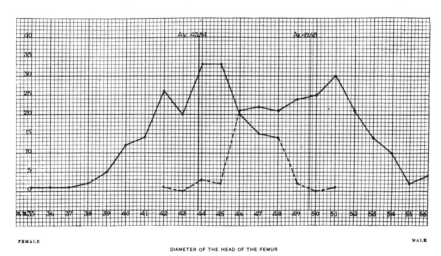

FEMALE   MALE

DIAMETER OF THE HEAD OF THE FEMUR

Fig. 42.   Diameters of the head of the femur.

ago I took a single known male and a single known female skeleton, both with statures at the respective sex averages, and observed as follows (dimensions in mm. are total lengths of long bones) (Krogman, '55):

Dimension	*Male* WRU 989	*Female* WRU 604	*Ratio*
Humerus	336.0	317.0	94.5
Radius	255.0	220.0	86.4
Ulna	276.0	236.0	85.5
Femur	491.0	434.0	88.5
Tibia	409.0	359.0	88.0
Fibula	388.0	351.0	90.5

The *femur* is the most-studied of all human long bones.   In 1917–1919 Pearson presented the following data on what was

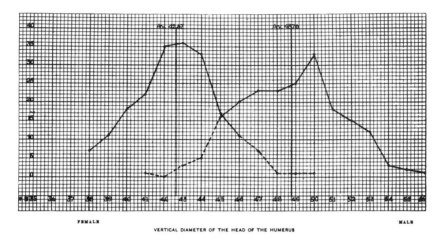

FEMALE   MALE

VERTICAL DIAMETER OF THE HEAD OF THE HUMERUS

Fig. 43.   Vertical diameter of the head of the humerus.

termed "the mathematic sexing of the femur."   These data have
been widely quoted and extensively used.

	Female (mm.)	Female? (mm.)	Sex? (mm.)	Male? (mm.)	Male (mm.)
Vertical diameter of head	< 41.5	41.5– 43.5	43.5– 44.5	44.5– 45.5	> 45.5
Popliteal length	<106	106 –114.5	114.5–132	132 –145	>145
Bicondylar width	< 72	72 – 74	74 – 76	76 – 78	> 78
Trochanteric oblique length	<390	390 –405	405 –430	430 –450	>450

In 1904–1905, Dwight stated that "it is very evident that the
differences between the bones of the arm and thigh in the matter
of length are much less important sexually than those of the diameters of the heads."   Accordingly he studied the *femur* and the
humerus of 200 male and 200 female adult whites.   The data on the
diameters of the heads of the humerus and femur are as follows
(in mm.):

	Humerus		Femur,
	Vert.	Trans.	Vert.
Male	48.76	44.66	49.68
Female	42.67	36.98	43.84
Diff.	6.09	5.68	5.84

The foregoing data are graphed in Figs. 42, 43 and 44, for vertical
diam. of humeral head, transverse diam. of humeral head, and vertical diam. of femoral head, respectively.

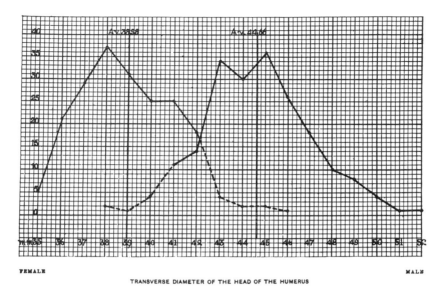

FEMALE   MALE

TRANSVERSE DIAMETER OF THE HEAD OF THE HUMERUS

Fig. 44.   Transverse diameter of the head of the humerus.

In 1913–1914 and 1914–1915, Parsons suggested certain sex categories for the *femur* as follows (31 male, 14 female femora):

Maximum length
  450 mm. + = male
  400 mm. − = female
Condylar breadth
  75 mm. + = male
  70 mm. − = female
Width of lower end (sic)
  72 mm. + = probably male
  71 mm. − = probably female
  71–72 mm. = male or female
Diameter of head
  48 mm. + = male
  44 mm. − = female

In 1917–1918, Maltby gave *femoral* head diameters (white) as follows (in mm.):

	———Male———		———Female———	
	R	L	R	L
Average	48.0	49.6	42.0	41.5
Range	43.0–51.0	44.0–56.0	37.5–45.5	37.0–46.0

Sex differences in the long bones, over and above heads or condyles, is reported by Godycki ('57), who considers femur, humerus, and ulna.

In the *femur* the angle formed by neck axis and shaft axis is sexually differentiated as follows:

	Values of the angle			
	I	*II*	*III*	*IV*
	35°–40°	*41°–45°*	*46°–50°*	*50°+*
Male femora	10%	51%	26%	11%
Female femora	2%	28%	38%	33%

	Groups			
	I	*II*	*III*	*IV*
Male femora	83.4%	65%	40.6%	25%
Female femora	16.6%	35%	59.3%	75%

A low angle is in a masculine direction, a high angle in a feminine direction.

In the *humerus* Godycki feels that a perforated olecranon fossa occurs more frequently in female humeri, and more often in left humeri. A perforated fossa shows a 1:3.7 ratio in favor of the female.

In the *ulna* Godycki cites Martin that the surface of the sigmoid notch is divided by a groove into two parts in 66.2% of ulnae, partially divided in 10.3%, and not divided in 25.5%. A divided notch, says Godycki, is male, an undivided notch is female; it is claimed that this holds true for 95% of male ulnae, 85% of female ulnae.

Of all the three bones studied by Godycki I think the data upon the femur are the most valid and the most useful. I doubt the value of the olecranon fossa perforation as a sex indicator. As for the ulna we may note a recent study by Maia Neto ('59) who found that of 407 ulnae with the groove (theoretically male) 286 were male, 121 female; of 204 ulnae without the groove (theoretically female) 52 were male, 152 were female.

Bainbridge and Genovese ('56) have studied sex differences in the *scapula*, using both morphological and dimensional criteria. The dimensions taken are defined as follows:

a. ScL—Max. lgth. of scapula between sup. and inf. angles.

b. ScB—Max. of scapula from base of spine to glenoid cavity.

c. ScLs—Max. lgth. of spine.

d. Sc Lax—Lgth. of axillary border between infrascapular and infraglenoid points.

e. Sc Wte.—Max. width or projection of process of teres major.

f. ScLc—Max. lgth. of coracoid in any direction between its apex and a terminal on the base.

g. ScLg—Length of glenoid cavity between supraglenoid and infraglenoid points.

h. ScBg—Max. lgth. of glenoid cavity outside the articular border, perpendicular to glenoid length.

i. ScWs—Max. width of crest of spine at level of deltoid tubercle in any direction perpendicular to the long axis of the crest.

j. ScWs°—minimum width of crest of spine between the deltoid tubercle and the acromion.

k. ScWax—Width of axillary border 3 c.m. below infraglenoid point.

TABLE 41

SUMMARY OF LIMITS OF MALE AND FEMALE GROUPS FOR SCAPULAR DIMENSIONS*

Character and Sex		99.87% Limits (mm.)	Character and Sex		97.80% Limits (mm.)	"84.20%" Limits (mm.)
ScBg'	♂	29.3	ScL'	♂	151.0	149.0
	♀	23.3		♀	139.7	143.8
ScB	♂	104.8	ScB	♂	100.7	100.5
	♀	90.7		♀	95.6	96.7
ScL'	♂	158.2	ScLs'	♂	132.6	
	♀	130.4		♀	127.3	128.3
ScWax	♂	14.4	ScLax	♂	129.2	126.2
	♀	8.8		♀	118.1	122.2
ScLs'	♂	141.3	ScLc'	♂	45.3	43.6
	♀	119.7		♀	40.2	42.6
ScLax	♂	135.5	ScBg'	♂	27.6	27.5
	♀	110.1		♀	25.4	26.0
			ScWs°	♂		10.4
				♀		6.9
			ScWax	♂	13.0	11.7
				♀	10.2	11.6

* From Bainbridge and Genovese, '59, Table XI.

In Table 41 the results are presented, at both the 99.87% limits and the 84.20% limits.

Discriminant functions have been employed in sexing long bones by Hanihara ('58; also on the scapula, '59), Pons ('55), Thieme ('57) and Thieme and Schull ('57a,b). Hanihara used humerus, radius, ulna, femur, and tibia. If all five bones were present the error is 3.41% (he missed three of 88). Pons gives data on femur and sternum. Using Fisher's method on the femur he

TABLE 42

Statistical Values Derived from Various Measurements taken from Male and Female American Negro Skeletons of Known Sex*

Measurement	Sex	Number	Mean (mm.)	Standard Deviation	Standard Error of Mean	Critical Ratio ("t")
A. Femur length	M	98	477.34	28.37	2.866	10.13
	F	100	439.10	24.55	2.456	
B. Femur head diameter	M	98	47.17	2.75	0.278	16.17
	F	100	41.52	2.12	0.212	
C. Humerus length	M	98	338.98	18.55	1.874	12.51
	F	100	305.89	18.66	1.866	
D. Epicondylar width of humerus	M	98	63.89	3.59	0.363	14.50
	F	100	56.76	3.32	0.332	
E. Clavicle length	M	98	158.24	10.06	1.158	13.90
	F	100	140.28	7.99	0.800	
F. Ischium length	M	98	90.55	5.06	0.511	13.52
	F	100	81.80	4.00	0.400	
G. Pubis length	M	98	74.14	5.11	0.516	6.39
	F	100	78.21	4.34	0.434	
H. Sternum length	M	99	36.15	3.91	0.393	9.66
	F	98	30.96	3.63	0.367	

* From Thieme, '57, Table 1.

TABLE 43

Discriminant Analysis Results Giving Multipliers and Limit Values for Various Combinations of Long Bone Measurements*

Measurements and Their Multipliers for Use in Sex Discriminations				
	7 × 7	6 × 6	4 × 4	3 × 3
A. Femur length	0.07	1.00	1.00	1.98
B. Femur head diameter	58.14	31.40	16.53	
F. Ischium	16.25	11.12	6.10	1.00
G. Pubic length	−63.64	−34.47	−13.80	−1.39
C. Humerus length	2.68	2.45		
D. Epicondylar width of humerus	27.68	16.24		
E. Clavicle length	16.09			

Discriminating Values			
Measurement Combination	Value Separating the Sexes (Females Less Than the Value)	Probability of Error in Classification (%)	Range Within Which 99% Will Fall
7 × 7	4099	1.5	2664–5533
6 × 6	1953	2.5	1205–2701
4 × 4	665	3.1	367–963
3 × 3	68	6.5	50–86

* From Thieme, '57, Table 2.

achieved an accuracy "approaching 95%"; using Penrose' method on the sternum the accuracy was 89%.

Thieme's data (on 99 Negro males, 101 Negro females) may be presented at greater length. In Table 42 pertinent data on sex differences in dimensions of femur, humerus, clavicle, ischium, pubis, and sternum are given.

In Table 43, Thieme presents the results of discriminant analysis of the measurements, giving multipliers and limit values.

Here is an example (from Thieme) of an actual case:

1.	Femur lgth.	429 mm.
2.	Femur head diam.	44 mm.
3.	Ischium lgth.	84 mm.
4.	Pubis lgth.	73 mm.

Multipliers from Table 43, give:

1.	1.00×429	429.00
2.	16.53×44	727.32
3.	6.10×84	512.40
4.	-13.80×73	-1007.40
	Total	661.32

Since the limiting value is 665, and all below 665 are female, the skeleton represented by the bones, is diagnosed as *female*.

Thieme says that "the maximum discrimination can be obtained from seven measurements. With this method the probability of error can be reduced to 1.5%, giving 98.5% expectation of accuracy in known material and double this, or 3% error, when the material is unknown."

Summarizing Statement

1. The sexing of unknown skeletal material depends, of course, upon relative completeness of the skeleton. Percentage of accuracy, for *adult* material, is about as follows: entire skeleton = 100%; skull alone = 90%; pelvis alone = 95%; skull plus pelvis = 98%; long bones alone = 80%; long bones plus skull = 90–95%; long bones plus pelvis = 95% +. In immature (prepuberal) material the situation is about 50-50, unless pelvic remains are present; then a 75–80% accuracy is a reasonable expectation.

2. The foregoing estimates are based on morphology plus morphometry (description, plus dimensions and proportions). Elab-

orate statistical analysis does not raise the averages appreciably. There seems to be this difference: to paraphrase, "with statistics you can be sure"; or, at least, more sure in an individual case.

3. Standards of morphological and morphometric sex differences in the skeleton may differ with the population samples involved. This is especially true with reference to dimensions and indices (average and range). As a general rule standards should be used with reference to the group from which they were drawn and upon which they are based: they are not ordinarily interchangeable.

REFERENCES

BAINBRIDGE, D. and GENOVESE, S.:   A study of the sex differences in the scapula. *JRAI, 86(2)*:109–134, 1956.

BOUCHER, B. J.:   Sex differences in the foetal sciatic notch.   *J. Forensic Med., 2(1)*: 51–54, 1955.

BOUCHER, B. J.:   Sex differences in the foetal pelvis.   *AJPA n.s., 15(4)*:581–600, 1957.

CALDWELL, W. E. and MOLOY, H. C.:   Anatomical variations in the female pelvis and their effect on labor with a suggested classification.   *AJOG, 26*:479–505, 1933.

DERRY, D. E.:   Note on the innominate bone as a factor in the determination of sex: with special reference to the sulcus preauricularis.   *JAP, 43*(3rd series, vol. 4): 266–276, 1909.

DERRY, D. E.:   The influence of sex on the position and composition of the human sacrum.   *JAP, 46*(3rd ser., vol. 7):184–192, 1912.

DERRY, D. E.:   On the sexual and racial characters of the ilium.   *JA, 58*:71–83, 1923/24.

DWIGHT, THOMAS: The size of the articular surfaces of the long bones as characteristic of sex; an anthropological study.   *AJA, 4(1)*:19–31, 1904/05.

GENOVESE, S. T.:   Diferencias sexuales en el hueso coxal.   U. Nacional Autonoma de Mexico.   Public. del Inst. de Hist. Primera serie, Num. 49,   1959, Mexico City, D.F.

GODYCKI, M.:   Sur la certitude de détermination de sexe d' aprés le fémur, le cubitus, et l' humérus.   *Bull. et Mem. de la Soc. d' Anth de Paris*, T. 8, Ser. 10, pp. 405–410, Masson, Paris, 1957.

GREULICH, W. W. and THOMS, H.:   The dimensions of the pelvic inlet of 789 white females.   *Anat. Rec., 72*:45–51, 1938.

GREULICH, W. W. and THOMS, H.:   An x-ray study of the male pelvis.   *Anat. Rec., 75*:289–299, 1939.

GREULICH, W. W. and PYLE, S. I.:   1958 (see *Refs.* Chap. II).

HAEUSERMANN, E.:   Zur Bestimmung von Geschlechts—und Rassen—unterscheiden am menschlichen Os ilium.   *ZMA, 25*:465–474, 1925/26.

HANIHARA, K.: Sexual diagnosis of Japanese long bones by means of discriminant functions. *J. Anth. Soc. Nippon.*, *66(717)*:39–48, 1958.

HANIHARA, K.: Sex diagnosis of Japanese skulls and scapulae by means of discriminant functions. *J. Anth. Soc. Nippon.* *67(722)*:21–27, 1959.

HANNA, R. E. and WASHBURN, S. L.: The determination of the sex of skeletons, as illustrated by a study of the Eskimo pelvis. *HB, 25*:21–27, 1953.

HOYME, L. E.: The earliest use of indices for sexing pelves. *AJPA n.s., 15(4)*: 537–546, 1957.

HUG, E.: Die Schädel der frühmittelalterlichen Gräber aus dem solothurmischen Aaregebiet in ihrer Stellung zur Reihengräberbevölkerung Mitteleuropas. Ein Beitrag zum problem der europaischen Brachycephalie. *ZMA, 38*:359–528, 1939/40.

HUNT, JR. E. E. and GLEISER, I.: The estimation of age and sex of preadolescent children from bones and teeth. *AJPA n.s., 13(3)*:479–487, 1955.

HURME, V. O.: Standards of variation in the eruption of the first six permanent teeth. *Child Dev., 19*:213–231, 1948.

KEEN, J. A.: Sex differences in skulls. *AJPA n.s., 8(1)*:65–79, 1950.

KEIL, E.: Uber das Grössenverhaltnis der Hüftgelenkpfanne zum Hüftbein. *Anth. Anzeig., 6(4)*:344–353, 1930.

KROGMAN, W. M.: 1939 (see *Refs.*, Chap. II).

KROGMAN, W. M.: 1955 (see *Refs.*, Chap. II).

KRUKIEREK, S.: The sexual differences in the human pelvis. *Gynaecologia, 132*: 92–110, 1951.

MAIA NETO, M. A.: Acerca do valor de grande cavidade sigmóide do cúbito como carácter sexual. *Contrib. paro o Estudo da Antropol. Portug. 8(1)*: 12 pp., reprint, 1959, (Engl. Summary.) Inst. Anth., U. Coimbra., Portugal.

MALTBY, J. R. D.: Some indices and measurements of the modern femur. *JA, 52*(3rd ser. vol. 13):363-382, 1917/18.

MOBIUS, P. J.: Über die Verschiedenheit männlicher und weiblicher Schädel. *Arch f. Anth. N.F., 6*:1–7, 1907.

MORTON, D. G.: Observations of the development of pelvic conformation. *AJOG, 44*:799–816, 1942.

PARSONS, F. G.: The characters of the English thigh-bone. Pt.I. *JAP, 48* (3rd Ser., vol. 9):238–267, 1913/14.

PARSONS, F. G.: The characters of the English thigh-bone. Pt. II. The difficulty of sexing. *JAP, 49*(Ser. 10):335–361, 1914/15.

PARSONS, F. G.: Sexual differences in the skull. *JA, 54*:58–65, 1920.

PEARSON, K.: A study of the long bones of the English skeleton. I. The femur. Chaps 1–4 in Draper's Co. Research Mem. U. of London. Biom. Series X, 1917–1919.

PEARSON, K.: On the problem of sexing osteometric material. *Biom., 10*:479-487, 1914/15.

PFITZNER, W.: Der Einfluss des Geschlechts auf die anthropologischen charaktere. *ZMA, 3*:385–575, 1901.

PITTARD, E.: Quelques comparisons sexuelles de crânes anciens. *L'Anth., 11:* 179–192, 1900.

PONS, J.: The sexual diagnosis of isolated bones of the skeleton. *HB, 27:*12–21, 1955.

REYNOLDS, E. L.: The bony pelvic girdle in early infancy. A roentgenometric study. *AJPA n.s., 3(4):*321–354, 1945.

REYNOLDS, E. L.: The bony pelvis in prepuberal childhood. *AJPA n.s., 5(2):* 165–200, 1947.

SAUTER, M. R. and PRIVAT, F.: Une nouvelle méthode de détermination sexuelle de l'os coxal: l' indice cotylo sciatique. *Bull. Schweiz Gesellsch. f. Anthropol. u. Ethnol., 28:*12–13, 1952.

SCHULTZ, A. H.: Proportions, variability, and asymmetries of the long bones of the limbs and the clavicles in man and apes. *HB, 9:*281–328, 1937.

SHIIHO, K.: Über die Hüftpfanne. *ZMA, 17:*325–56, 1914/15.

STEWART, T. D.: Medico-legal aspects of the skeleton. I. Age, sex, race, and stature. *AJPA n.s., 6(3):*315–321, 1948.

STEWART, T. D.: 1951 (see *Refs.*, Chap. I).

STEWART, T. D.: 1954 (see *Refs.*, Chap. II).

STRAUS, W. L.: The human ilium: sex and stock. *AJPA, 11(1):*1–28, 1927.

THIEME, F. P.: Sex in Negro skeletons. *J. Forensic Med., 4(2):*72–81, 1957.

THIEME, F. P. and SCHULL, W. J.: Sex determination from the skeleton. *HB, 29(3):*242–273, 1957.

THOMS, H., and GREULICH, W. W.: A comparative study of male and female pelves. *AJOG, 39:*56–62, 1940.

TÖRÖK, A. VON: Über den Trochanter tertius und die Fossa hypotrochanterica (Houzé) in ihrer sexuellen Bedeutung. *Anat. Anzeig., 1:*169–178, 1886.

WASHBURN, S. L.: Sex differences in the pubic bone. *AJPA, n.s., 6(2):*199–208, 1948.

WASHBURN, S. L.: Sex differences in the pubic bone of Bantu and Bushman. *AJPA, n.s., 7(3):*425–432, 1949.

WEISBACH, A.: Der deutsche Weiberschädel. *Arch. f. Anth., 3:*59–85, 1868.

WILLIAMS, J. T.: Normal variations in type of the female pelvis and their obstetrical significance. *AJOG, 3:*345–351, 1922.

VI

The Calculation of Stature from Long Bones

1. INTRODUCTORY REMARKS: HISTORICAL

I have excavated many human skeletons, chiefly those of prehistoric American Indians. It is impressive (and instructive)
how the lay person tends to *over-estimate* the stature represented
by the gleaming skeleton as it is being progressively and carefully
exhumed. The leg bones are especially impressive. Time and
again I've heard a bystander exclaim, "that one must have been
a giant!" On the other hand there is a reverse situation. As one
looks at medieval armor one has the feeling, "why, those suits of
armor would not fit any average man of today." The fact is that
we *are* taller today than ever before. The bearing of these two
contrasting impressions of size upon statural reconstruction will
be emergent as we go along.

In 1888, Rollet published the earliest formal tables, using the
humerus, radius, ulna, femur, tibia, and fibula of 50 male and 50
female French cadavera. The bones were measured first in the
"fresh state," and 10 months later in the "dry state"; in this time
they had lost two mm. in over-all length.

In 1892–93, Manouvrier re-assessed Rollet's data, but he excluded all subjects (26 male, 25 female) over 60 years of age, for
in old age, he said some three cm. of calculated stature has been
lost.* Thus, his tables were based on 24 male, 25 female, French
skeletons. There were two methodological differences between

* Pearson ('99) felt that this was unnecessary: "it would appear that whatever shrinkage may be due to old age, it is not a very marked character in these [Rollet] data, or
largely disappears after death on a flat table; the senile stoop may then be largely
eliminated."

153

Rollet and Manouvrier that must be noted: Manouvrier determined the average stature of individuals who presented the same length for a given long bone; Rollet determined the average length of a given long bone from individuals with the same stature.

In 1899, Pearson, using Rollet's data, developed regression formulae, based on bones from the right side only.

During this period the anthropologists held an international meeting at Geneva, Switzerland. There emerged the "Geneva Agreement": "For the reconstruction of the stature with the aid of the long bones, the maximum length shall be measured in all cases, save in those of the femur which is to be measured in the oblique position, and the tibia which is also to be measured in an oblique position, the spine being excluded." This has not always been followed in the many different tables that have been developed; departures from the Agreement will be noted as we present the data.

In Table 44 Manouvrier's data on French long bones and stature are shown (see Hrdlička, '39):

To calculate stature from these data Manouvrier added two mm. to the length of each bone, and then subtracted two mm. from the height thus obtained.

Pearson laid down certain basic rules for stature reconstruction, as follows ('99, p. 170). (it should be noted that he was oriented more toward prehistoric and racial reconstructions than he was to forensic problems):

> (a) The mean sizes, standard deviations and correlations of as many organs in an extant allied race as it is possible conveniently to measure (should be secured). When the correlations of the organs under consideration are high (e.g., the long bones in Man), fifty to a hundred individuals may be sufficient; in other cases it is desireable that several hundred at least should be measured.

> (b) The like sizes or characters for as many individual organs or bones of the extinct race should then be measured as it is possible to collect. It will be found always possible to reconstruct the *mean* racial type with greater accuracy than to reconstruct a single individual.

> (c) An appreciation must be made of the effect of time and climate in producing changes in the dimensions of the organs which have survived from the extinct race.

TABLE 44

Manouvrier's Tables Showing the Correspondence of Bone Lengths Among Themselves and with Stature, in White People*

Humerus mm.	Radius mm.	Ulna mm.	Stature mm.	Femur mm.	Tibia mm.	Fibula mm.
			Males			
295	213	227	1,530	392	319	318
298	216	231	1,552	398	324	323
302	219	235	1,571	404	330	328
306	222	239	1,590	410	335	333
309	225	243	1,605	416	340	338
313	229	246	1,625	422	346	344
316	232	249	1,634	428	351	349
320	236	253	1,644	434	357	353
324	239	257	1,654	440	362	358
328	243	260	1,666	446	368	363
332	246	263	1,677	453	373	368
336	249	266	1,686	460	378	373
340	252	270	1,697	467	383	378
344	255	273	1,716	475	389	383
348	258	276	1,730	482	394	388
352	261	280	1,754	490	400	393
356	264	283	1,767	497	405	398
360	267	287	1,785	504	410	403
364	270	290	1,812	512	415	408
368	273	293	1,830	519	420	413

Mean coefficients for bones shorter than those shown in the table:

5.25	7.11	6.66	—	3.92	4.80	4.82

Mean coefficients for bones longer than those shown in the table:

4.93	6.70	6.26	—	3.53	4.32	4.37

Humerus	Radius	Ulna	Stature	Femur	Tibia	Fibula
			Females			
263	193	203	1,400	363	284	283
266	195	206	1,420	368	289	288
270	197	209	1,440	373	294	293
273	199	212	1,455	378	299	298
276	201	215	1,470	383	304	303
279	203	217	1,488	388	309	307
282	205	219	1,497	393	314	311
285	207	222	1,513	398	319	316
289	209	225	1,528	403	324	320
292	211	228	1,543	408	329	325
297	214	231	1,556	415	334	330
302	218	235	1,568	422	340	336
307	222	239	1,582	429	346	341
313	226	243	1,595	436	352	346
318	230	247	1,612	443	358	351
324	234	251	1,630	450	364	356
329	238	254	1,650	457	370	361
334	242	258	1,670	464	376	366
339	246	261	1,692	471	382	371
344	250	264	1,715	478	388	376

Mean coefficients for bones shorter than those shown in the table:

5.41	7.44	7.00	—	3.87	4.85	4.88

Mean coefficients for bones longer than those shown in the table:

4.98	7.00	6.49	—	3.58	4.42	4.52

* From Hrdlička, '39.

TABLE 45
LIVING STATURE FROM DEAD LONG BONES*

Male

(a) S = 81.306 + 1.880 F.
(b) S = 70.641 + 2.894 H.
(c) S = 78.664 + 2.376 T.
(d) S = 85.925 + 3.271 R.
(e) S = 71.272 + 1.159 (F + T).
(f) S = 71.443 + 1.220 F + 1.080 T.
(g) S = 66.855 + 1.730 (H + R).
(h) S = 69.788 + 2.769 H + .195 R.
(i) S = 68.397 + 1.030 F + 1.557 H.
(k) S = 67.049 + .913 F + .600 T + 1.225 H − .187 R.

Female

(a) S = 72.844 + 1.945 F.
(b) S = 71.475 + 2.754 H.
(c) S = 74.774 + 2.352 T.
(d) S = 81.224 + 3.343 R.
(e) S = 69.154 + 1.126 (F + T).
(g) S = 69.561 + 1.117 F + 1.125 T.
(g) S = 69.911 + 1.628 (H + R).
(h) S = 70.542 + 2.582 H + .281 R.
(i) S = 67.435 + 1.339 F + 1.027 H.
(k) S = 67.469 + .782 F + 1.120 T + 1.059 H − .711 R.

* From Pearson, '99, Tables XIV and XV.

In Table 45, for male and for female, Pearson's regression formulae are given, based on dead long bones (dead = "a bone from which all animal matter has disappeared, and which is in a dry state"; S = stature; F = femur; H = humerus; T = tibia; R = radius).

2. MODERN STUDIES IN STATURE RECONSTRUCTION: AMERICAN WHITES AND NEGROES

Before proceeding to current data it is instructive to note that in 1898–1902 Hrdlička (see '39) measured the long bones of miscellaneous American whites and Negroes in a dissecting-room population. From this sample, with cadaver statures measured, and with long bones measured, he calculated long bone/stature ratios. Specifically, we may note the humerus/stature index and the femur/stature index.

The researches of Trotter and Gleser ('51, '52, '58) and of Dupertuis and Hadden ('51) are basic, not only for American whites and Negroes, but for the whole problem of statural reconstruction as well. Trotter and Gleser first considered the problem of temporal changes in stature, using data from the Terry Collection, and data on military personnel. Table 46 summarizes their findings:

HUMERUS/STATURE PROPORTION*

Misc.	Males				Females		
	Subjects	Stature (cm.)	Length of Humeri (cm.)	Humerus: Stature Index	Subjects	Stature (cm.)	Length of Humeri (cm.)	Humerus: Stature Index

Misc.	Subjects	Stature (cm.)	Length of Humeri (cm.)	Humerus: Stature Index	Subjects	Stature (cm.)	Length of Humeri (cm.)	Humerus: Stature Index
American Whites	(354)	168.3	32.50	19.31	(82)	156.9	29.77	18.97
American Negroes	(32)	168.6	33.34	19.80	(20)	151.9	30.91	20.34

FEMUR/STATURE PROPORTIONS*

	Male				Female			
	Subjects	Stature (cm.)	Femur (cm.)	Femur: Stature Index	Subjects	Stature (cm.)	Femur (cm.)	Femur: Stature Index
U.S. Whites (misc.)	(271) (23–60 y.)	168.1	44.8	26.60	(89) (23–60 y.)	157.6	41.9	26.60
U.S. Negro	(19) (19–60 y.)	169.2	46.1	27.27	(16) (22–60 y.)	160.6	43.8	27.29

* From Hrdlička ('39). Note that slightly different samples were used for each bone.

On the basis of the foregoing data it was concluded (pp. 438–439):

> There obtains a relatively constant average stature devoid of trend for all 4 groups born between 1840 and 1895. There is a tendency for the Negroes (both males and females) to increase slightly in stature from 1895 to 1905. A significant increase in male stature is present in individuals born between 1905 and 1924 (data for Negroes are less conclusive than for Whites because of the smaller sample). Stature trend in American White and Negro populations thus presents minor fluctuations in the nineteenth century followed by a rapid increase in the twentieth century. This total picture of stature trend over a period of 85 consecutive years refutes the hypothesis that stature increases progressively from decade to decade.
>
> The length of the long bones in all four groups showed fluctuations consistent with stature changes in the corresponding time periods. Thus, the feasibility of utilizing such measures in the study of stature trends is demonstrated and even recommended since the effect of the aging factor and the need for recorded stature of the subject are eliminated. The scope of accessible data for studies of stature trend is enlarged by means of documented skeletal collections.

In 1952, Trotter and Gleser published a definitive study on stature calculation of American whites and Negroes. Data used were from the dead of World War II, from which stature data were available at the time of induction, and from the Terry Collection. All six long bones were measured for max. length; in addition bicondylar length of the femur was taken, as was also the length of the tibia between upper and lower articulating surfaces. Table 47 gives the basic data for stature and for long bone lengths.

Negroes of both sexes have longer arm and leg bones than whites. Also, they have longer forearm and leg bones, relative to upper arm and thigh. In general Negroes have longer limb bones relative to stature. Hence, different equations for the estimation of stature must be established, for whites and Negroes, male and female. This has been achieved, as in Table 48.

In Figure 45 (Stewart, '54) regression lines for American whites and American Negroes are graphically shown. (Chinese have been added; see Section 3.)

TABLE 46

AVERAGES OF STATURE AND SELECTED LONG BONES (IN CMS.) ACCORDING TO YEAR OF
BIRTH, SOURCE, RACE AND SEX*

Year of Birth	No.	Av. Age When Stature Was Measured	Stature as Measured	Corrected Stature**	Femur	Tibia	Femur and Tibia
			WHITE MALES				
			Terry Collection				
1840–49	9	83.9	171.6	172.8	46.5	36.5	83.0
1850–59	29	76.0	168.2	168.9	45.2	34.8	80.0
1860–69	79	68.3	170.0	170.3	45.8	35.6	81.4
1870–79	68	58.9	171.2	170.9	45.8	35.4	81.2
1880–89	51	49.3	170.3	169.5	45.4	34.9	80.4
1890–99	15	38.9	171.4	169.9	45.4	35.0	80.4
1900–09	4	33.2	175.8	173.9	47.5	37.2	84.7
			Military Personnel				
1905–09	33	32.8	171.2		46.1	35.6	81.7
1910–14	77	29.1	172.9		47.1	36.5	83.6
1915–19	171	24.5	173.3		47.1	36.7	83.8
1920–24	249	20.3	174.8		47.5	37.1	84.6
			NEGRO MALES				
			Terry Collection				
1840–49	5	85.8	166.2	167.6	45.2	35.9	81.1
1850–59	14	77.1	169.6	170.4	46.9	37.0	83.9
1860–69	45	67.6	171.7	172.0	47.6	37.6	85.2
1870–79	67	59.9	172.5	172.3	47.6	37.9	85.5
1880–89	83	50.0	172.0	171.2	47.2	37.3	84.5
1890–99	65	39.0	172.2	170.7	47.2	37.4	84.6
1900–09	72	29.8	175.6	173.6	48.1	38.3	86.4
1910–19	9	24.3	176.6	174.6	48.0	38.4	86.4
			Military Personnel				
1905–09	8	32.1	168.5		46.5	36.5	83.0
1910–14	15	29.8	173.8		48.5	39.0	87.5
1915–19	25	24.8	171.2		48.3	38.4	86.7
1920–24	33	20.1	173.2		48.5	38.9	87.4
			WHITE FEMALES				
			Terry Collection				
1840–49	2	87.0	150.5	151.9	40.3	30.2	70.5
1850–59	11	79.9	156.0	157.0	42.1	32.9	75.0
1860–69	22	71.2	161.8	162.3	43.2	33.3	76.5
1870–79	10	61.2	162.6	162.5	43.4	33.8	77.2
1880–89	8	52.2	160.1	159.4	43.4	33.5	76.9
1890–99	4	38.0	166.5	165.0	44.4	34.3	78.7
1900–09	6	32.3	162.2	160.3	42.0	32.0	74.0
			NEGRO FEMALES				
			Terry Collection				
1840–49	3	87.0	155.0	156.4	43.1	34.9	78.0
1850–59	8	80.0	155.2	156.2	42.7	33.3	76.0
1860–69	18	71.0	158.7	159.2	43.7	34.7	78.4
1870–79	23	62.0	162.0	161.9	43.9	34.6	78.5
1880–89	32	49.0	160.9	160.0	43.5	34.5	78.0
1890–99	40	40.3	161.1	159.7	43.6	34.3	77.9
1900–09	38	29.7	161.7	159.7	43.7	34.5	78.2
1910–19	15	23.4	163.3	161.3	44.9	35.6	80.5

* From Trotter and Gleser, '51, Table 1.
** Corrections were made by adding 0.06 cm. per year (above 30 years) for age and
by subtracting 2.0 cm. to make cadaver stature comparable with living stature.
Statures of military personnel were measured on the living at an age providing approximate maximum stature, thus no correction was needed.

TABLE 47

MEAN (WITH STANDARD ERROR) AND STANDARD DEVIATION OF AGE (YEARS), STATURE* AND LONG BONE MEASUREMENTS (CM.) ACCORDING TO RACE, SEX AND SOURCE OF DATA**

White Males

	Military Complete (545)		Military Incomplete (165)		Terry Collection (255)	
	Mean	S.D.	Mean	S.D.	Mean	S.D.
Age	23.14 ± .18	4.31	22.65 ± .35	4.46	61.66 ± .77	12.25
Stature	173.899 ± .284	6.626	174.442 ± .476	6.091	170.392 ± .461	7.343
Humerus	33.618 ± .072	1.672	33.678 ± .124	1.582	32.998 ± .112	1.787
Radius	25.151 ± .055	1.280	25.099 ± .103	1.316	24.403 ± .084	1.334
Ulna	27.035 ± .055	1.283			26.218 ± .088	1.402
Femur	46.908 ± .099	2.306	47.179 ± .187	2.391	45.415 ± .151	2.411
Femur$_m$	47.261 ± .100	2.346	47.525 ± .188	2.410	45.660 ± .154	2.447
Tibia$_m$	37.826 ± .093	2.179	37.991 ± .181	2.316	36.374 ± .136	2.170
Tibia	36.848 ± .091	2.113	37.059 ± .180	2.307	35.345 ± .134	2.139
Fibula	38.135 ± .089	2.084			36.782 ± .132	2.103

Negro Males

	Military (54)		Terry Collection (360)	
	Mean	S.D.	Mean	S.D.
Age	25.07 ± .68	4.98	49.46 ± .82	15.51
Stature	172.111 ± .843	6.139	172.729 ± .412	7.807
Humerus	33.793 ± .184	1.337	33.777 ± .099	1.883
Radius	26.568 ± .170	1.240	26.332 ± .084	1.597
Ulna	28.509 ± .182	1.323	28.164 ± .086	1.623
Femur	47.930 ± .307	2.234	47.073 ± .153	2.903
Femur$_m$	48.337 ± .310	2.256	47.424 ± .157	2.969
Tibia$_m$	39.554 ± .316	2.298	38.721 ± .134	2.533
Tibia	38.606 ± .322	2.344	37.667 ± .131	2.486
Fibula	39.763 ± .315	2.295	38.950 ± .130	2.456

| | *Females (Terry Collection)* | | | |
| | *White (63)* | | *Negro (177)* | |
	Mean	*S.D.*	*Mean*	*S.D.*
Age	63.93 ± 2.02	16.07	47.21 ± 1.55	17.64
Stature	160.682 ± .946	7.508	160.892 ± .574	6.534
Humerus	30.430 ± .218	1.728	30.764 ± .139	1.578
Radius	22.211 ± .156	1.240	23.602 ± .130	1.477
Ulna	23.994 ± .173	1.372	25.390 ± .115	1.305
Femur	42.654 ± .315	2.503	43.273 ± .205	2.335
Femur$_m$	42.959 ± .319	2.531	43.712 ± .210	2.391
Tibia$_m$	34.029 ± .271	2.151	35.415 ± .188	2.135
Tibia	33.181 ± .263	2.091	34.538 ± .184	2.098
Fibula	34.335 ± .270	2.143	35.549 ± .184	2.099

* Stature indicates measurement of the living for military personnel and of the cadaver for the Terry Collection subjects.
** From Trotter and Gleser, '52, Table 5.

TABLE 48*

EQUATIONS FOR ESTIMATION OF LIVING STATURE (CM.) (WITH STANDARD ERRORS) FROM
LONG BONES FOR AMERICAN WHITES AND NEGROES BETWEEN 18 AND 30

*Years of Age***			
White Males		*Negro Males*	
3.08 Hum + 70.45	±4.05	3.26 Hum + 62.10	±4.43
3.78 Rad + 79.01	±4.32	3.42 Rad + 81.56	±4.30
3.70 Ulna + 74.05	±4.32	3.26 Ulna + 79.29	±4.42
2.38 Fem_m + 61.41	±3.27	2.11 Fem_m + 70.35	±3.94
2.52 Tib_m + 78.62	±3.37	2.19 Tib_m + 86.02	±3.78
2.68 Fib + 71.78	±3.29	2.19 Fib + 85.65	±4.08
1.30 (Fem_m + Tib_m) + 63.29	±2.99	1.15 (Fem_m + Tib_m) + 71.04	±3.53
1.42 Fem_m + 1.24 Tib_m + 59.88	±2.99	0.66 Fem_m + 1.62 Tib_m + 76.13	±3.49
0.93 Hum + 1.94 Tib_m + 69.30	±3.26	0.90 Hum + 1.78 Tib_m + 71.29	±3.49
0.27 Hum + 1.32 Fem_m + 1.16 Tib_m + 58.57†	±2.99	0.89 Hum − 1.01 Rad + 0.38 Fem_m + 1.92 Tib_m + 74.56	±3.38
White Females		*Negro Females*	
3.36 Hum + 57.97	±4.45	3.08 Hum + 64.67	±4.25
4.74 Rad + 54.93	±4.24	2.75 Rad + 94.51	±5.05
4.27 Ulna + 57.76	±4.30	3.31 Ulna + 75.38	±4.83
2.47 Fem_m + 54.10	±3.72	2.28 Fem_m + 59.76	±3.41
2.90 Tib_m + 61.53	±3.66	2.45 Tib_m + 72.65	±3.70
2.93 Fib + 59.61	±3.57	2.49 Fib + 70.90	±3.80
1.39 (Fem_m + Tib_m) + 53.20	±3.55	1.26 (Fem_m + Tib_m) + 59.72	±3.28
1.48 Fem_m + 1.28 Tib_m + 53.07	±3.55	1.53 Fem_m + 0.96 Tib_m + 58.54	±3.23
1.35 Hum + 1.95 Tib_m + 52.77	±3.67	1.08 Hum + 1.79 Tib_m + 62.80	±3.58
0.68 Hum + 1.17 Fem_m + 1.15 Tib_m + 50.122	±3.51	0.44 Hum − 0.20 Rad + 1.46 Fem_m + 0.86 Tib_m + 56.33	±3.22

* From Trotter and Gleser, '52, Table 13.
** To estimate stature of older individuals subtract .06 (age in years—30) cm; to estimate cadaver stature add 2.5 cm.
† This equation is presented in preference to that involving the radius since the weight of the radius is essentially zero.

In 1958, Trotter and Gleser re-evaluated the entire problem of skeletal reconstruction from long bones. The skeletal material was from casualties of the Korean War. Here, larger series of whites and Negroes were available, plus a small series of Mongoloids, Mexicans, and Puerto Ricans.

In Table 49 the regression formulae for American white, American Negro, Mongoloid, and Mexican males are given.

The conclusions of this study by Trotter and Gleser merit quoting in full (pp. 121–122):

TABLE 49*

REGRESSION EQUATIONS FOR ESTIMATION OF MAXIMUM, LIVING STATURE (CM.) OF AMERICAN MALE WHITES, NEGROES, MONGOLOIDS AND MEXICANS IN ORDER OF PREFERENCE ACCORDING TO STANDARD ERRORS OF ESTIMATE**

White		Negro	
1.31 (Fem + Fib) + 63.05	±3.62	1.20 (Fem + Fib) + 67.77	±3.63
1.26 (Fem + Tib) + 67.09	±3.74	1.15 (Fem + Tib) + 71.75	±3.68
2.60 Fib + 75.50	±3.86	2.10 Fem + 72.22	±3.91
2.32 Fem + 65.53	±3.94	2.19 Tib + 85.36	±3.96
2.42 Tib + 81.93	±4.00	2.34 Fib + 80.07	±4.02
1.82 (Hum + Rad) + 67.97	±4.31	1.66 (Hum + Rad) + 73.08	±4.18
1.78 (Hum + Ulna) + 66.98	±4.37	1.65 (Hum + Ulna) + 70.67	±4.23
2.89 Hum + 78.10	±4.57	2.88 Hum + 75.48	±4.23
3.79 Rad + 79.42	±4.66	3.32 Rad + 85.43	±4.57
3.76 Ulna + 75.55	±4.72	3.20 Ulna + 82.77	±4.74

Mongoloid		Mexican	
1.22 (Fem + Fib) + 70.24	±3.18		
1.22 (Fem + Tib) + 70.37	±3.24		
2.40 Fib + 80.56	±3.24	2.44 Fem + 58.67	±2.99
2.39 Tib + 81.45	±3.27	2.50 Fib + 75.44	±3.52
2.15 Fem + 72.57	±3.80	2.36 Tib + 80.62	±3.73
1.68 (Hum + Ulna) + 71.18	±4.14		
1.67 (Hum + Rad) + 74.83	±4.16		
2.68 Hum + 83.19	±4.25	3.55 Rad + 80.71	±4.04
3.54 Rad + 82.00	±4.60	3.56 Ulna + 74.56	±4.05
3.48 Ulna + 77.45	±4.66	2.92 Hum + 73.94	±4.24

* From Trotter and Gleser, '58, Table 12.
** When a stature estimate of a White male is to be compared with a stature measurement taken before the individual was 21 years of age the measured stature should be increased according to the time lapse between measurement and death.

When stature is estimated for an individual over 30 years of age the estimate should be reduced by the amount of 0.06 (age in years — 30) cm.

The relationships of stature to length of long limb bones differ sufficiently among the three major races (White, Negro, Mongoloid) to require different regression equations from which to derive the most precise estimates of stature for individuals belonging to each of these groups. The Puerto Rican group, although of shorter stature than the American Negro, presents in this series of data approximately the same relationship of stature to length of long bones as does the Negro group, and thus the equations for estimation of stature derived from the data of the Negro series are applicable to Puerto Ricans. The proportions found in the small sample of Mexicans differ sufficiently from those of any of the other four groups to indicate that more precise estimates of stature for Mexicans will be determined from equations derived from the data of the Mexican series than from any of the other four series.

The standard errors of estimates of stature from lengths of long bones are larger in the present series of White males than in the series of the previous study. The primary reason for this difference is attributed to the evidence that stature and its relationship to long bone lengths are in a state of flux, since some individuals over 21 years of age with given bone lengths are taller today than were individuals six to ten years ago with the same bone lengths.

American White males of the present generation are continuing to grow up to at least 21, and possibly 23, years of age before maximum stature is attained. This finding is in contrast to that obtained from extensive World War II data in which there was no significant increase in stature after 18 years of age. The longer period of growth in stature of the present military series than of World War I, series and the nature of the growth curve for this terminal period were substantiated in two sets of longitudinal growth data, wholly unrelated to the military series.

It is probable that growth in stature is occurring after 18 years of age in all groups in the U.S.A. at the present time. By using the theoretical growth curve with constants computed from the American White military data, averages of the amount of increase in stature for each one-half year interval are provided from age 17 to 21 years. These averages should be applied, when appropriate, to observed or "presumed stature." The application is indicated in identification problems which involve a time lapse between the measuring of stature and the completion of growth in stature.

On the basis of the difference found in stature-long bone length relationships between the World War II and Korean War series, it is indicated that equations for estimation of stature should be derived anew at opportune intervals.

The 1951 study of Dupertuis and Hadden on American whites and Negroes was on a cadaver population, the stature of which was measured while the bodies, with Achilles tendons severed, were

TABLE 50
RATIOS, LONG BONES TO STATURE*

	Male			Female		
	White	*Negro*	*Pearson*	*White*	*Negro*	*Pearson*
F/S	26.2	27.1	27.0	26.2	26.8	26.8
T/S	21.3	22.6	22.0	21.0	22.2	21.6
H/S	19.0	19.3	19.8	18.8	18.9	19.3
R/S	14.1	15.0	14.6	13.5	14.4	14.0
F + T/S	47.5	49.7	49.0	47.3	49.0	48.5
H + R/S	33.1	34.3	34.4	32.3	33.3	33.2

* From Dupertuis and Hadden, '51, Table 9.

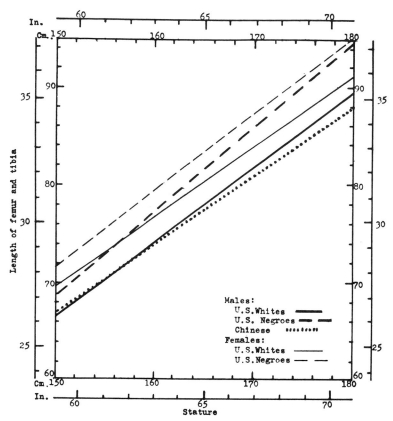

Fig. 45.   Regression lines showing combined lengths of femur and tibia (cm. and in.) plotted against stature (cm. and in.) for whites, Negroes, Chinese.   This is a rapid method of estimating stature from femoral and tibial lengths.

suspended in a vertical position via tongs in the ears (Todd Collection).   Maximum length of humerus, radius, femur and tibia (H, R, F, T) was taken as in Martin ('28).   The sample consisted of 100 skeletons for each sex and for each race.   The study was designed primarily as a test of the validity of the Pearsonian formulae.

In Table 50 the ratios of long bones to stature are given on a comparative basis.

The Pearson white ratios are consistently higher than the Dupertuis and Hadden white ratios.

TABLE 51

	Probable Error cm.
A. WRU male Whites	
a. $S = 77.048 + 2.116F$	0.2308
b. $S = 92.766 + 2.178T$	0.2436
c. $S = 98.341 + 2.270H$	0.3094
d. $S = 88.881 + 3.449R$	0.2907
e. $S = 84.898 + 1.072(F + T)$	0.2508
f. $S = 87.543 + 1.492(H + R)$	0.2889
g. $S = 76.201 + 1.330F + 0.991T$	0.2173
h. $S = 82.831 + 0.907H + 2.474R$	0.2835
i. $S = 78.261 + 2.129F - 0.055H$	0.2328
j. $S = 88.581 + 1.945T + 0.524R$	0.2385
k. $S = 52.618 + 1.512F + 0.927T - 0.490H + 1.386R$	0.1582
B. WRU female Whites	
a. $S = 62.872 + 2.322F$	0.2256
b. $S = 71.652 + 2.635T$	0.2433
c. $S = 56.727 + 3.448H$	0.2762
d. $S = 68.238 + 4.258R$	0.2963
e. $S = 57.872 + 1.354(F + T)$	0.2016
f. $S = 42.386 + 2.280(H + R)$	0.2134
g. $S = 60.377 + 1.472F + 1.133T$	0.2063
h. $S = 53.187 + 2.213H + 1.877R$	0.2632
i. $S = 55.179 + 1.835F + 0.935H$	0.1827
j $S = 64.702 + 2.089T + 1.169R$	0.2328
k. $S = 56.660 - 1.267F + 0.992T + 0.449H + 0.164R$	0.2068
C. WRU male Negroes	
a. $S = 55.021 + 2.540F$	0.2819
b. $S = 72.123 + 2.614T$	0.2983
c. $S = 50.263 + 3.709H$	0.3445
d. $S = 69.168 + 4.040R$	0.3522
e. $S = 52.702 + 1.411(F + T)$	0.2485
f. $S = 57.601 + 1.962(H + R)$	0.3564
g. $S = 54.438 + 1.615F + 1.123T$	0.2559
h. $S = 48.275 + 2.182H + 2.032R$	0.3251
i. $S = 48.802 + 2.175F + 0.696H$	0.2749
j. $S = 67.964 + 2.260T + 0.689R$	0.2964
k. $S = 53.873 + 1.637F + 1.101T + 0.084H - 0.093R$	0.2626
D. WRU female Negroes	
a. $S = 54.235 + 2.498F$	0.2419
b. $S = 72.391 + 2.521T$	0.2867
c. $S = 69.978 + 3.035H$	0.3189
d. $S = 74.906 + 3.761R$	0.3277
e. $S = 70.584 + 1.165(F + T)$	0.2953
f. $S = 61.982 + 1.866(H + R)$	0.2926
g. $S = 52.989 + 2.112F + 0.501T$	0.2397
h. $S = 62.402 + 1.906H + 1.796R$	0.3082
i. $S = 55.103 + 2.517F - 0.033H$	0.2380
j. $S = 66.005 + 2.076T + 0.952R$	0.2832
k. $S = 53.342 + 2.201F + 0.359T - 0.663H + 0.930R$	0.2365
E. Pearson's male Whites	
a. $S = 81.306 + 1.880F$	0.3047
b. $S = 78.664 + 2.376T$	0.3275
c. $S = 70.641 + 2.894H$	0.3056
d. $S = 85.925 + 3.271R$	0.3728
e. $S = 71.272 + 1.159(F + T)$	0.2835
f. $S = 66.855 + 1.730(H + R)$	0.3139

	Probable Error c.m.
E. Pearson's male Whites (*Continued*)	
g. S = 71.443 + 1.220F + 1.080T	0.2845
h. S = 69.788 + 2.769H + 0.195R	0.3054
i. S = 68.397 + 1.030F + 1.557H	0.2750
j. (not calculated)	
k. S = 67.049 + 0.913F + 0.600T + 1.225H − 0.187R	0.2748
F. Pearson's female Whites	
a. S = 72.844 + 1.945F	0.3058
b. S = 74.774 + 2.352T	0.3146
c. S = 71.475 + 2.754H	0.3284
d. S = 81.224 + 3.343R	0.3816
e. S = 69.154 + 1.126(F + T)	0.2898
f. S = 69.911 + 1.628(H + R)	0.3380
g. S = 69.561 + 1.117F + 1.125T	0.2922
h. S = 70.542 + 2.582H + 0.281R	0.3279
i. S = 67.435 + 1.339F + 1.027H	0.2971
j. (not calculated)	
k. S = 67.469 + 0.782F + 1.120T + 1.059H − 0.711R	0.2836

* From Dupertuis and Hadden, '51, Table 15.

TABLE 52

General Formulae for Reconstruction of Stature from Long Bone Lengths*

Male

    a. S = 69.089 + 2.238F
    b. S = 81.688 + 2.392T
    c. S = 73.570 + 2.970H
    d. S = 80.405 + 3.650R
    e. S = 69.294 + 1.225(F + T)
    f. S = 71.429 + 1.728(H + R)
    g. S = 66.544 + 1.422F + 1.062T
    h. S = 66.400 + 1.789H + 1.841R
    i. S = 64.505 + 1.928F + 0.568H
    j. S = 78.272 + 2.102T + 0.606R**
    k. S = 56.006 + 1.442F + 0.931T + 0.083H + 0.480R

Female

    a. S = 61.412 + 2.317F
    b. S = 72.572 + 2.533T
    c. S = 64.977 + 3.144H
    d. S = 73.502 + 3.876R
    e. S = 65 213 + 1.233(F + T)
    f. S = 55.729 + 1.984(H + R)
    g. S = 59.259 + 1.657F + 0.879T
    h. S = 60.344 + 2.164H + 1.525R
    i. S = 57.600 + 2.009F + 0.566H
    j. S = 65.354 + 2.082T + 1.060R**
    k. S = 57.495 + 1.544F + 0.764T + 0.126H + 0.295R

* From Dupertuis and Hadden, '51, Table 20.
** Formula "j" includes only the data of our series. Pearson did not construct **any** of this type.

In Table 51 Dupertuis and Hadden present their formulae, again on a comparative basis including the Pearson formulae.

The stature of the WRU cadaver population (Todd Collection) averaged as follows: male whites close to means of good series of living whites; female whites ca. one cm. shorter than means of good series of living whites; Negro males and females four to six cm. taller than means of good series of living whites; the male and female whites averaged eight and one-half cm. taller than Pearson's whites.

Dupertuis and Hadden suggest the calculation of stature, where possible, from a combination of two or more long bones. Leg long bones give a closer estimate than do arm long bones. In every instance the WRU white formulae indicate taller statures than those calculated by Pearson. In a final evaluation the authors recommend "general formulae," non-racial, for males and females, as given in Table 52.

3. MODERN STUDIES IN STATURE RECONSTRUCTION: VARIOUS ETHNIC AND RACIAL GROUPS

I am here using "ethnic" more in the sense of a national sub-group of whites. "Racial" will contrast White, Negro, Mongoloid (these three are often called "stocks" and their subdivisions are called "races").

As we did in Section 2 we note first Hrdlička's 1898–1902 studies ('39). Here, for misc. U.S. whites, German, Irish, Italian, he gave femur/stature ratios, by sex and by age. His data are given in Table 53.

The femur/stature index is higher in females and it increases a bit with age.

We may now turn to reconstruction formulae for *European* groups (other than those already given). Of passing historic note is Beddoe's (1887–1888) attempt, on a very small sample, to estimate the stature of the "Older Races of England." Where X = living stature and F = femur lgth. in inches, he formulated as follows:

$$X = 4\{F - \tfrac{1}{8}(F - 13) - \tfrac{1}{8}(F - 13 - [F - 19])\}$$
$$= 3F + F - \tfrac{1}{2}(F - 13) - \tfrac{1}{2}(F - 13 - [F - 19])$$
$$= 3F + 13 + \tfrac{1}{2}(F - 19)$$

TABLE 53

FEMUR:STATURE PROPORTIONS IN WHITES*

Paired Bones	23-30			31-45			46-60			Above 60		
	Stature	Bicond. Length of Femur	F:S Index	Stature	Bicond. Length of Femur	F:S Index	Stature	Bicond. Length of Femur	F:S Index	Stature	Bicond. Length of Femur	F:S Index
Males												
Subjects: U.S.A. Misc.	169.6	(20) 44.8	26.43	169.3	(68) 45.2	26.73	167.9	(42) 45.25	26.94	166.9	(18) 45.3	27.14
German	—	—	—	166.4	(8) 45.3	27.23	168.0	(13) 45.05	26.81	162.6	(14) 44.5	27.37
Irish	—	—	—	169.0	(7) 44.6	26.42	166.6	(12) 44.1	26.47	163.2	(9) 45.5	27.09
Italian	166.4	(5) 43.55	26.16	166.4	(15) 43.4	26.09	163.1	(10) 43.7	26.81	162.4	(6) 42.7	26.29
Misc. Whites	—	(35)	—	162.7	(5) 42.7	26.25	167.1	(7) 44.3	26.52	—	(63)	—
Total subjects:					(123)			(113)				
Totals, paired and single bones												
Aver.	169.09	44.82	26.51	168.26	44.78	26.62	167.7	44.87	26.75	165.14	44.86	27.17
Min.	146.5	39.5	24.82	145.5	38.25	24.55	150.2	40.4	24.79	148.2	38.95	25.00
Max.	184.5	50.91	28.37	185.2	50.25	30.62	183.1	50.4	28.80	181.5	50.8	30.77
Females												
Subjects: U.S.A. Misc.	158.68	(12) 42.28	26.65	159.37	(23) 42.22	26.49	157.95	(20) 42.15	26.67	151.8	(12) 40.79	26.91
German	—	—	—	—	—	—	150.9	(2) 41.75	27.67	160.06	(5) 43.64	27.28
Irish	—	—	—	—	—	—	—	—	—	—	—	—
Italian	—	—	—	—	—	—	157.02	(9) 41.68	26.55	155.28	(10) 42.61	27.47
Misc. Whites	—	(17)	—	148.53	(3) 38.47	25.86	—	(39)	—	—	(41)	—
Total subjects:					(33)							
Totals, paired and single bones												
Aver.	158.96	42.46	26.71	157.41	41.86	26.59	157.11	41.73	26.56	154.70	41.83	27.04
Min.	152.4	39.8	25.69	141.3	34.55	24.45	146.95	36.85	24.78	137.2	35.6	25.22
Max.	171.1	45.2	28.85	172.3	47.9	28.53	171.5	47.45	28.14	168.4	47.05	28.71

* From Hrdlička ('39).

TABLE 54

LONG BONE LENGTHS IN GERMAN MALES, RELATED TO STATURE*

Humerus		Radius		Femur	Tibia
Max. Length mm.	Head Length mm.	Max. Length mm.	Stature cm.	Max. Length mm.	Medial Length mm.
268	261	192	154	363	294
272	264	195	155	369	299
276	268	198	156	375	304
279	272	202	157	381	309
283	275	205	158	387	314
287	279	209	159	393	319
291	283	212	160	399	324
294	287	215	161	405	329
298	290	219	162	412	334
302	294	222	163	418	339
305	298	225	164	424	344
309	301	229	165	430	349
313	305	232	166	436	354
316	309	236	167	442	359
320	312	239	168	448	364
324	316	242	169	454	369
328	320	246	170	460	374
331	323	249	171	466	379
335	327	252	172	472	384
338	331	256	173	478	389
342	334	259	174	485	394
346	338	262	175	491	399
349	342	266	176	497	404
353	345	269	177	503	409
357	349	273	178	509	415
361	353	276	179	515	420
364	356	279	180	521	425
368	360	283	181	527	430
372	364	286	182	533	435
375	368	289	183	539	440
379	371	293	184	545	445
383	375	296	185	551	450
387	379	300	186	557	455

* From Breitinger ('37).

This is for males; for females substitute 12 for 13 and 17.5 for 19.

For *Germans* Breitinger ('37) offers formulae based on 2400 *male* skeletons. He based his work on maximum lengths of humerus, radius, femur, and tibia (H, R, F, T).

$$\text{Stature} = 83.21 + 2.715 \, (H) \pm 4.9 \text{ cm.}$$
$$\text{''} = 97.09 + 2.968 \, (R) \pm 5.4 \text{ ''}$$
$$\text{''} = 94.31 + 1.645 \, (F) \pm 4.8 \text{ ''}$$
$$\text{''} = 95.59 + 1.988 \, (T) \pm 4.7 \text{ ''}$$

Breitinger's formulae give consistently higher statures than do those of Manouvrier and Pearson. For a series of medieval

TABLE 55

THE STATURES CORRESPONDING TO GIVEN BONE LENGTHS—MALE*

Humerus Max. Length mm.	Radius Phys. Length mm.	Ulna Phys. Length mm.	Stature cm.	Femur Max. Length mm.	Tibia Whole Length mm.	Fibula Max. Length mm.
278	185	186	155	387	293	303
281	188	189	156	391	298	307
285	191	192	157	396	302	311
288	194	195	158	401	307	315
292	197	198	159	406	312	319
296	199	202	160	410	317	323
299	202	205	161	415	322	327
303	205	208	162	420	327	331
306	208	211	163	425	332	335
310	211	214	164	430	336	339
313	214	217	165	434	341	343
317	217	220	166	439	346	348
320	220	224	167	444	350	352
324	223	227	168	448	355	356
328	226	230	169	453	360	360
331	229	233	170	458	365	364
335	232	236	171	463	370	368
338	235	239	172	468	375	372
342	238	242	173	472	379	376
346	241	245	174	477	384	380
349	244	249	175	482	389	384
353	246	252	176	487	394	388
356	249	255	177	492	398	392
360	252	258	178	496	403	396
363	255	261	179	501	408	400
367	258	264	180	506	412	404
371	261	267	181	511	417	408
374	264	270	182	515	422	412
378	267	274	183	520	426	416
381	270	277	184	525	431	420
385	273	280	185	529	435	424

* From Telkkä, '50, Table 3.

German skeletons the stature was calculated as 168.2 cm. (Manouvrier), 169.0 (Pearson), and 171.7 (Breitinger). In Table 54 bone lengths associated with stated statures are given (in this Table for humerus max. length and head-capitellum lgth. are given; for radius max. lgth.; for femur max. lgth.; for tibia medial lgth., from medial margin of condyle to tip of malleolus).

For *Finns* Telkkä ('50) studied 115 male and 39 female dry skeletons: humerus, max. lgth; radius, physiological lgth. (styloid proc. omitted); ulna, physiol. lgth. (omitting much of olecranon proc. and styloid proc.); femur, tibia, fibula, all max. lgths.

He re-stated certain principles: if bones are measured "wet," or "fresh," or "green," two mm. must be deducted from the lgth.

TABLE 56

THE STATURES CORRESPONDING TO GIVEN BONE LENGTHS—FEMALE*

Humerus Max. Length mm.	Radius Phys. Length mm.	Ulna Phys. Length mm.	Stature cm.	Femur Max. Length mm.	Tibia Whole Length mm.	Fibula Max. Length mm.
263	170	177	145	352	268	276
267	173	180	146	357	274	280
271	176	183	147	363	280	284
274	180	186	148	369	285	289
278	183	189	149	375	290	293
282	186	192	150	380	295	298
285	189	195	151	386	300	302
289	192	198	152	392	306	306
293	196	202	153	397	311	311
297	199	205	154	403	316	315
300	202	208	155	408	321	320
304	205	211	156	414	327	324
308	209	214	157	419	332	328
312	212	217	158	425	337	332
315	215	220	159	430	343	337
319	218	223	160	436	348	341
323	222	226	161	441	353	345
326	225	229	162	447	358	350
330	228	232	163	453	364	354
334	231	235	164	458	369	358
337	235	238	165	463	374	363
341	238	241	166	469	380	367
345	241	244	167	474	385	372
348	244	247	168	480	390	376
352	247	250	169	485	395	381
356	251	253	170	491	400	385
360	254	256	171	496	405	389
363	257	259	172	502	411	394
367	260	262	173	508	416	398
371	264	265	174	513	421	403
374	267	268	175	518	426	407

* From Telkkä, '50, Table 4.

of each bone; supine cadaver lgth. is 2 cm. greater than standing (living) stature. His formulae are as follows:

Male

Stature S = 169.4 + 2.8 × (humerus-32.9) ± 5.0 cm.
169.4 + 3.4 × (radius-22.7) ± 5.0 cm.
169.4 + 3.2 × (ulna-23.1) ± 5.2 cm.
169.4 + 2.1 × (femur-45.5) ± 4.9 cm.
169.4 + 2.1 × (tibia-36.2) ± 4.6 cm.
169.4 + 2.5 × (fibula-36.1) ± 4.4 cm.

Female

Stature S = 156.8 + 2.7 × (humerus-30.7) ± 3.9 cm.
156.8 + 3.1 × (radius-20.8) ± 4.5 cm.
156.8 + 3.3 × (ulna-21.3) ± 4.4 cm.
156.8 + 1.8 × (femur-41.8) ± 4.0 cm.
156.8 + 1.9 × (tibia-33.1) ± 4.6 cm.
156.8 + 2.3 × (fibula-32.7) ± 4.5 cm

TABLE 57
STATURE CALCULATION IN PORTUGUESE*

		Av. Length mm.	Stature According to the Table		Stature Calculated by Interpolation	
			Cadaver m.	Living m.	Cadaver m.	Living m.
			Male			
Humerus	R	317.75	1.644	1.624	1.642	1.622
	L	316.25	1.644	1.624	1.640	1.620
Radius	R	235.96	1.654	1.634	1.651	1.631
	L	235.64	1.654	1.634	1.649	1.629
Ulna	R	254.80	1.654	1.634	1.653	1.633
	L	260.21	1.677	1.657	1.674	1.654
Femur	R	438.73	1.654	1.634	1.655	1.635
	L	433.06	1.644	1.624	1.646	1.626
Tibia	R	358.06	1.654	1.634	1.650	1.630
	L	356.72	1.644	1.624	1.647	1.627
Fibula	R	347.27	1.634	1.614	1.635	1.615
	L	346.29	1.634	1.614	1.633	1.613
			Female			
Humerus	R	293.41	1.556	1.536	1.551	1.531
	L	290.42	1.543	1.523	1.544	1.524
Radius	R	207.81	1.528	1.508	1.534	1.514
	L	211.68	1.556	1.536	1.555	1.535
Ulna	R	231.38	1.568	1.548	1.563	1.543
	L	225.44	1.543	1.523	1.540	1.520
Femur	R	400.96	1.528	1.508	1.528	1.508
	L	399.67	1.528	1.508	1.524	1.504
Tibia	R	327.13	1.543	1.523	1.543	1.523
	L	327.08	1.543	1.523	1.543	1.523
Fibula	R	324.09	1.543	1.523	1.546	1.526
	L	327.08	1.556	1.536	1.552	1.532

* From Mendes-Corrêa, '32.

In Tables 55 and 56, for males and females, Telkkä presents bone lengths associated with stated statures.

In 1932, Mendes-Corrêa carried out a study on *Portuguese*. He used maximum lengths of humerus, radius, ulna, femur, tibia, and fibula, and related his calculations to both a cadaver and a living population sample, the latter consistently 20 mm. shorter than the former. He used Manouvrier's data and came out with a pretty good agreement, as can be seen in Table 57.

For *Chinese* Stevenson ('29) reports on data derived from measurements of cadaver length and dry bone lengths of 48 Chinese male skeletons. He compared his findings with samples of acient Egyptian (Naqada), French, and Aino (aborigines of Japan). In Table 58 these data are given for stature and for max. lgths. of humerus, radius, femur, and tibia. Means, standard deviations, and coefficients of variation (standard deviation/mean) are given.

	Body	Femur		Tibia		Fibula		Humerus		Radius		Ulna	
	L.	L.	P.	L.	P.	L.	P.	L.	P.	L.	P.	L.	P.
Males	63.8	16.7	26.2	14.2	22.3	14.3	22.4	12.0	18.8	9.4	15.1	10.5	16.4
Females	59.0	15.5	—	13.2	—	13.3	—	11.1	—	8.8	—	9.7	—
Both sexes	62.0	16.2	—	13.8	—	13.9	—	11.6	—	9.0	—	10.2	—

(From Pan, '24.)

Stevenson's formulae for Chinese males, based on cadaver lengths (C), are as follows (for femur (F), humerus (H), Tibia (T), and radius (R):

$$
\begin{aligned}
\text{(a)}\quad C &= 61.7207 + 2.4378\ F & \pm\ 2.1756 \\
\text{(b)}\quad &= 81.5115 + 2.8131\ H & \pm\ 2.8903 \\
\text{(c)}\quad &= 59.2256 + 3.0263\ T & \pm\ 1.8916 \\
\text{(d)}\quad &= 80.0276 + 3.7384\ R & \pm\ 2.6791 \\
\text{(e)}\quad &= 54.2522 + 1.4294\ (F + T) & \pm\ 1.9214 \\
\text{(f)}\quad &= 55.3865 + 0.6024\ F + 2.4014\ T & \pm\ 1.8605 \\
\text{(g)}\quad &= 63.4865 + 1.9222\ (H + R) & \pm\ 2.6529 \\
\text{(h)}\quad &= 64.4272 + 1.3052\ H + 2.6889\ R & \pm\ 2.5691 \\
\text{(i)}\quad &= 59.7828 + 2.3397\ F + 0.2012\ H & \pm\ 2.1747 \\
\text{(j)}\quad &= 57.1954 + 2.8594\ T + 0.3398\ R & \pm\ 1.8838 \\
\text{(k)}\quad &= 52.2596 + 0.6640\ F + 2.2065\ T & \\
& \quad - 0.1008\ H + 0.4464\ R & \pm\ 1.8201
\end{aligned}
$$

For *East Indians* (Hindus) Pan ('24) measured 142 male and female cadavera: stature, and max. lgth. of humerus, radius, ulna, femur, tibia, fibula (inches). The bones were measured "wet," with cartilage. Pan presented his data in terms of the length (L) of a given long bone in % stature (P = proportion).

(See page opposite for data.)

Also for *East Indians* (United Provinces) Nat ('31) offers data based on the max. lgth. of dry bones: humerus, radius, ulna, femur, tibia, fibula. The bones are measured in inches, and for each a "multiplying factor" (M.F.) has been derived as follows:

Bone	*M.F.*
Humerus	5.3
Radius	6.9
Ulna	6.3
Femur	3.7
Tibia	4.48
Fibula	4.48

Nat observes that these data are applicable only to people of the United Provinces. He reports an accuracy of $\pm 1''$.

It remains but to mention several other studies in which *stature is estimated from other than long bone lengths*. Actually, the formulae are mainly based on proportions in living subjects. Macdonnel ('01) studied 3000 English criminals (English, Welsh, Irish, "and a few Scots"). No "foreigners" or individuals under 21 were included. He took stature (to nearest $1/8''$) head ht., head brdth., face brdth., finger III lgth., cubit lgth. (from elbow to tip of finger III), and foot lgth. (all to nearest mm.). For finger III lgth.,

TABLE 58

STATURE (CADAVER) AND DRY LONG BONE MEASUREMENTS: CHINESE MALES*

(Absolute Measurements in cms.)

	Naqada	French	Chinese	Aino
Means:				
Stature	—	166.260 ± 0.525	168.923 ± 0.528	157.900
Femur	45.930 ± 0.170	44.578 ± 0.226	43.975 ± 0.174	40.770 ± 0.193
Tibia	37.970 ± 0.137	36.336 ± 0.172	36.248 ± 0.149	33.895 ± 0.183
Humerus	32.618 ± 0.146	32.600 ± 0.147	31.073 ± 0.115	29.502 ± 0.135
Radius	25.697 ± 0.127	24.174 ± 0.112	23.779 ± 0.096	22.913 ± 0.121
Standard Deviations:				
Stature	—	5.502 ± 0.371	5.424 ± 0.373	—
Femur	2.519 ± 0.134	2.372 ± 0.160	1.788 ± 0.123	1.898 ± 0.136
Tibia	1.877 ± 0.097	1.799 ± 0.121	1.535 ± 0.106	1.668 ± 0.129
Humerus	1.701 ± 0.103	1.538 ± 0.104	1.182 ± 0.081	1.343 ± 0.095
Radius	1.290 ± 0.090	1.170 ± 0.079	0.987 ± 0.068	1.117 ± 0.086
Coefficients of Variation:				
Stature	—	3.309 ± 0.223	3.211 ± 0.221	4.655 ± 0.336
Femur	5.484 ± 0.293	5.425 ± 0.354	4.066 ± 0.280	4.921 ± 0.381
Tibia	4.943 ± 0.256	4.888 ± 0.330	4.234 ± 0.291	4.552 ± 0.322
Humerus	5.216 ± 0.317	4.659 ± 0.314	3.802 ± 0.262	4.875 ± 0.375
Radius	5.021 ± 0.350	4.796 ± 0.323	4.150 ± 0.286	

* From Stevenson, '29, Table 1.

cubit lgth., and foot lgth, or combinations, he derived the following formulae:

$H = 166.45716 + 7.7849$ (Finger III—11.54737)
$H = 166.45716 + 2.6301$ (Cubit—45.05864)
$H = 166.45716 + 4.0301$ (Foot—25.68770)
$H = 166.45716 - .6703$ (Finger III—11.54737) $+ 2.7886$ (Cubit—45.05864)
$H = 166.45716 + 2.8360$ (Finger III—11.54737) $+ 3.0304$ (Foot—25.68770).

The probable errors of the stature reconstruction based on these formulae are as follows:

Reconstruction from:	*Probable Error*
Finger	3.2671
Cubit	2.6127
Foot	2.9453
Finger and Cubit	2.6094
Finger and Foot	2.8651

Smith ('39) employed diaphyseal length of *fetal long bones* to calculate *fetal length* as follows:

Lgth. $= 11.30 \times$ clavicle
" $= 7.60 \times$ humerus
" $= 9.20 \times$ radius
" $= 6.71 \times$ femur
" $= 7.63 \times$ tibia

The *vertebral column*, if intact, can be used in calculating adult stature. The column defined is from odontoid tip of second cervical to lower border of fifth lumbar. Here are the data:

C2-L5 LENGTH

Male		*Female*	
Lgth.	*Coeff.*	*Lgth.*	*Coeff.*
X–569 mm.	2.93	X–539 mm.	2.94
570–599 mm.	2.84	540–569 mm.	2.82
600–629 mm.	2.78	570–599 mm.	2.79
630–659 mm.	2.79	600–X mm.	2.76
660–X mm.	2.65		

This gives a rather crude approximation.

4. THE USE OF IMMATURE OR FRAGMENTARY LONG BONES IN STATURE RECONSTRUCTION

The relation between epiphyseal and diaphyseal dimensions focusses upon the problem of how much an epiphysis contributes to the total length of the bone. For example, in skeletal remains estimated to be about 10 years old there will be many long bones sans epiphyses. The problem then is: how much should be added

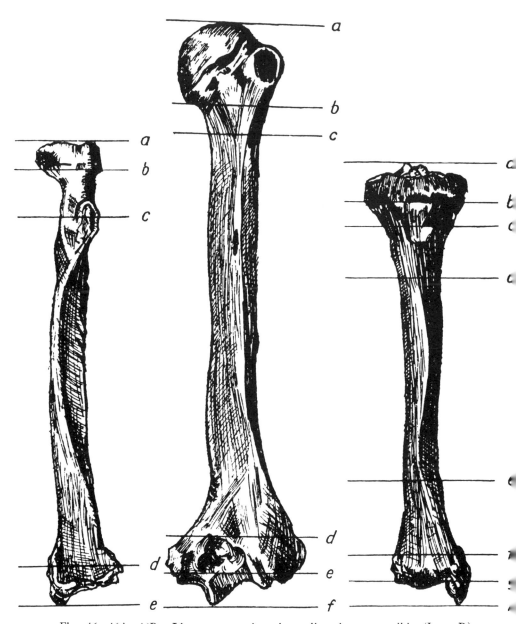

Fig. 46, 46A, 46B. Linear proportions in radius, humerus, tibia (L to R).

to diaphyseal length to give total length?   This is not for the purpose of use in statural formulae, but rather to aid in age estimation, for there are tables available that will give average bone lengths on a chronological age basis (See Martin and Bach, '26; Krogman, '41).

Seitz ('23) is about the only reference here, and the data are partial, i.e., for humerus and tibia only.   In the humerus the height of the proximal epiphysis is from the greatest prominence on the head to the epiphyseal line; the total length is from the same prominence to the lateral trochlear surface.   In the tibia the height of the proximal epiphysis is from a point just posterior to the intercondyloid eminence to the epiphyseal line; the height of the distal ephiphysis is from the inferior articular surface to the epiphyseal line; the total length is from the most prominent point of the intercondyloid eminence to the tip of the medial malleolus.   All measurements were on sagittally-sectioned adult white humeri and tibiae, 84 (44 right, 40 left) humeri, 58 proximal tibial epiphyses, 55 distal tibial epiphyses, on 38 right and 37 left tibiae.

In the humerus the proximal epiphysis varied from 1.3% to 2.2% of the total length of the bone.   In the tibia the proximal epiphysis varied from 2.4% to 3.9%, and the distal epiphysis varied from 1.8% to 2.9%, of the total length of the bone.   In none of the epiphyses was there any correlation with the total length of the respective bones.

What can be done with fragmentary bones?   First, to estimate their total length, second, to then employ them in statural formulae.   Here reference must be made to the studies of Müller ('35), who made available useful data on 50 radii, 100 humeri, and 100 tibiae (see Figures 46, 46A, 46B for all measurements).

In the *humerus* (middle bone) *a* is at the most proximal point in the head; *b* is at the most distal point of the circumference of the head; *c* is at the convergence of two areas of muscle attachment just below the major tubercle; *d* is at the upper margin of the olecranon fossa; *e* is at the lower margin of the olecranon fossa; *f* is at the most distal point on the trochlea.

These dimensions are proportionately related to total humeral length as follows:

$$
\begin{aligned}
\text{a–f} &= 100\% \\
\text{a–b} &= 11.44\% \pm 1.71\% \\
\text{b–c} &= 7.60\% \pm 1.67\% \\
\text{c–d} &= 69.62\% \pm 1.74\% \\
\text{d–e} &= 6.26\% \pm 0.90\% \\
\text{e–f} &= 5.47\% \pm 0.86\%
\end{aligned}
$$

In the *radius* (bone to the left) *a* is at the most proximal point of the head; *b* is at the distal margin of the head; *c* is through the mid-point of the radial tuberosity; *d* is at the distal epiphyseal line; and *e* is at the tip of the styloid process.

These dimensions are proportionately related to total radial length as follows:

$$
\begin{aligned}
\text{a–e} &= 100\% \\
\text{a–b} &= 5.35\% \pm 1.31\% \\
\text{b–c} &= 8.96\% \pm 1.95\% \\
\text{c–d} &= 78.72\% \pm 0.25\% \\
\text{d–e} &= 7.46\% \pm 1.10\%
\end{aligned}
$$

In the *tibia* (bone to the right) *a* is at the most proximal point of the intercondyloid eminences; *b* is at the proximal epiphyseal line, near the proximal end of the tibial tuberosity; *c* is through the most elevated point of the tuberosity; *d* is at the proximal end of the anterior tibial crest; *e* is at the level of minimum circumference; *f* is at the distal epiphyseal line; *g* is at the level of the distal articular surface; *h* is at the most distal point on the medial malleolus.

These dimensions are proportionately related to total tibial length as follows:

$$
\begin{aligned}
\text{a–h} &= 100\% \\
\text{a–b} &= 7.88\% \pm 1.31\% \\
\text{b–c} &= 4.84\% \pm 1.31\% \\
\text{c–d} &= 8.86\% \pm 0.93\% \\
\text{d–e} &= 48.54\% \pm 4.27\% \\
\text{e–f} &= 22.09\% \pm 3.35\% \\
\text{f–g} &= 3.29\% \pm 0.74\% \\
\text{g–h} &= 5.03\% \pm 0.92\%
\end{aligned}
$$

Obviously the foregoing data cannot cover *all* fragmentation, nor are all long bones included. But for the three bones specified the data are extremely worth-while in the hands of a competent osteologist.

5. THE INTERPRETATION OF STATURAL RECONSTRUCTION FORMULAE

The wealth of tabular data in this area is a veritable "embarrassment of riches." Which is the best formula? When should a

TABLE 59

Age	No.	Stature	Femur	Tibia	Humerus
		Negro Male			
20–29	46	176.54	48.05	38.65	34.34
30–39	66	174.17	47.14	37.82	33.81
40–49	69	172.58	46.59	37.37	33.42
50–59	76	172.20	47.12	37.59	33.79
60–69	65	171.77	47.13	37.58	33.78
70–89	38	169.84	46.60	37.07	33.66
Total	360	172.73	47.07	37.67	33.78
		White Male			
28–49	49	170.92	45.36	36.07	32.79
50–59	53	170.76	45.26	35.14	32.96
60–64	39	171.54	45.65	35.58	32.94
65–69	47	169.79	45.38	35.54	33.30
70–87	67	169.48	45.47	35.44	33.00
Total	255	170.39	45.42	35.35	33.00
		Negro Female			
19–29	33	161.76	43.71	34.81	31.00
30–39	38	161.71	43.10	34.51	30.57
40–49	36	161.50	43.37	34.58	30.78
50–59	26	161.19	43.42	34.40	30.70
60–69	16	162.06	43.66	34.83	30.86
70–91	28	157.04	42.77	34.16	30.74
Total	177	160.89	43.27	34.54	30.76
		White Female			
27–39	9	162.44	43.21	32.39	30.33
40–59	11	163.09	43.52	34.05	31.08
60–69	16	162.00	42.80	33.49	30.28
70–79	18	161.28	43.01	33.43	30.71
80–87	9	152.44	41.08	31.87	29.43
Total	63	160.68	42.65	33.18	30.43

* From Trotter and Gleser, '51a, Table 1.

given formula be used? What factor, or factors, should be taken into consideration? How does a group derived formula apply to an individual?

In 1939, Hrdlička said that the correlation of long bones to stature differs with sex, race, and side of body. He might well have omitted sidedness (for it is not a significant factor) and have, instead, mentioned *age*, a factor properly evaluated by Trotter and Gleser ('51a). Their work is based on the skeletons of 255 American white males, 63 females, and 360 American Negro males, 177 females. The first data to be noted are age-changes in lengths of humerus, femur, tibia (Table 59).

There is a consistent tendency, especially in the femur, and notably in that of the Negro male, for the several long bones to show a length decrease with age. This will, of course, be registered in stature itself, and in estimates of stature (Table 60).

TABLE 60

COMPARISON OF ESTIMATED STATURE AT AGE 30 WITH OBSERVED STATURE ACCORDING TO RACE, SEX, AND AGE*

Age	Estimated Stature at Age 30	Observed Stature	Estimated Minus Observed Stature
	Negro Male		
20–29	176.46 ± .52	176.54	− .08
30–39	174.20 ± .43	174.17	.03
40–49	172.92 ± .43	172.58	.34
50–59	173.78 ± .40	172.20	1.58
60–69	173.77 ± .44	171.77	2.00
70–89	172.41 ± .58	169.84	2.57
	White Male		
28–49	171.84 ± .52	170.92	.92
50–59	171.73 ± .50	170.76	.97
60–64	172.40 ± .59	171.54	.86
65–69	172.36 ± .53	169.79	2.57
70–87	172.42 ± .45	169.48	2.94
	Negro Female		
19–29	162.65 ± .59	161.76	.89
30–39	161.43 ± .55	161.71	− .28
40–49	161.91 ± .56	161.50	.41
50–59	161.79 ± .67	161.19	.60
60–69	162.60 ± .86	162.06	.54
70–91	160.58 ± .64	157.04	3.54
	White Female		
27–39	163.87 ± 1.16	162.44	1.43
40–59	166.83 ± .99	163.09	3.74
60–69	165.01 ± .85	162.00	3.01
70–79	165.20 ± .79	161.28	3.92
80–87	160.22 ± 1.16	152.44	7.78

* From Trotter and Gleser, '51, Table 4.

In all groups there is a statural decrement of the order of about 1.2 cm. per 20 years. Trotter and Gleser tested this for Rollet's data (50 male, 50 female French cadavera) and found the same estimate of 1.2 cm. per 20 years.

There are certainly *racial* factors to be considered. Stevenson ('29) switched Chinese and French formulae and came up with the following:

Formula	Chinese from French	French from Chinese
True Value	168.923 ± .528	166.260 ± .525
(a) F	165.239 ± .314	170.247 ± .307
(b) H	161.841 ± .318	173.218 ± .408
(c) T	166.051 ± .307	169.190 ± .267
(d) R	164.968 ± .384	170.400 ± .378
(e) F + T	165.536 ± .291	169.825 ± .271
(f) F and T	165.502 ± .293	169.461 ± .263
(g) H + R	162.997 ± .323	172.617 ± .375
(h) H and R	161.955 ± .314	171.978 ± .363
(i) F and H	163.323 ± .283	170.501 ± .307
(j) T and R	165.675 ± .328	169.309 ± .266
(k) F, T, H, and R	163.915 ± .283	169.500 ± .257
Mean (a)–(k)	164.273 ± .312	170.568 ± .315

Telkkä ('50) applied four different formulae, based on French, German, and Finnish bones to the same set of (Finnish) long bones and for humerus and femur reported as follows:

	mm.	Manouvrier cm.	Pearson cm.	Breitinger cm.	Telkkä cm.
Male Humerus	300	155.1	157.3	163.0	159.2
	330	165.7	166.0	171.2	167.6
	360	177.9	174.7	179.3	176.0
	380	186.3	180.5	184.8	181.6
Male Femur	400	155.4	156.5	160.5	155.8
	440	164.4	164.0	167.0	164.2
	480	171.9	171.5	173.6	172.6
	520	183.3	179.1	180.1	181.0
Female Humerus	270	143.0	145.8		144.8
	300	154.8	154.1		153.0
	330	163.6	162.4		161.0
	360	177.3	170.6		169.0
Female Femur	360	138.8	142.9		144.5
	400	151.4	150.6		151.5
	440	159.7	158.4		158.8
	480	169.8	166.2		166.0

Trotter and Gleser ('52) found the Pearson formulae to be 3.67 cm. too low on 100 American white femora, and 6.22 cm. too low on the humeri.

In differing racial samples there are two sets of factors to be considered, viz., differences in stature and differences in stature-limb, limb-limb, and intra-limb proportions.

In 1899, Pearson said that "the probable error of the reconstruction of the stature of a single individual is never sensibly less than two cm., and if we have only the radius to predict from may amount to 2.66 cm. . . . Hence, no attempt to reconstruct the stature of an individual from the four long bones can possibly exceed this degree of accuracy on the average, at any rate, no *linear* formula." Pearson also noted that such formulae could not apply to persons of extreme stature limits (dwarfs or giants).

From the formulae that have been presented the standard errors (S.E.) may be tabulated as follows (in cm.):

Author	Humerus		Femur	
	Male	*Female*	*Male*	*Female*
Pearson ('99)	3.2	3.4	3.2	3.2
Telkkä ('50)	5.0	3.9	4.9	4.0
Dupertuis and Hadden ('51)				
White	4.6	4.1	3.4	3.3
Negro	5.1	4.7	4.3	3.6
Trotter and Gleser ('52)				
White	4.0	4.5	3.3	3.7
Negro	4.4	4.3	3.9	3.4

In handling a statural reconstruction in a single case, based on a femur, what are the limits or chances of being correct? (see Keen, '53). As an example take the 3.2 cm. S.E. for the femur in Pearson's formula; let us assume that the best estimate of stature is 180 cm. then:

$$\pm 1 \quad \text{S.E.} = 176.8–183.2 \text{ cm. chances are } 1:3$$
$$\pm 2 \quad \text{S.E.} = 173.6–186.4 \text{ cm.} \quad \text{`` `` } 1:22$$
$$\pm 2^1/_2 \text{ S.E.} = 172.0–188.0 \text{ cm.} \quad \text{`` `` } 1:100$$
$$\pm 3 \quad \text{S.E.} = 170.4–189.6 \text{ cm.} \quad \text{`` `` } 1:1000$$

This assumes the probability that the calculated individual stature is *correct within a certain range.* We may accept ±2 S.E. (1:22) as a safe bet. The individual estimate of 180 cm. must yield to the likelihood that the calculated stature is somewhere between 173.6–186.4 cm., a spread of 12.8 cm., or a little over 5″.

Another variable factor to be evaluated is that of the rate and amount of drying in long bones. In 1927, Ingalls calculated the shrinkage in the right femur as follows:

Dimension	Av. Lgth.* (mm.)	Av. Loss (mm.)	% Loss	Range of Loss (mm.)
1. Oblique lgth.				
W. male	458	6.89	1.50	4.25–8.75
N. male	469	7.25	1.55	6.00–9.25
N. female	441	6.61	1.50	5.50–8.00
2. Vert. diam. head				
W. male	52	2.56	4.93	1.75–3.75
N. male	50	2.90	5.76	2.25–3.50
N. female	44	2.54	5.81	1.50–3.25
3. Horiz. diam. head				
W. male	51	3.04	5.91	2.25–4.25
N. male	50	3.12	6.22	2.75–4.00
N. female	44	3.04	6.97	2.50–3.50

* I have given av. lgths. to the nearest whole mm. W = white, N = Negro.

The per cent loss in femoral length is less than in head dimensions, but loss in the latter is proportional, i.e., vertical and horizontal diameters both lose about 5–7%. There are no real race or sex differences.

In evaluating the several formulae which have been discussed certain strictures must be made: those based on small samples of cadaveral stature are limited in their application (Pearson, Telkkä, Dupertuis and Hadden); those with no allowance for the age factor should be carefully used (same series); those in which dry-wet bones are combined or in which palpable body landmarks have been used in lieu of long bone lengths, have inherent errors (Pearson, Breitinger). Hence the Trotter and Gleser data emerge as the single, most useful set of formulae; I would add to this that the general formulae of Dupertuis and Hadden are also acceptable.

Finally, these words of caution by Trotter and Gleser ('58, p. 119) are worth noting:

1. Do not combine formulae obtained by different investigators, based on different races or populations in different geographical areas, nor pertinent to different generations.
2. Do not estimate stature by determining the average of estimates obtained from several equations, each of which is based on a different bone or on a combination of bones.
3. Do not plot estimated stature against observed stature in order to test the precision of regression equations.

Summarizing Statement

1. In the estimation of stature from the measurement of long bones care should be taken to ascertain how the long bones were measured in the formula it is proposed to use. The bone, or bones, in an individual case should be measured in exactly the same way as by the author(s) of a given formula.

2. It is advisable in the calculation of stature to use more than one long bone, wherever this is possible; also leg bone lengths (tibia and femur) give better estimates than arm bone lengths (radius and humerus).

3. In using comparative tabulations care should be taken to consider: temporal changes (use the most recent data); sex differences; race differences; age differences (correct for stature loss in old age).

4. In an over-all stature reconstruction problem I suggest use of the data of Trotter and Gleser on American male and female whites and Negroes (Table 48 of this Chapter), plus a check by the "general formulae" of Dupertuis and Hadden (Table 52 of this Chapter).

5. Immature and fragmentary bones may be used to estimate the total length of a given bone. The immature lengths may be referred to tables of length-for-age to give an idea of chronological age; this, in turn, may fit into a height-for-age category. Restored lengths (fragmentary adult bones) may, of course, be referred to tabulations of formulae.

6. The use of formulae must recognize that a mean stature calculation refers only to a central tendency. The error (standard error) must be used to estimate the chance that the true stature is within certain limits.

7. The rate and amount of drying in long bones is not enough of a factor to play any significant role in the reconstruction of stature.

REFERENCES

BACH, F. and MARTIN, R.: (See *Refs.*, Chap. II).

BEDDOE, J.: On the stature of the older races of England, as estimated from the long bones. *JRAI, 17*:202–207, 1887/88.

BREITINGER, E.: Zur Berechnung der Körperhöhe aus den längen Gliedmassen-knochen. *Anth. Anzeig., 14*:249–274, 1937.

DUPERTUIS, C. W. and HADDEN, Jr., J. A.: On the reconstruction of stature from long bones. *AJPA n.s., 9(1)*:15–54, 1951.

HRDLIČKA, A.: 1939 (see *Refs.*, Chap. II).

INGALLS, N. W.: Studies on the femur. III. Effects of maceration and drying in the white and the Negro. *AJPA, 10(2)*:297–321, 1927.

KEEN, E. N.: Estimation of stature from the long bones. *J. Forensic Med., 1(1)*: 46–51, 1953.

KROGMAN, W. M.: Growth of Man. *Tab. Biol., 20*:1–967, Junk, Den Haag. 1941.

MACDONNEL, W. R.: On criminal anthropometry and the identification of criminals. *Biom. 1*:177–227, 1901.

MANOUVRIER, L.: Determination de la taille d'apres les grands os des membres. *Rev. Mem. de l'Ecole d'Anth., 2*:227–233, 1892; *Mem. Soc. d'Anth. 2e ser. 4*:347–402, 1893.

MARTIN, R.: *Lehrbuch der Anthropologie* (2nd ed., 3 vols.). Fischer, Jena., 1928.

MATIEGKA, H.: Über den körperwuchs der prähistorischen Bevölkerung Böhmens und Mährens. *MAGW, 41*:348–387, 1911.

MENDES-CORRÊA, A. A.: La taille des Portugais d'apres les os longes. *Anthroplogie, Prague.*, *10*:268–272, 1932.

MÜLLER, G.: Zur Bestimmung der Länge beschädigter Extremitätenknochen. *Anth. Anzeig.*, *12*:70–72, 1935.

NAT, B. S.: Estimation of stature from long bones in Indians of the United Provinces: A medico-legal inquiry in anthropometry. *Indian J. Med. Res.*, Calcutta, *18*:1245–1253, 1931.

PAN, N.: Length of long bones and their proportion to body height in Hindus. *JA*, *58(4)*:374–378, 1924.

PEARSON, KARL: Mathematical contributions to the theory of evolution. V. On the reconstruction of the stature of prehistoric races. *Phil. Trans. Roy. Soc. London.*, 192:169–244, 1899.

ROLLET, F.: De la mensuration de os longs du membres. *Thesis* pour le doc. en med., 1st series, *43*:1–128, Paris, 1899.

SEITZ, R. P.: Relation of epiphyseal length to bone length. *AJPA*, *6(1)*:37–49, 1923.

SMITH, S.: *Forensic Medicine* (ed. 6). Little, Brown Co., Boston, 1939.

STEVENSON, P. H.: On racial differences in stature long bone regression formulae, with special reference to stature reconstruction formulae for the Chinese. *Biom.*, *21(1–4)*:303–318, 1929.

STEWART, T. D.: 1954 (See *Refs.*, Chap. II).

TELKKÄ, A.: On the prediction of human stature from the long bones. *Acta Anat.*, *9*:103–117, 1950.

TROTTER, M. and GLESER, G. C.: The effect of ageing on stature. *AJPA n.s.*, *9(3)*:311–324, 1951a.

TROTTER, M. and GLESER, G. C.: Trends in stature of American whites and Negroes born between 1840 and 1924. *AJPA, n.s.*, *9(4)*:427–440, 1951b.

TROTTER, M. and GLESER, G. C.: Estimation of stature from long bones of American whites and Negroes. *AJPA, n.s.*, *10(4)*:463–514, 1952.

TROTTER, M. and GLESER, G. C.: A re-evaluation of estimation of stature based on measurements of stature taken during life and of long bones after death. *AJPA n.s.*, *16(1)*:79–123, 1958.

WELLS, L. H.: Estimation of stature from longbones: a reassessment. *J. Forensic Med.*, *6(4)*:171–177, 1959.

VII

Race Differences in the Human Skeleton

1. THE AMERICAN PICTURE: WHITE AND NEGRO

In the United States problems of skeletal identification center around two major groups of peoples: whites of European origin, Negroes, ultimately of West African origin. Neither group is biologically homogeneous: the American whites are a composite of all the sub-groups (races) of European and Asia Minor; the American Negro is a trihybrid blend of his African ancestry, plus white intermixture, plus admixture with the American Indian (who represents a third major group in the United States, the Mongoloid, for the American Indian traces back to Asia).

There are three major references of use in giving an overall Negro-white comparison: Todd and Lindala ('28); Cobb ('34, '42); Lewis ('42). The first reference is a major contribution to the somatic morphometry of the two groups, though it is based on cadaver body measurements (100 male white, 100 male Negro, 36 female white, 32 female Negro, Todd collection). Cobb and Lewis offer compendia on the biology of the American Negro. In Table 61 is presented a list of the major bodily dimensions which may be of some use when skeletal material is to be studied on a comparative basis (racial, and/or sexual).

The real problem is not so much *dimensional*, for the S.D.'s show that there is a marked over-lap. (The pelvis may form an exception to this generalization, as later noted.) The basic problem is *proportional*, e.g., in ratios of limb to stature, in inter-membral ratios (arm to leg), and in intra-membral ratios (forearm to upper arm, leg to thigh, the first called the "brachial index," the second

TABLE 61

SELECTED BODY, HEAD. AND FACE DIMENSIONS IN AMERICAN WHITES AND NEGROES, MALE AND FEMALE*

Dimension	White				Negro			
	Male		Female		Male		Female	
	M	S.D.	M	S.D.	M	S.D.	M	S.D.
1. Body								
Stature	1706	60.54	1597	78.01	1744	60.80	1586	64.91
Arm L, total	760	30.19	695	38.08	798	41.20	713	32.66
Upper arm L	333	16.43	302	22.78	340	21.85	303	15.62
Forearm L	249	12.35	225	16.66	269	15.03	237	14.74
Hand L	187	9.29	172	11.31	199	12.33	179	10.17
Leg L (ant. sup. sp.)	938	40.04	871	51.20	984	49.12	892	41.79
Thigh L	497	24.34	461	31.57	515	27.49	467	24.92
Lower leg L	376	19.77	352	25.84	401	23.77	365	19.78
Foot L	244	11.86	215	13.56	256	13.88	231	11.78
Bi-iliac B	292	16.86	287	22.47	270	16.45	267	24.74
Bi-spinous B	246	17.16	242	25.06	227	18.08	220	22.52
2. Head								
Max. L	188	7.52	182	6.54	193	6.08	186	7.66
Max. B	154	6.46	145	5.62	149	6.10	144	6.18
Auric. H	120	5.08	118	5.27	124	5.27	120	4.80
3. Face								
Bizyg. B	139	6.73	130	7.04	139	6.09	132	8.72
Mand. B	110	7.43	103	8.89	109	8.67	105	11.97
Interoc. B	33	3.49	31	2.83	35	2.71	34	2.86
Total morph. H	122	9.67	113	9.46	125	7.63	116	11.59
Upper face H	69	6.26	66	6.18	71	5.56	67	4.51
Nasal H	54	4.72	52	3.84	52	4.84	50	4.37
Nasal B	35	3.68	32	4.87	43	3.68	40	4.14

* From Todd and Lindala ('28). I have rounded off all means to the nearest whole mm. (M = mean, S.D. = standard deviation; L = length, B = breadth, H = height).

the "crural index"*). The likelihood of discerning skeletal racial difference must be looked for in skull, in pelvis, and in long bone proportions.

In the discussion of race differences in the skeleton it is impossible to do more than sketch in the broad outline. This is a difficult, and, indeed, a controversial area, and had better be left to the physical anthropologist. Texts in physical anthropology, as Comas ('60), Martin ('28), Hooton ('46), Montagu ('60), and Martin-Saller ('58/'61), will provide necessary details. What I propose to undertake, in the following pages, is a general presentation of race differences in skull (including mandible), pelvis, and long bones. I plan to give useful general information, but shall include a few specific studies covering areas not generally used in racial identification.

* In the skeleton the inter-membral ratio is humerus + radius/femur + tibia; the intra-membral ratios are radius/humerus and tibia/femur.

TABLE 62

CRANIOFACIAL TRAITS OF THE THREE MAIN HUMAN STOCKS*

	Caucasoid			Negroid	Mongoloid
	Nordic (North European)	Alpine (Central European)	Mediterranean (South European)		
Skull length	Long	Short	Long	Long	Long
Skull breadth	Narrow	Broad	Narrow	Narrow	Broad
Skull height	High	High	Moderately high	Low	Middle
Sagittal contour	Rounded	Arched	Rounded	Flat	Arched
Face breadth	Narrow	Wide	Narrow	Narrow	Very wide
Face height	High	High	Moderately high	Low	High
Orbital opening	Angular	Rounded	Angular	Rectangular	Rounded
Nasal opening	Narrow	Moderately wide	Narrow	Wide	Narrow
Lower nasal margin	Sharp	Sharp	Sharp	"Troughed" or "guttered"	Sharp
Facial profile	Straight	Straight	Straight	Downward slant	Straight
Palate shape	Narrow	Moderately wide	Narrow	Wide	Moderately wide
General impression of the skull	Massive, rugged, elongate, ovoid	Large, moderately rugged, rounded	Small, smooth, elongated, pentagonoid to ovoid	Massive, smooth, elongate, constricted oval	Large, smooth, rounded

* From Krogman, '55, Table 13.

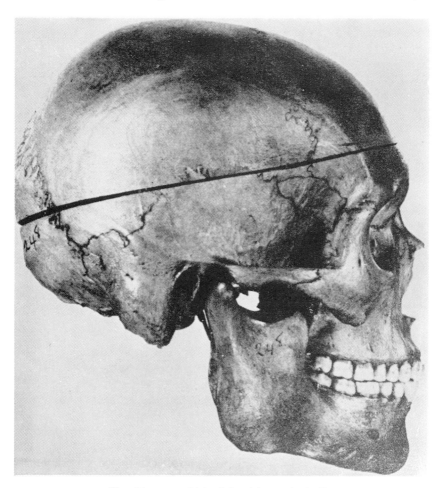

Fig. 47. A typical adult white male skull.

2. RACIAL DIFFERENCES IN THE SKULL AND MANDIBLE

In Table 62 I have outlined (Krogman, '55) the essential descriptive morphology* of the *skull* in the three main human stocks: Caucasoid (European); Negroid (African); Mongoloid (Asiatic). For the Caucasoid I present three major races: N. European (Nordic); C. European (Alpine); S. European (Mediterranean).

In a very real sense the data of Table 62 represent an arch-type

* Jones ('30/'31) points out that "non-metric" traits of the skull are exceedingly useful in diagnosis of race.

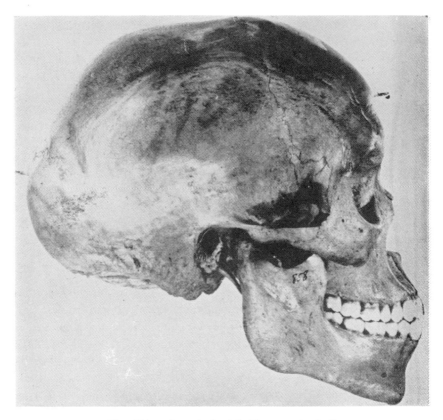

Fig. 47A.   A typical adult Negro male skull.

to the point of stereotypy.   (See Figures 47-47A.)   There really are
no "pure" races and, hence (certainly as far as the U.S. is concerned) no "pure" Negro skulls, or "pure" Mediterranean skulls,
and so forth.   There are only skulls which, to a greater or lesser
degree, present a *combination* of traits that suggests stock or race
category.   As far as mixture is concerned, as I said in Chapter I we
simply do not know enough of human genetics to do more than hint
at racial trait-dominance or trait-recessiveness in the skeleton
(see Todd, '29, and Krogman, '36).*

* Hauschild ('37) discerns racial differences in the skull at the third fetal month, as
between European and Negro fetuses.   The differences are to be found mainly in the
cranial base relations of the occipito-spheno-ethmoid areas.   It is suggested that the
definitive facial prognathism of the Negro skull is already manifest.

Todd and Tracy ('30) studied the morphological traits of 398 adult American Negro skulls (Todd Collection), 64 white Anglo-Saxon skulls (Parsons, London) and 277 African Negro skulls (von Luschan Collection, American Museum of Natural History, New York City). The skulls were studied in norma frontalis (facial view) and in norma lateralis sinistra (left lateral view); 100 of the American Negro skulls were further studied via lateral orthodiagraphic tracings made in the Reserve Craniostat.

The authors focussed on five descriptive traits, seen in *frontal view*, as follows:*

(1) Supra-orbital ridges
    *M*esa-like
    *U*ndulating
(2) Upper orbital margins
    *S*harp
    *B*lunt

(3) Glabella
    *R*ounded
    *D*epressed
(4) Fronto-nasal junction
    *P*lain
    *B*eetling
(5) Inter-orbital distance
    *N*arrow
    *W*ide

The two variants of each trait are contrasting characters and are, presumably, race-linked. The African and American Negroes seem to form two groups. The more typically negroid has undulating supra-orbital ridges, sharp upper orbital margins, a rounded glabella, a plain fronto-nasal junction, and a wide inter-orbital distance. This gives the formula of *USRPW*, or a *U-type* skull. The white skulls have mesa-like supra-orbital ridges, blunt upper orbital margins, a depressed glabella, a "beetling" fronto-nasal junction, and a narrow inter-orbital distance. This gives the formula of *MBDBN*, or an *M-type* skull. The less typically negroid type (usually American) may be expressed by the formula M (B/S) D B N, i.e., an equivalence in the blunt-sharp upper orbital margin dichotomy, suggestive of the presence of white admixture. The distribution of U-types and M-types, in all groups, is shown at top of page 194.

In *lateral view*, studied via orthodiagraphic tracings, the negroid U-type skull has a full rounded frontal contour (rounded forehead), a sagittal plateau (more or less horizontal or "flat" sagittal con-

---

* The supra-orbital ridges are the bony prominences above the orbits; glabella is the most forward projecting midline part of the frontal bone, at a level with the supra-orbital ridges; fronto-nasal junction refers to intersection of internasal and naso-frontal sutures; upper orbital margins and inter-orbital distance are self-explanatory.

Modal Characters	Supra-Orb. Ridges		Upper-Orb. Margins		Glabella		F-N Junction		Inter-Orb. Distance	
	U.	*M.*	*S.*	*B.*	*R.*	*D.*	*P.*	*B.*	*W.*	*N.*
White M-type		+	+	+	+	+		+		+
Am. Negroes M-type		+	+	+		+		+		+
East Africans M-type		+	+	+	+	+	+	+	+	
West Africans M-type		+	+				+	+	+	
White U-type	+		+		+		+	+		+
Am. Negroes U-type	+		+		+		+		+	
East Africans U-type	+		+		+		+		+	
West Africans U-type	+		+		+		+		+	

tour), often with a post-bregmatic depression (just behind where sagittal and coronal sutures intersect), and a fully rounded occipital contour. Contrariwise the M-type white skulls, and to a less extent, the hybrid Negro skulls, have a steeper frontal curve, no sagittal plateau, and a variable occipital curve. It is worthy of note that this lateral-view cranial analysis is directly applicable to tracings of lateral x-ray films of skull and head (see discussion of use of radiography in identification, Chapter X).

The cranial base has been studied in its racial aspect by several authors, but the results are rather equivocal. Ecker (1870) stated that the flexure of the cranial base (angle formed by line from anterior margin of foramen magnum to sella turcica, and from sella through floor of anterior cerebral fossa) is greater in Negroes. Kramp ('36) reported variable racial difference in the position of the condyles and mastoid processes relative to a line through the ear-holes, perpendicular to the mid-sagittal plane.

In 1955, Ray reported possible racial differences (530 white and Negro skulls, male and female) in the configuration of the superior orbital fissure as in Table 63.

His conclusions are as follows:

> The degree of similarity between fissures of the same cranium is noted. Interrelationships of the variations with race and sex are demonstrated. The greatest divergence shown between any groups, as to configuration and closure, is found between Negro males and White females. The former group shows the greatest number of widened configurations; the latter, the greatest number of narrowed, pointed, configurations. Similarly this divergence is noted in lateral closure.

It is difficult for me to evaluate just *how* a single skull is classified as white, or Negro, or Mongoloid. Each one of the items in Table 62 is carefully noted; the lateral view is studied, for frontal, sagittal, occipital contours, and for facial or profile orthognathism (straightness) or prognathism (downward and forward slant). This is, of course, largely inspectional. Certain measurements and proportions may be further useful: for example, the breadth/length index of the skull: the Negro tends to be long-headed, the Mongoloid round-headed, whites run the gamut of long- to round-headedness; the height/breadth index of the orbit: the Negro orbit tends to be lower, wider, the Mongoloid higher, more rounded, the whites in between; the breadth/height index of the nasal aperture: the Negro nasal aperture tends to be broad, the white narrow, the Mongoloid in between.

TABLE 63

SUPERIOR ORBITAL FISSURE CONFIGURATIONS IN 530 CRANIA GIVEN AS PERCENTAGES ACCORDING TO RACE AND SEX*

Race	Sex	Configuration of Superior Orbital Fissures						Similarity in R. and L. Orbits		
		P	S	R	O	C	W/B	S	Dm	D
W	M	38.7	31.5	17.3	7.6	5.2	9.2	66.2	17.7	16.1
W	F	57.7	18.6	11.5	3.2	7.7	2.6	74.4	18.0	7.7
N	M	30.4	21.2	36.8	4.6	6.2	9.7	62.5	10.3	27.2
N	F	41.6	24.7	25.2	1.9	7.0	5.8	60.0	11.5	28.8
Means		42.1	22.8	24.0	4.4	6.6	6.8	65.8	14.4	20.0

Configurations: P = point, S = square, R = round, O = oval, C = cul-de-sac. Overall configuration, W/B = wide blunt.
Similarity in orbits: S = similar, Dm = differ only to a minor degree, D = markedly different.

* From Ray, '55, Table 1.

Fortunately there is available the precise statistical tool of discriminant analysis.* In 1960, Giles and Elliot reported on discriminant functions in 408 skulls of known race (Negro or white) from the Todd and Terry Collections: 108 white male; 79 white female; 113 Negro male; 108 Negro female; average age 43.31 years, standard deviation 13.21 years. In actual calculations 75 skulls of each sex and race were randomly chosen to give a sample

* I have not used this technique personally, but have ascertained results from the literature (see Chap. V). Available texts are Rao ('52), Kendall ('57), and Williams ('59). A recent short article by McKern and Munroe is very helpful ('59).

of 300; the remaining 108 were used as an independent control series.

The skull measurements chosen were as follows:

1. Maximum length (gl-op)
2. Maximum breadth (eu-eu)
3. Baso-facial length, upper (ba–na)
4. Baso-facial length, mid (ba–pr)
5. Upper face height (na–alv. pt.)
6. Baso-frontal diam. (opis-forehead)
7. Nasal breadth

The application of discriminant function is given by Giles and Elliot as follows:

> In applying a discriminant function, we first assume on inde-
> pendent evidence that the cranial specimen came from a Negro or
> a white population. These two populations overlap to some degree
> in all of the measurements which we use to describe their skulls.
> If they did not, we would have no need for a discriminant function:
> any single non-overlapping measurement could easily place any
> skull in either the white or the Negro population. What we are
> seeking is some way of interpreting our measurements so that the
> chance of placing a white skull in the Negro population or a Negro
> skull in the white population is minimized. To do this we deter-
> mine the linear function for our 5 or 7 measurements, or variable,
> that best separates the white skulls from the Negro ones on the
> basis of these variables. Then when a skull is to be classified, it
> will give to the function a value somewhere between the two poles
> of Negroes and whites. If we have no *a priori* reason to suspect
> that the skull is more likely to be white, say, than Negro, half the
> "distance" between the mean for the Negroes and the mean for
> the whites will be the sectioning point. If the skull falls on the
> Negro side of this point it would be called Negro, if on the white
> side, it would be called white.

In practice the relative importance of the seven dimensions in both races was for *males* 7, 4, 6, 1, 3, 5, 2; for *females* 1, 6, 2, 4, 7 (nos. 3 and 5 not used in females).

In *males* of both races the seven-variate discriminant function was: baso-facial lgth., mid. + 3.457 nasal breadth + .745 max. lgth. + .663 upper face ht. − 1.178 baso-frontal diam. − 1.120 baso-facial length, upper − . 447 max. brdth. + 11.005.

In *males* of both races the five-variate discriminant function (almost as good as the preceding) was: baso-facial lgth., mid. + 4.110 nasal brdth. + 1.043 max. lgth. − 2.049 baso-frontal diam. − .579 max. brdth. + 32.750.

In *females* of both races the five-variate discriminant function was: baso-facial lgth., mid. + 2.542 nasal brdth. + 1.248 max. lgth. − 1.509 baso-frontal diam. − .958 max. brdth. + 2.336.

The authors "successfully classified over 90% of (the) sample of 408 individuals," distributed as follows (in % correct):

	Total Sample	*300 Series*	*108 Series*
7-variate male	91.0%	90.0%	93.0%
5- " "	89.1%	87.3%	93.0%
5- " female	92.5%	94.0%	86.5%

Race differences in the *mandible* is a moot question. Biometrically Morant ('36) says that racial differences in the mandible are virtually non-existent. Jankowsky ('30) studied two indices (ramal H/corpal L, and min. ramal B/min. corpal B) and concluded that dimensions and angles of the mandible were so variable that race differences are not demonstrable. Schultz ('33) feels that there are, however, morphological differences between white and Negro mandibles. The white mandible, he says, has larger breadth measures; a higher, narrower ramus; a greater gonial (mandibular) angle; ramal surfaces more parallel to the median sagittal plane; a more protrusive chin with mental tubercles more lateral in position; a higher corpal body, which is short relative to bigonial breadth; gonial angle laterally directed (some eversion); strong masseteric attachment relative to the pterygoidic attachments. In contrast, the Negro mandible has a lower, wider, and more vertical ramus; greater corpal and dental arch length (a long, U-shaped dental arch); relatively smaller breadth dimensions; a less dominant chin (i.e., mental tubercles more medial in position and smaller).

3. RACIAL DIFFERENCES IN THE PELVIS

There have been quite a few studies on the pelvic structure of *living females* of different races: Adair ('21) on French and American whites; Thoms ('46) on the American Negro; Torpin ('51) on the American white, American Negro, and Mexican. These

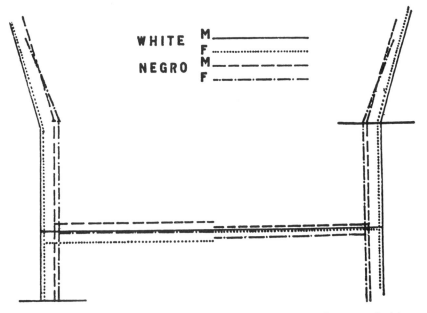

Fig. 48. Pelvic form in white and Negro. The vertical lines are fictitious, emphasizing bispinous diameter.   Horizontal line is at upper end of symphysis. Left side is erected on ischial tuberosity, right on anterior superior spine.   White pelvis is broader, white symphysis is low.   Sex differences slight.

studies have been based on both direct bodily measurements and roentgenographic pelvimetry.

Adair ('21) gives some useful racial data on the *bony pelvis*. (female only, in mm.) :

Race	Interspinous Diameter*	Intercristal Diameter*
Amerind	22.6	25.7
Javanese	20.2	21.8
Chinese	20.5–22.6	22.0–25.2
Mexican	18.0	22.1
Peruvian	21.7	25.4
European	22.2	26.6
"Aryan"	26.0	27.0
Egyptian	22.4	26.2
Bengalese	17.9	21.6
Negro (misc.)	17.4–21.7	21.4–26.9
New Caledonian	20.4	26.2
Australian	18.2	23.7
Bushman	17.0	21.5

* In Table 61 these are bi-spinous B and bi-iliac B, respectively.

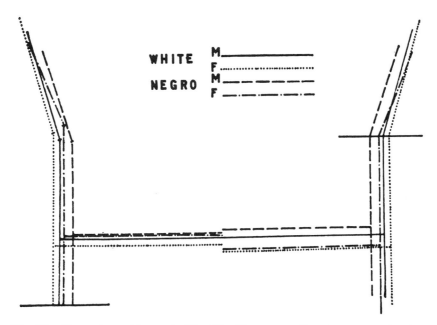

Fig. 49. General graphing as in Fig. 48. Transverse diameters proportional to torso length, vertical measurements to leg length. White pelvis relatively broader, symphysis lower, than Negro. Female relatively broader, symphysis lower, than male.

Todd's 1929 study on the American white and the American Negro pelvis is the best reference in this area. It can best be summarized by observing that the white pelvis is a wide basin for a broad torso, while the Negro pelvis is a pedestal for a narrow torso. In Figures 48 and 49 Todd's data (see also Todd and Lindala, '28) are graphically shown. It is noteworthy that Todd observed that "for individual discrimination the pelvis may be unreliable for its dimensions and ratios are not very firmly entrenched" (p. 61).

4. RACIAL DIFFERENCES IN THE LONG BONES AND SCAPULA

The four *long bones* almost invariably employed in the study of race differences are humerus, radius, femur and tibia, in terms of absolute dimensions and in terms of proportions. In 1955, I presented the following data for American whites and Negroes, male and female, as follows (in mm.) :

Traits	White		Negro	
	Male	*Female*	*Male*	*Female*
Max. L humerus	321	292	329	303
	(276–371)	(240–328)	(278–364)	(265–348)
Max. L femur	434	399	449	416
	(377–480)	(338–455)	(379–480)	(355–473)
Intermembral index	70.5	69.0	70.3	69.2
(H + R/F + T)	(65.3–75.7)	(64.5–74.4)	(66.5–74.5)	(65.6–73.6)
Brachial index	74.5	73.2	78.5	77.0
(R/H)	(67.2–79.1)	(64.9–79.3)	(70.2–84.6)	(68.1–84.1)
Crural index	83.3	83.5	86.2	86.1
(T/F)	(78.1–90.0)	(77.8–89.3)	(80.0–91.1)	(80.5–92.4)

Male bones are absolutely longer than female bones, and a bit longer in Negroes than in whites.   The intermembral index shows no real differences.   The brachial index is higher in Negroes (relatively long radius), as is also the crural index (relatively long tibia).   These are group values.   I have given the *range* for each dimension and each index.   The ranges are so great (such great over-lap) that individual identification as to race via these bones is extremely hazardous.   At best they may be corroborative; rarely are they diagnostic.

Modi ('57, p. 23) offers data similar to the foregoing for Indians of the United Provinces, Europeans, and Negroes.   He gives only average values, as follows:

Indices	U.P. Indians (Compiled by Khan)	Europeans	Negroes
1. Brachial Index (Radio-humeral Index) $\dfrac{\text{Length of Radius} \times 100}{\text{Length of Humerus}}$	76.49	74.5	78.5
2. Crural Index (Tibio-femoral Index) $\dfrac{\text{Length of Tibia} \times 100}{\text{Length of Femur}}$	86.49	83.3	86.2
3. Intermembral Index $\dfrac{\text{Length of Humerus} + \text{Length of Radius} \times 100}{\text{Length of Femur} + \text{Length of Tibia}}$	67.27	70.4	70.3
4. Humero-femoral Index $\dfrac{\text{Length of Humerus} \times 100}{\text{Length of Femur}}$	71.11	69.0	72.4

These data emphasize the non-discriminatory nature of the indices.   In the brachial index Indians are intermediate, in the crural

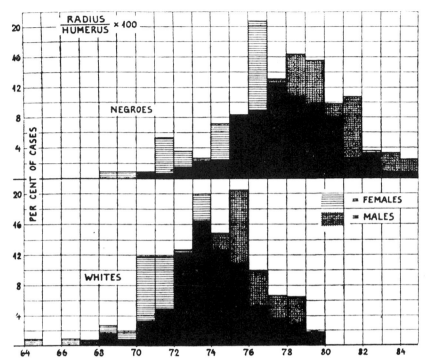

Fig. 50. Frequency diagrams showing percentage distribution of variation in brachial index, male and female, adult whites and Negroes.

index nearest Negroes, in the intermembral index set apart from both Europeans and Negroes, and in the humero-femoral index they are nearest Negroes.

Münter ('36) offers comparative racial data on the radio-humeral and humero-femoral indices (Table 64). Here, too, inter-racial over-lap is seen.

Schultz ('37) offers the most complete data in this area. In Tables 65–68 his data on the claviculo-humeral index, the inter-membral, index, the brachial index (see also Figure 50), and the crural index, are given (no. in sample, total range, mean, standard deviation, coefficient of variation, the last three with their standard errors).

The *scapula*, the principal bone of the pectoral girdle, just as the pelvis is of the pelvic girdle, has been the object of much study. Flower (1879) credits Broca, in 1878, with devising the scapular

TABLE 64

MEANS OF INDICES DERIVED FROM LENGTHS OF LONG BONES*

Series	Author	Side	$100 \times \dfrac{\text{Radius Max.}}{\text{Humerus Max.}}$		$100 \times \dfrac{\text{Humerus Max.}}{\text{Femur Obl.}}$	
			Male	Female	Male	Female
Anglo-Saxon	Munter	R	74.6 ± .19 (62)	73.5 ± .22 (31)	73.5 ± .14 (100)	73.6 ± .25 (36)
		L	75.4 ± .23 (48)	74.2 ± .21 (26)	72.2 ± .15 (77)	72.7 ± .22 (36)
Swiss	Schwerz	R + L	74.8 ± .22 (63)	73.3 ± .35 (38)	72.0 ± .17 (57)	72.1 ± .19 (52)
Norwegian	Wagner	R + L	{75.3 ± .12* (182)}	{75.1 ± .12* (172)}	{72.7 ± .09* (314)}	{74.4 ± .09* (312)}
U.S.A. (White)	Hrdlička	R	73.8 ± .12* (182)	72.8 ± .20* (62)	72.2 ± .11* (200)	71.8 ± .19* (63)
		L	73.9 ± .12* (182)	72.9 ± .20* (62)	71.7 ± .11* (200)	70.9 ± .19* (63)
Irish	"	R	73.5 ± .15* (109)	72.8 ± .16* (97)		71.7 ± .26* (35)
		L	73.5 ± .15* (109)	73.1 ± .16* (97)		70.6 ± .26* (35)
German	"	R	73.2 ± .16* (93)	72.0 ± .29* (30)	72.8 ± .17* (86)	—
		L	73.5 ± .16* (93)	71.8 ± .29* (30)	72.0 ± .17* (86)	—
Italian	"	R	74.5 ± .22* (53)		72.5 ± .25* (39)	—
		L	74.6 ± .22* (53)		72.3 ± .25* (39)	—
White of other countries	"	R	73.4 ± .17* (89)		73.9 ± .21* (53)	—
		L	73.3 ± .17* (89)		73.0 ± .21* (53)	—
French	Rollet	R	74.0 ± .18 (47)	72.2 ± .20 (48)	73.5 ± .20 (48)	72.3 ± .19 (48)
		L	74.0 ± .20 (45)	72.9 ± .24 (43)	72.4 ± .20 (47)	71.0 ± .19 (48)
Lapp	Schreiner	R + L	73.9 ± .11 (216)	73.3 ± .11 (179)	75.5 ± .09 (257)	74.3 ± .10 (215)
Predynastic Egyptian	Warren	R + L	79.3 ± .22* (52)	78.6 ± .17* (84)	70.9 ± .16* (80)	70.7 ± .13* (111)
American Indian	Hrdlička	R	77.8 ± .18* (81)	76.6 ± .22* (50)	72.4 ± .16* (99)	72.7 ± .20* (61)
		L	77.6 ± .18* (81)	76.8 ± .22* (50)	71.6 ± .16* (99)	71.8 ± .20* (61)
Pueblo Indian	Hooton	R	{77.2 ± .17* (91)}	{75.9 ± .19* (68)}	73.2 ± .15 (114)	73.8 ± .14 (85)
		L	{77.3 ± .16* (100)}	{76.0 ± .21* (57)}	72.7 ± .15 (116)	72.7 ± .16 (78)
Western Eskimo	Hrdlička	R + L	75.0 ± .14* (135)	73.1 ± .14* (133)	72.0 ± .10* (243)	71.8 ± .13* (153)
American Negro	"	R + L	77.3 ± .18* (74)	77.2 ± .27* (34)	71.6 ± .22* (50)	70.2 ± .21* (52)
Chinese	Stevenson	R	76.6 ± .23 (48)			

* The means in curled braces were found from the means of the component lengths and all others are for indices of individual skeletons. The probable errors marked with an asterisk were found by using the pooled standard deviations given in Table XIV. From Münter, '36, Table XV. No. in parentheses is size of sample.

TABLE 65

THE ADULT CLAVICULO-HUMERAL INDEX (LENGTH OF CLAVICLE IN PERCENTAGE OF
LENGTH OF HUMERUS)*

Group	Sex	Number of Skeletons	Range of Variations	$M \pm E(A)$	$S.D. \pm E(\sigma)$	$C.V. \pm E(C)$
White	♂	122	41.4–54.6	47.6 ± 0.13	2.19 ± 0.09	4.60 ± 0.20
White	♀	110	41.8–52.9	46.8 ± 0.16	2.52 ± 0.11	5.38 ± 0.24
Negro	♂	122	41.8–54.7	47.0 ± 0.15	2.43 ± 0.10	5.17 ± 0.22
Negro	♀	111	39.9–52.2	46.3 ± 0.16	2.49 ± 0.11	5.38 ± 0.24
Eskimo	♂	73	42.8–58.2	49.1 ± 0.22	2.76 ± 0.15	5.62 ± 0.31
Eskimo	♀	49	43.8–54.6	48.5 ± 0.24	2.50 ± 0.17	5.15 ± 0.35
Indian	♂	64	42.3–53.2	49.0 ± 0.18	2.10 ± 0.13	4.29 ± 0.26
Indian	♀	54	41.9–53.4	47.8 ± 0.20	2.18 ± 0.14	4.56 ± 0.30
Chinese	♂	39	44.6–55.2	48.2 ± 0.25	2.35 ± 0.18	4.88 ± 0.37
Australian	♂♀	7	39.4–45.5	43.0	—	—	—

* From Schultz, '37, Table 7. Reprinted from *Human Biology* by permission of the Wayne State University Press.

TABLE 66

THE ADULT INTERMEMBRAL INDEX (LENGTH OF HUMERUS + RADIUS IN PERCENTAGE
OF LENGTH OF FEMUR + TIBIA)*

Group	Sex	Number of Skeletons	Range of Variations	$M \pm E(A)$	$S.D. \pm E(\sigma)$	$C.V. \pm E(C)$
White	♂	122	65.3–75.7	70.5 ± 0.12	1.89 ± 0.08	2.68 ± 0.12
White	♀	110	64.5–74.4	69.0 ± 0.13	2.05 ± 0.09	2.97 ± 0.13
Negro	♂	122	66.5–74.5	70.3 ± 0.10	1.62 ± 0.07	2.30 ± 0.10
Negro	♀	111	65.6–73.6	69.2 ± 0.10	1.62 ± 0.07	2.34 ± 0.11
Eskimo	♂	73	65.9–78.0	71.7 ± 0.19	2.41 ± 0.13	3.36 ± 0.19
Eskimo	♀	49	64.9–75.0	70.2 ± 0.20	2.13 ± 0.14	3.03 ± 0.21
Indian	♂	64	67.3–75.5	71.5 ± 0.14	1.67 ± 0.10	2.34 ± 0.14
Indian	♀	54	68.9–79.2	71.3 ± 0.15	1.65 ± 0.11	2.31 ± 0.15
Chinese	♂	39	67.1–74.0	71.1 ± 0.18	1.70 ± 0.13	2.39 ± 0.18
Australian	♀♂	7	68.0–72.0	70.2	—	—	—

* From Schultz, '37, Table 8. Reprinted from *Human Biology* by permission of the Wayne State University Press.

TABLE 67

THE ADULT BRACHIAL INDEX (LENGTH OF RADIUS IN PERCENTAGE OF LENGTH OF
HUMERUS)*

Group	Sex	Number of Skeletons	Range of Variations	$M \pm E(A)$	$S.D. \pm E(\sigma)$	$C.V. \pm E(C)$
White	♂	122	67.2–79.1	74.5 ± 0.14	2.29 ± 0.10	3.07 ± 0.13
White	♀	110	64.9–79.3	73.2 ± 0.16	2.57 ± 0.12	3.51 ± 0.16
Negro	♂	122	70.2–84.6	78.5 + 0.17	2.73 ± 0.12	3.48 ± 0.15
Negro	♀	111	68.1–84.1	77.0 ± 0.19	3.04 ± 0.14	3.95 ± 0.18
Eskimo	♂	73	67.0–82.1	74.7 ± 0.21	2.64 ± 0.15	3.53 ± 0.20
Eskimo	♀	49	66.4–79.0	72.7 ± 0.24	2.52 ± 0.17	3.47 ± 0.24
Indian	♂	64	71.6–83.7	78.2 ± 0.22	2.58 ± 0.15	3.30 ± 0.20
Indian	♀	54	71.1–82.9	76.9 ± 0.22	2.38 ± 0.15	3.09 ± 0.20
Chinese	♂	39	72.5–82.0	77.3 ± 0.23	2.11 ± 0.16	2.73 ± 0.21
Australian	♂♀	7	76.0–80.7	78.3	—	—	—

* From Schultz, '37, Table 9. Reprinted from *Human Biology* by permission of the Wayne State University Press.

TABLE 68

The Adult Crural Index (Length of Tibia in Percentage of Length of Femur)*

Group	Sex	Number of Skeletons	Range of Variations	$M \pm E(A)$	$S.D. \pm E(\sigma)$	$C.V. \pm E(C)$
White	♂	122	78.1–90.0	83.3 ± 0.13	2.12 ± 0.09	2.55 ± 0.11
White	♀	110	77.8–89.3	83.5 ± 0.15	2.37 ± 0.11	2.84 ± 0.13
Negro	♂	122	80.0–91.1	86.2 ± 0.16	2.59 ± 0.11	3.00 ± 0.13
Negro	♀	111	80.5–92.4	86.1 ± 0.15	2.38 ± 0.11	2.76 ± 0.12
Eskimo	♂	73	76.0–90.1	83.0 ± 0.22	2.80 ± 0.16	3.37 ± 0.19
Eskimo	♀	49	77.4–86.8	82.3 ± 0.24	2.48 ± 0.17	3.01 ± 0.20
Indian	♂	64	80.2–92.4	85.9 ± 0.20	2.39 ± 0.14	2.78 ± 0.17
Indian	♀	54	80.3–89.8	85.2 ± 0.20	2.18 ± 0.14	2.56 ± 0.17
Chinese	♂	39	80.6–88.7	83.6 ± 0.20	1.82 ± 0.14	2.18 ± 0.17
Australian	♂ ♀	7	84.8–92.6	88.8	—	—

* From Schultz, '37, Table 10.   Reprinted from *Human Biology* by permission of the Wayne State University Press.

and infraspinous indices.   Flower stated that "when we examine the individual cases, as many of the Negroes have indices as low as some Europeans, and vice versa.   The general peculiarities of race are only developed by an extensive series" (p. 14).   Flower measured 200 European adult scapulae; his other racial samples ranged in size from 2–12 adult specimens.*

Hrdlička ('42) has studied the scapula in great detail.   I have chosen two of his Tables for presentation here (all on adult scapulae).   Table 69 gives racial data on scapular height and breadth, and the scapular index, in males and females (measurements in cm.).

In Table 70 are presented data on adult scapulae, male and female, for whites, American Indians, American Negroes, and Alaskan Eskimo.   The data are of especial value since total ranges of variation are given (dimensions in cm.).

Hrdlička concluded (p. 401) as follows:

> The racial and group differences in both the descriptive features and the dimensions of the scapula are, on the whole, but moderate and do not in any case amount to safe criteria for distinguishing the groups.   The basic proportions of the bone are throughout much alike.   What differences crop out are evidently mainly those due to stature, sex, side, and muscular variation or activity.†

* The height of the scapula is from superior to inferior angles; the breadth is from margin of glenoid fossa to base of spine on vertebral border; the scapular index is B/H × 100.   The infraspinous fossa height is from base of spine on vertebral border to inferior angle; the infraspinous index is infraspinous H/scapular H × 100.

† With respect to scapular shape and muscle function the studies of Wolffson ('50) suggest that dimensions and proportions of the scapula are in part related to muscular development and function.

TABLE 69

SCAPULAE: MAIN EARLIER DATA

(Principally after Vallois, Arranged on Basis of Scapular Index in Males by A. H)*

Group	Specimens** M F†	Male			Female			Author
		Height Total	Breadth	Scapular Index	Height Total	Breadth	Scapular Index	
Fuegian	35–28	16.02	9.90	61.8	14.33	9.22	64.3	Vallois
Eskimo	4–4	15.70	9.72	61.9	(15.87)	(9.85)	62.0	Vallois
Finn	72–14	16.55	10.25	62.4	14.80	9.32	63.9	Kajava
New Caledonia	10–5	14.83	9.60	63.6	12.86	8.94	69.5	Sarasin
Europ. White	146–102	16.76	10.65	63.7	13.55	9.05	66.8	Livon
Old Peruv. Indian	55–39	15.83	10.17	64.2	13.78	9.17	66.5	Hrdlička
Fuegian	7–2	15.38	9.88	64.3	14.20	9.40	66.1	Garson
N. W. Indian	10–14	16.52	10.48	64.3	14.07	9.37	66.1	Dorsey
Portuguese	37–20	15.92	10.21	64.4	13.62	9.04	66.5	Correa
Fuegian	4–6			64.8			65.7	Martin
French	78–68	15.92	10.37	65.2	14.11	9.28	65.9	Vallois
U. S. White	70–44	16.40	10.70	65.3	14.40	9.60	66.7	Hrdlička
Mex. Indian	9–12	15.80	10.40	65.5	13.75	9.75	70.7	Hrdlička
Egyptian	6–9			65.9			68.0	Warren
Egyptian	11–6	15.78	10.42	66.5	13.0	9.31	68.6	Vallois
Afr. Black	58–15	15.23	11.19	66.6	13.46	9.01	68.2	Vallois
Amer. Negro	46–18	16.25	10.90	66.8	14.20	9.25	65.0	Hrdlička
So. Mongol	20–4			66.9			(65.1)	Vallois
So. Utah Indian	18–10	15.10	10.15	67.4	13.70	9.70	70.6	Hrdlička
Pecos Indian	79–24	14.74	10.11	68.3	13.42	9.67	73.5	Hooton
Melanesian	20–11			68.6			69.1	Vallois
Melanesian	10–12	14.90	10.29	69.1	13.42	9.20	68.6	Sarasin
Lenape Indian	4–9	15.20	10.60	69.5	13.90	9.90	70.7	Hrdlička
Pima and Pueblo	5–5	15.50	11.05	71.0	13.80	9.95	72.0	Hrdlička
Negrillo	4–6	13.15	10.03	77.1	12.10	8.93	73.8	Vallois

* From Hrdlička, '42, p. 381.

** Number of specimens not equal for all the measurements, but nearly so.

† First figure denotes male, second female specimens.

The Human Skeleton in Forensic Medicine

TABLE 70

SCAPULAR DIMENSIONS AND INDICES: RANGES OF VARIATION*

		Height, Total	Height, Infra-spinous	Breadth (Broca's)	Indexes Scapular Total	Infra-spinous
			Male			
All Whites	Range	13.7–19.0	9.8–14.7	8.6–12.4	53.8–85.4	68.1–111.1
(1200)	Means	16.04	12.08	10.49	65.0	86.9
	R.A.**	32.8	40.6	36.2	48.6	49.5
N. A. Indian	(229)	13.0–18.4	9.9–14.8	8.9–12.0	57.3–75.9	66.2–101.3
		15.36	11.69	10.115	65.86	86.52
		35.2	41.9	30.6	28.2	40.6
Alaskan	(239)	13.1–18.4	10.0–15.0	8.7–12.2	54.2–72.5	67.4–94.6
Eskimo		16.22	12.77	10.12	62.4	79.2
		32.7	39.2	34.6	27.7	34.3
Amer. Negro	(126)	14.1–18.7	9.9–14.3	9.0–12.4	58.9–76.9	76.8–111.1
		15.98	11.66	10.66	66.7	91.4
		28.8	36.9	31.9	27.0	37.5
			Female			
All Whites	(457)	11.7–16.8	8.5–13.0	8.1–11.3	55.6–84.7	71.4–116.7
		14.19	10.67	9.39	66.3	88.1
		35.9	42.2	34.1	43.9	51.4
Indian	(179)	11.4–16.4	8.4–13.0	8.3–10.9	58.4–86.8	72.3–114.3
		13.73	10.535	9.615	70.0	91.245
		36.4	43.7	27.0	40.6	46.0
Alaskan	(197)	12.3–17.1	9.2–14.2	8.0–10.3	56.7–76.6	65.0–98.0
Eskimo		14.10	11.06	9.25	65.6	83.6
		34.0	45.2	24.9	30.3	39.5
Amer. Negro	(46)	12.6–16.1	8.8–12.4	8.7–10.6	57.7–76.3	75.6–112.8
		14.17	10.23	9.51	67.2	93.0
		24.7	35.2	20.0	27.7	40.0

* From Hrdlička, '42, p. 399.
** R.A. = Range/Average Index.

Summarizing Statement

1. Race differences in the skeleton are best known for American studies in detail, i.e., American whites and American Negroes. The Todd and Terry Collections are our basic sources of study material.

2. On the basis of the usual morphological and morphometric studies the race of the *skull* should be determined in 85–90% of cases; on the basis of discriminant analysis the accuracy (white vs. Negro) should be 90%+.

3. The *mandible* (not considering the dentition) cannot be racially classified.

4. The *pelvis*, using Todd, and Todd and Lindala, should be correctly classified (white vs. Negro) in 70–75% of cases.

5. The *long bones* are too variable to be little more than corroborative.

6. The *scapula* cannot be accurately classified with reference to racial differences.

REFERENCES

ADAIR, F.: A comparison by statistical methods of certain external pelvic measurements of French and American women. *AJOG*, *2*:256–278, 1921.

BARTH, G.: Die Volumina der längen Extremitätenknochen. *Anth. Anzeig.*, *16*: 245–259, 1939.

COBB, W. M.: The physical constitution of the American Negro. *J. Negro Educ.*, 1934, pp. 340–388.

COBB, W. M.: Physical anthropology of the American Negro. *AJPA*, *29(2)*: 113–223, 1942.

COMAS, J.: *A Manual of Physical Anthropology.* Thomas, Springfield, 1960.

ECKER, A.: Ueber die verschiedene Krümmung des Schädelrohres und über die Stellung des Schädels auf der Wirbelsäule beim Neger und beim Europäer. *Arch. f. Anth.*, *4*:287–311, 1870.

FLOWER, W. H.: On the scapular index as a race character in man. *JA*, *14*: 13–17, 1879.

GILES, E. and ELLIOT, O.: Negro-white identification from the skull. *Proc. 6th Internat. Anth. Cong.* Paris, 1960 (unpubl.).

HAUSCHILD, R.: Rassenunterscheide zwischen negriden und europiden Primordial-cränien des 3. Fetalmonats. *ZMA*, *36*:215–279, 1937.

HENNIG, C.: Das Rassenbecken. *Arch f. Anth.*, *16*:161–228, 1886.

HOOTON, E. A.: *Up from the Ape.* (ed. 2). Macmillan, 1946.

HRDLIČKA, A.: The adult scapula; additional observations and measurements. *AJPA*, *29(3)*:363–415, 1942.

JANKOWSKY, W.: Uber Unterkiefermasse und ihren rassendiagnostischen Wert. *ZMA*, *28*:347–359, 1930.

JONES, F. WOOD: The non-metric morphological characters of the skull as criteria for racial diagnosis. Pt. I. General considerations. *JA 65*:179–195 1930/31. Pt. II. Hawaiian skull. *JA*, *65*:368–378, 1930/31. Pt. III. Prehistoric inhabitants of Guam. *JA*, *65*:438–445, 1930/31.

KENDALL, M. G.: *A Course in Multivariate Analysis.* Griffin Co., London, 1957.

KIEFFER, J.: Beiträge zur Kenntniss der Veränderungen am Unterkiefer und Kiefer-gelenk des Menschen durch Alter und Zahnverlust. *ZMA*, *11*:1–82, 1907/08.

KRAMP, P.: Die topographischen Verhältnisse der menschlichen Schädelbäsis. *Anth. Anzeig.*, *13*:112–130, 1936.

KROGMAN, W. M.: 1936 (see *Refs.* Chap. I).

KROGMAN, W. M.: 1949 (see *Refs.*, Chap. II).

KROGMAN, W. M.: 1955 (see *Refs.*, Chap. II).

LEWIS, J. H.: *The Biology of the Negro.* Univ. of Chicago Press, 1942.

MARTIN, R.: 1928 (see *Refs.*, Chap. VI).

MARTIN, R. and SALLER, K.: *Lehrbuch der Anthropologie* (3rd ed.). (11 Sections now available). Urban und Schwarzenburg, Stuttgart. 1958/61.

McKERN, T. W. and MUNROE, E. H.: A statistical method for classifying human skeletal remains. *Antiquity, 24(4)*:375–382, 1959.

MICHELSON, N.: Studies in the physical development of Negroes III. Cephalic index. *AJPA n.s., 1(4)*:417–424, 1953.

MODI, J. P.: (See *Refs.*, Chap. II).

MONTAGU, M. F. A.: *Introduction to Physical Anthropology* (3rd ed.). Thomas, Springfield, 1960.

MORANT, G. M.: A biometric study of the human mandible. *Biom., 28*:84–122, 1936.

MUNTER, A. H.: A study of the lengths of the long bones of the arms and legs in man, with special reference to Anglo Saxon skeletons. *Biom., 28*:258–294, 1936.

RAO, C. R.: *Advanced Statistical Methods in Biometric Research.* Wiley Sons, N. Y., 1952.

RAY, C. D.: Configuration and lateral closure of the superior orbital fissure. Whites and American Negroes of both sexes. *AJPA n.s., 13(2)*:309–321, 1955.

SCHULTZ, A. H.: Proportions, variability and asymmetries of the long bones of the limbs and the clavicles in man and apes. *HB, 9(3)*:281–328, 1937.

SCHULZ, H. E.: Ein Beitrag zur Rassenmorphologie des Unterkiefers. *ZMA, 32*:275–366, 1933.

THOMS, H.: A discussion of pelvic variation and a report on the findings in 100 Negro women. *AJOG, 52*:248–254, 1946.

TODD, T. W.: 1929 (see *Refs.* Chap. I).

TODD, T. W. and LINDALA, A.: Dimensions of the body; Whites and American Negroes of both sexes. *AJPA, 12(1)*:35–119, 1928.

TODD, T. W. and TRACY, B.: Racial features in the American Negro cranium. *AJPA, 15(1)*:53–110, 1930.

TORPIN, R.: Roentgenpelvimetric measurements of 3604 female pelves, white, Negro, and Mexican, compared with direct measurements of Todd Anatomy Collections. *AJOG, 62*:279–293, 1951.

WILLIAMS, E. J.: *Regression Analysis.* Wiley Sons, N. Y., 1959.

WOLFFSON, D. M.: Scapula shape and muscle function, with special reference to vertebral border. *AJPA n.s., 8(3)*:331–342, 1950.

VIII

Additional Data in the Direction of Individualization and Limitation

1. GENERAL NOTE

There are certain additional data to be considered, over and beyond problems of age, sex, race, etc., on the skeleton and its parts. Also, there are several bones, e.g., ribs, sternum, sacrum, that have not been adequately covered. In a sense this Chapter is a sort of catch-all, a discussion of limiting factors, a presentation of correlative data, and a possible contribution to a further individualization of the material being identified.

2. DATA ON THE SKULL

When a skull or its parts are exhumed and received for study it must be assumed that it has undergone *alternate drying and wetting* in the earth. This raises the problem of changes that are possibly significant in relation to the cranial dimensions that existed in the actual skull of the living individual. What is the amount of change and to what extent must it be corrected? The work of Todd ('25, '26) on male and female American white, male and female American Negroes, holds the answer.

Skulls from the dissecting-table were dried (mummification) and then were wetted by live steam and by immersion in a tank (maceration). Careful measurements were taken during and after each process.

Here, as typical, I present Todd's Tables I–II ('25,) on 49 male white skulls. Mummification proceeded as follows:

		Mean	*S.D.*	*C. of V.*
(A)	Length, S.R.	184.32 ± .770	7.99 ± .544	4.33 ± .295
Cleaned, wet,	Length, glab.	183.73 ± .759	7.88 ± .537	4.29 ± .292
not macer-	Breadth	146.39 ± .549	5.70 ± .388	3.90 ± .266
ated, not cut	Aur. Height	117.18 ± .426	4.42 ± .301	3.77 ± .257
(B)	Length, S.R.	184.45 ± .771	8.00 ± .545	4.34 ± .296
Immediately	Length, glab.	183.84 ± .760	7.89 ± .537	4.29 ± .292
after section,	Breadth	146.31 ± .546	5.67 ± .386	3.92 ± .267
wet	Aur. Height	117.16 ± .432	4.48 ± .305	3.82 ± .260
(C)	Length, S.R.	183.13 ± .768	7.97 ± .543	4.35 ± .296
Final dry	Length, glab.	182.41 ± .766	7.95 ± .542	4.36 ± .297
dimensions	Breadth	145.43 ± .534	5.54 ± .377	3.81 ± .260
	Aur. Height	116.28 ± .419	4.35 ± .296	3.74 ± .255
(D)	Length, S.R.	1.34 ± .568	0.590 ± .402	44.03 ± 3.540
Total shrinkage	Length, glab.	1.40 ± .514	0.534 ± .364	38.14 ± 2.962
	Breadth	0.88 ± .620	0.643 ± .438	73.07 ± 7.169
	Aur. Height	0.89 ± 284	0.295 ± .201	33.15 ± 2.484

On the same skulls maceration was as follows:

		Mean	*S.D.*	*C. of V.*
(F)	Length, S.R.	184.26 ± .771	8.00 ± .545	4.34 ± .296
Macerated wet	Length, glab.	183.56 ± .764	7.93 ± .540	4.32 ± .294
	Breadth	146.12 ± .539	5.59 ± .381	3.82 ± .260
	Aur. Height	117.16 ± .425	4.41 ± .300	3.76 ± .256
(G)	Length, S.R.	182.97 ± .772	8.01 ± .546	4.38 ± .298
Final dry	Length, glab.	182.31 ± .769	7.98 ± .544	4.38 ± .298
dimensions	Breadth	145.04 ± .546	5.67 ± .386	3.91 ± .266
	Aur. Height	116.06 ± .419	4.35 ± .296	3.75 ± .255
(H)	Length, S.R.	1.29 ± .435	0.452 ± .308	35.04 ± 2.674
Total shrinkage	Length, glab.	1.26 ± .473	0.491 ± .334	38.97 ± 3.027
	Breadth	1.08 ± .619	0.642 ± .437	59.44 ± 5.305
	Aur. Height	1.10 ± .404	0.419 ± .285	38.09 ± 2.958
(I)	Length, S.R.	1.48		
Complete	Length, glab.	1.53		
shrinkage,	Breadth	1.27		
i.e., B to G	Aur. Height	1.10		

It was found that shrinkage in mummification was complete in eight weeks, and equalled 0.6–0.8% of the final cranial dimension (length, breadth, auricular height). After maceration dimensions are restored to within 0.3% of their "green" or original wet state. After maceration shrinkage is complete by four weeks; here the dried dimensions are within 0.8–1.0% of the green dimensions (in his '26 study Todd went up to 1.0–1.2%). It was concluded ('25, p. 187):

> Mummification, maceration and drying after maceration represent, for practical purposes, merely variations in the water content of the bones. No unforeseen factors influence the cranial dimensions as a result of these procedures.

TABLE 71

NUMBER OF THE MEASURED NORMAL SELLAE AND THE SIZE OF THE SELLAR AREA IN
SQUARE MILLIMETERS IN THE DIFFERENT AGES AND SEXES (VARIATION AND MEAN)*

	Male			Female			Total		
	N	*Range*	*Mean*	*N*	*Range*	*Mean*	*N*	*Range*	*Mean*
– 4 wk.	4	11– 16	14.5	4	10– 19	13.5	8	10– 19	14.0
2– 6 mo.	22	13– 36	19.7	12	11– 28	18.7	34	11– 36	19.4
7–12 mo.	14	17– 38	26.0	13	18– 38	28.5	27	17– 38	27.2
13–18 mo.	15	20– 42	32.3	15	21– 46	33.1	30	20– 46	32.7
19–30 mo.	19	28– 54	38.8	14	27– 54	40.6	33	27– 54	39.6
3– 5 yr.	40	30– 69	48.0	27	29– 69	46.0	67	29– 69	47.2
6– 8 yr.	33	37– 79	58.9	27	37– 72	51.3	60	37– 79	55.5
9–11 yr.	31	43– 86	65.0	19	43– 80	64.0	50	43– 86	64.5
12–14 yr.	29	47– 89	71.8	22	46– 98	69.5	51	46– 89	70.7
15–17 yr.	30	46–104	80.6	17	45– 92	78.8	47	45–104	80.0
18–20 yr.	33	54–121	83.2	28	58–113	84.4	61	54–121	83.8
21–50 yr.	244	59–125	86.1	247	58–120	87.2	491	58–125	86.7
51–60 yr.	54	60–118	88.0	46	59–119	87.0	100	59–119	87.5
61– yr.	40	58–118	86.5	30	78–114	90.4	70	58–118	88.6

* From Haas, '54, Table I.

In its dry stage the cranium is sensitive to changes in atmospheric humidity, but the alteration in dimension due to this cause is negligible.

The problem of *cranial capacity* (endocranial or "brain" volume), is not a critical one in identification. It is too variable, and, additionally, is of little import. It may be measured directly (see, e.g. Todd and Kuenzel, '25), or it may be calculated by formulae. (See Chapter X for further discussion.)

The *thickness* of the skull has been studied by Todd ('24) on male whites. He found 11.26 mm. at glabella (frontal bone), 5.75 mm. at opisthocranion (occipital bone), 5.88 mm. at vertex (parietal bone, top), and 3.56 mm. at euryon (parietal bone, side). There is a slight increase in thickness up to 60 years of age. Bone thickness is *"extremely variable."** Certainly, there are no group differences that would make for thicker- or thinner-skulled races.

Age and sex differences in the *sella turcica* have been considered by Haas ('54) (see also Francis, '48). In Table 71 and in Figure 51 Haas' data are presented.

Kadanoff ('39) reports a positive correlation between sellar di-

* Froriep ('10/'11) reported for total skull length a range of 7–8 mm. taken up by bone, for total breadth a range of 6–12 mm., and for height a range of 4–8 mm.

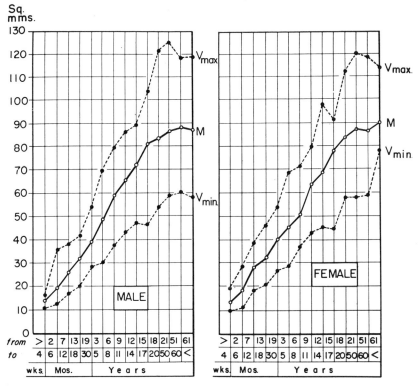

Fig. 51.   Development of male and female sellar size, showing mean and range at different ages.

mensions (length, breadth, depth) and total skull size.   There are no racial studies that I know of.

3. THE VERTEBRAL COLUMN AND THE SACRUM

The effects of *maceration* and *drying* have been noted by Todd and Pyle ('28).   For each vertebra ventral, mid-centrum, and dorsal heights were secured.   A total of 106 vertebral columns was studied: (1) 10 columns, in which lateral x-ray films were taken prior to maceration;   (2) 71 columns, in which the "green" discs were measured, prior to maceration;   (3) 25 columns, in which lateral and a-p stereoscopic x-ray films were taken prior to maceration, and which were measured while drying.   In actually measuring the 24 pre-sacral vertebral heights (one vertebra at a time) an over-all error of 6 mm. was allowed.

It was found that drying of cancellous tissue occurred within 14 days. The total column shrinkage = 2.7% of final summated dry length. "There is no constant relation of the summation of measurements of individual vertebra lengths [heights] to articulate column length."

Age-changes in vertebral body height have been studied by All-brook ('56) in the lumbar vertebrae of 51 male, 21 female, East African skeletons (age 20–50 years). The combined L1-5 heights were as follows:

	Ant. ht.	*Post. ht.*
Male	130.5 mm. (S.D. 8.7)	132.6 mm. (S.D. 8.7)
Female	128.2 " (S.D. 2.0)	128.6 " (S.D. 1.8)

In Table 72 the ant. and post. heights are given for each lumbar vertebra.

TABLE 72
AVERAGE TOTAL HEIGHT OF EACH INDIVIDUAL VERTEBRA*

Segment	Sex	Posterior Height (P)	S.D.	Anterior Height (A)	S.D.	(P-A)
L 1	Male	27.37	1.70	25.19	1.76	+2.17
	Female	26.50	0.28	25.00	1.22	+1.50
L 2	Male	27.85	1.88	26.02	1.87	+1.82
	Female	27.10	1.45	25.81	1.42	+1.29
L 3	Male	27.64	2.00	26.30	1.94	+1.35
	Female	26.60	1.52	26.10	1.34	+0.50
L 4	Male	25.92	2.10	26.20	2.56	−0.27
	Female	25.10	1.77	25.50	1.42	−0.40
L 5	Male	23.90	2.18	26.78	2.72	−2.88
	Female	23.40	1.42	25.80	1.58	−2.40

* From Allbrook, '56, Table 3.

Apart from the longer L1-5 in males it is noteworthy that in males ant. and post. vertebral heights both increased in the 20-45 year age period. This did not occur in females.

A further useful age criterion in the vertebrae, in the form of *"lipping"* (osteophytosis), has been studied by Stewart ('58). The skeletons in the Terry Collection (87 male, 17 female, 38–84 yrs.) and of Korean War dead (368 male, 17–50 yrs.) were studied.

Stewart set up a scale of *o* (no lipping) to +++ (maximum

lipping).* Numerical ranking was given, e.g., $+ = 1$, $++ = 2$, $+++ = 3$; if there was a $+$ on an upper surface of a vertebral body, a $++$ on a lower surface, the value was $1^{1}/_{2}$. Stewart presents graphs for lumbar, cervical, and thoracic vertebrae separately. In Figure 52 I present his data on the lumbar series.

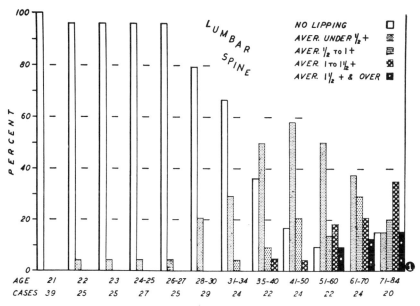

Fig. 52. Graphic occurrence of five categories of osteophytes in 306 lumbar spines of white American males, age 21–84 years.

He concludes (p. 149) that "osteophytosis by itself does not permit close ageing of skeletons. Nevertheless, in skeletons of the white race, the absence of grade $++$ vertebral lipping usually means an age under 30; and conversely, the presence of extensive lipping, including grades $++$ and $+++$ at some sites, usually means an age over 40."

For the *sacrum* Weisl ('54) has studied 62 sacro-iliac articular surfaces. The concavity of the dorsal border is more marked in females than in males. In younger subjects elevations on the articular surfaces are seen only at cranial and caudal ends (upper and

* The term "lipping" refers to the building up of bone in a sort of rampart around the periphery of the articular surfaces of the vertebral bodies.

lower). In older subjects (more frequently) size of these elevations increases, and other elevations appear just anterior to the dorsal border (posterior) and smaller ones on the ventral margin (anterior). Whether these elevations are analagous to lipping is not clear. Age variability is too extreme to be definitive.

4. THE STERNUM

At birth the sternum, or breastbone, is composed (see Girdany and Golden, '52) of five separate bones, the uppermost of which is called the manubrium, the lower four of which form the body. According to these authors segments three and four of the body fuse at 4–8 years, segments one and two at 8–25 years, by which time the body is in one piece. The manubrium fuses with the body "in old age." At the base of the sternal body there is a cartilage (ensiform or xiphoid) which may or may not calcify.

Race and sex differences in the sternum, based mainly on dimensions and proportions, have been studied by Dwight (1881 1889/90), by Stieve and Hintzsche ('23/'25), and by Hintzsche ('24).

Dwight stated a manubrium:body length ratio of 49:100 in males and 52:100 in females (49 or below, 52 or above). Union of body elements was complete by 20 years or so, but union of body and manubrium, and ossification of xiphoid cartilage, were extremely variable. In his 1881 article he concluded (p. 333) that "the breast bone is no trustworthy guide either to the sex or the age."

Stieve and Hintzsche offer dimensional data as follows (in indices):

	Male		*Female*	
	M (Range)	*S.D.*	*M (Range)*	*S.D.*
B/L of sternum	24.87 (15.1–38.7)	4.27	26.16 (11.0–37.0)	4.12
B/L of corpus	36.64 (21.7–57.4)	6.53	41.08 (18.1–61.7)	8.23
Corpus L/Manub. L	46.13 (35.4–61.4)	5.20	56.55 (40.8–83.8)	8.60

Two sex dichotomies are attempted: (1) max. corpal L over 110 mm. = male, under 85 = female; 2) a corpus L/manub. L ratio under 43.0 = male, over 58.0 = female. Variability is so great that individual definition is wholly unreliable. There are no race differences.

Age-changes in the sternum have been studied by Trotter ('33/'34), by Stewart ('54), and by McKern and Stewart ('57).

Trotter studied manubrial-corpal union in American whites and Negroes (435 male white, 307 male Negro, 45 female white, 90 female Negro, age 30–80 years). The incidence of union was about 10%; white females showed the condition twice as frequently as in males of either race. There is "no correlation between the incidence of the variation and age."

Stewart studied sterni (mostly archaeological material) in terms of age-changes in other skeletal areas, as follows (pp. 527–28):

1. *Up to the time the proximal epiphysis of the humerus is uniting (up to 17–18? year?).*

Component elements of the corpus sterni are still identifiable, although those in the inferior two-thirds may have fused. Joint surfaces here and in the manubrium are rounded, dimpled or billowed, and exhibit a matte-like surface texture.

2. *Coincident with, and somewhat following, the union of the proximal epiphysis of the humerus (about 19–20? years).*

Epiphyseal plates can be found in all stages of union on the clavicular facets. At the end of this period epiphyseal plates are beginning to unite on the rib facets, or failing the formation of plates, the articular surfaces are beginning to glaze over. Also, in most cases, the superior element of the corpus is fusing with the element next below.

3. *Coincident with the union of the epiphyses for the iliac crest and ischial ramus (about 20–23? years).*

The eminence marking the boundary between the articular areas of the clavicle and first rib gives way to a sharp transverse ridge. The last step in the formation of this ridge is the filling-in of a ventral interarticular notch. At this time the facets for the third ribs are usually divided by a transverse cleft, the last remaining sign of the recent fusion of the superior element of the corpus.

4. *Coincident with and immediately following union of the epiphysis at the sternal end of the clavicle (about 23–30? years).*

Raised rim is formed around the articular areas of the first and second ribs and those of the superior intersternal joint. By this time the superior intersternal joint has broadened so that the articular surfaces are rectangular. Facets for first ribs become slightly more porous. Clefts in facets for third ribs are being bridged across ventrally and dorsally.

5. *Just before or coincident with the appearance of arthritis in the vertebrae (about 35 years).*

Hypertrophic bone spurs appear around the margins of the facets for the first ribs, particularly ventrally and dorsally and more above than below. The other rib facets develop spurs much more slowly. Also, there may be progressive, disorderly break-down of the joint surfaces.

McKern and Stewart (368 Korean War dead, male, 17–50 years) found fusion of the component elements of the corpus sterni to be "essentially complete in most cases by 22–23 years, although rarely the uppermost segment was found still separate as late as 27 years." Signs of recent union were occasionally found in the depths of costal notches III and IV "throughout the third decade." The

TABLE 73

Exostoses Along the Margins of the Costal I Notch, by Size and According to Age* (in %)

Age	No. of Cases Observed**	No Exostoses	Slight (1)	Medium (2)	Moderate (3)	Large (4)
21–23	73	94.5	5.5	—	—	—
24–25	25	80.0	20.0	—	—	—
26–27	25	68.0	28.0	4.0	—	—
28–30	26	38.5	42.3	15.4	3.8	—
31–35	28	25.0	53.6	14.3	7.1	—
36–40	15	13.3	40.0	26.7	13.3	6.7
41–50	5	—	40.0	20.0	40.0	—

* From McKern and Stewart, '57, Table 47.
** Cases not recorded: 18 in 21–23 age group, 3 in 24–25 age group, 3 in 28–30 age group, 1 in 41–50 age group.

epiphyseal plate for the surface of the clavicular notch united between 18–22 years, "with greatest activity at 19 years." Obviously immature costal I notches were not found after 23 years; by 26 years all signs of immaturity had disappeared. Costal I notch showed a "slightly raised rim" (lipping?) at all ages between 21–50 years, "but cases with sizeable spurs or exostoses were rarely seen before 30 (see Table 73).

Upon the upper border of the manubrium sterni there occur small separate bones called "ossa suprasternialia." They have been studied in great detail by Cobb ('37) in 2204 skeletons of the

Todd Collection, American whites and Negroes, male and female. These bones ossify between 17–23 years of age. Average size is L = 10.4 mm., B = 10.4 mm., H = 7.3 mm., though over-all size varies from that of a small lead shot to that of a carpal bone (female lunate). They may occur singly or in pairs. "The ossicles appear three times more frequently in whites than in Negroes. They are more than twice as frequent in white males as in Negro males, and nearly eight times more frequent in white females than in Negro females."

5. THE RIBS

The 12 ribs that articulate posteriorly with the thoracic vertebrae have two sets of epiphyses: (1) on the head; (2) on the costal tubercle (often double). Stevenson ('24) grouped head and tubercle by observing that ribs were completely united after the 22nd year. McKern and Stewart ('57) offer data on rib heads only. Earliest union observed is in the 17th year, but ribs "complete their maturation in the 23rd year" (24 years of age).

The upper ribs, 1–3, and the lower ribs, 10–12, unite earliest ribs 4–9 latest. This upper-lower priority is found in the bodies of the vertebrae also.

Lanier ('44) studied the lengths of ribs 1, rib 12, and accessory ribs (cervical and lumbar) in American whites and Negroes. His data are given in Table 74.

The conclusions are as follows (p. 145):

1. The first ribs of Whites are longer than those of Negroes. The first ribs of White males, Negro males and White females are longer than those of Negro females; there is no difference in length of first ribs in the first three groups. There is no difference in variability in length of first ribs between the races; first ribs of White females and Negro males vary more in length than those of White males and Negro females.

2. There is no racial difference in length of twelfth ribs. Twelfth ribs of males are longer than those of females. Twelfth ribs are longer than first ribs in White males, Negro males, and Negro females. Twelfth and first ribs are of equal length only in White females. Twelfth ribs vary in length more than first ribs, and in Whites more than in Negroes.

TABLE 74

LENGTH (IN MM.) OF FIRST AND TWELFTH RIBS, SIDES COMBINED*

	First Ribs				Twelfth Ribs			
	No.	Mean	Standard Deviation	Coefficient of Variation	No.	Mean	Standard Deviation	Coefficient of Variation
W M	250	91.6 ± 0.4	6.4 ± 0.3	7.0 ± 0.3	221	107.7 ± 2.1	30.8 ± 1.5	28.6 ± 1.4
W F	176	89.5 ± 0.8	10.1 ± 0.5	11.2 ± 0.6	145	88.5 ± 2.8	34.2 ± 2.0	38.6 ± 2.3
W	426	90.7 ± 0.4	8.2 ± 0.3	9.0 ± 0.3	366	100.9 ± 1.7	33.0 ± 1.2	32.6 ± 1.2
N M	408	90.0 ± 0.4	9.1 ± 0.3	10.1 ± 0.4	400	111.0 ± 1.4	27.5 ± 1.0	24.8 ± 0.9
N F	206	85.4 ± 0.5	7.5 ± 0.4	8.8 ± 0.4	195	95.5 ± 1.8	25.6 ± 1.3	26.8 ± 1.3
N	614	88.5 ± 0.4	8.8 ± 0.3	10.0 ± 0.3	595	105.8 ± 1.2	28.1 ± 0.8	26.6 ± 0.8
W&N	1040	89.4 ± 0.3	8.7 ± 0.2	9.7 ± 0.2	961	103.9 ± 1.0	30.1 ± 0.7	29.0 ± 0.7

* From Lanier, '44, Table 3.

3. The length of the first ribs cannot be predicted from the length of the 12th rib and vice versa.

4. The incidence of certical ribs is 1.1% and lumbar ribs 8.8% in 559 subjects.

Michelson ('34) studied the calcification of the first costal cartilage in 5098 healthy (living) subjects, American white and Negro. Calcification does not occur before 11 years, and proceeds from the rib toward the sternum. There are no sex differences until 15 years, but at 16 years males of both races show more intensive calcification. The sex difference lasts until age 66 "when both sexes approach the final stage of calcification." The "most rapid increase of average calcification" is found at about 20 years, irrespective of race and sex; after 40 years the tempo drops markedly. In Negroes of both sexes the entire process proceeds more rapdily than in whites.

6. LONG BONES: NUTRIENT FORAMEN; HAVERSIAN SYSTEM

In fragmentary long bones it has been suggested that the position of the *nutrient foramen* might give a clue as to estimation of the total length of a given long bone. However it is far too variable in position. Pyle ('39) on the radius observed that on relatively longer bones the foramen is nearer the proximal end. Lütken ('50) on the humerus and femur concluded that "the position of the nutrient foramina on the shaft of these bones was so variable that it was not possible to determine one typical position" (p. 67).

It is possible that under the microscope bone fragments may be differentiated as to non-human and human, but I do not know of any such studies. For age and individual bone differences Tirelli ('10) offers micrometric data on the Haversian system of 27 skeletons (all measurements are in μ):

Age-Period	Femur	Tibia	Fibula	Clavicle	Rib
Up to 40 yrs.	48.2	60.9	63.6	47.5	51.6
40–70 yrs.	68.0	65.0	65.0	65.0	47.0
Over 70 yrs.	88.5	103.6	70.2	58.2	52.2

Tirelli additionally describes the histological picture of normal, healthy, long bones of persons of middle-age.

Hansen ('53/'54, see also William, '54) has demonstrated age-changes, seen roentgenologically, in the cancellous structure of proximal humerus and distal femur. Fazzari ('41) studied the pelvis similarly. Turkewitsch ('30) studied age and sex differences in the structure of the bony labyrinth of the auditory complex.

Deslypere and Baert ('58) published on human Haversian canals. (See also de Carvalho and Baillot, '33.) Two factors are stressed: (1) the canals show very great individual variation; (2) they are subject to repeated and extensive remodelling during life.

In general I feel at present that microscopic studies, especially of age-changes in trabeculation, may well be used sparingly. The procedures are elaborate and time-consuming and are very specialized. At best information gained may be corroborative, but not definitive.

7. BONE WEIGHTS

The use of bone weights in identification has four main possibilities: (1) differences in weight with sex; (2) with age; (3) with

TABLE 75
WEIGHTS OF ENTIRE SKELETON, AXIAL SKELETON*

	Mean in Grams	±	S.D.	±	C. of V.	±	Range Min.	Max.
Entire skeleton, except hyoid	4956.85	48.55	719.76	34.32	14.51	.71	2984	6976
Id. Teeth restored	4975.78							
1. Cranium	642.56	7.69	114.02	5.44	17.73	.87	388	983
1a. Teeth restored	652.03							
2. Mandible	81.98	1.11	16.48	.79	20.10	1.00	44	127
2a. Teeth restored	91.44							
3. Cranium and mandible	724.54	8.14	120.72	5.76	16.67	.82	435	1110
3a. Teeth restored	743.47							
4. Cervical vertebrae	73.1	.85	12.65	.60	17.33	.85	38	110
5. Thoracic vertebrae	217.28	2.60	38.58	1.84	17.78	.87	116	323
6. Lumbar vertebrae	173.13	2.40	35.52	1.69	20.54	1.02	106	282
7. Sacrum	111.48	2.10	31.18	1.49	28.10	1.44	41	189
8. Coccyx (82 cases)	1.77							
9. Spine (nos. 4–8)	576.76	7.31	108.40	5.17	18.79	.93	312	891
10. Sternum	32.5	.60	8.89	.42	27.79	1.42	13	56
11. Ribs, right	165.14						86	279
12. Ribs, left	165.04						87	285
13. Ribs, all	330.18	4.35	64.44	3.07	19.53	.97	173	564

* From Ingalls, '15, Table 1.

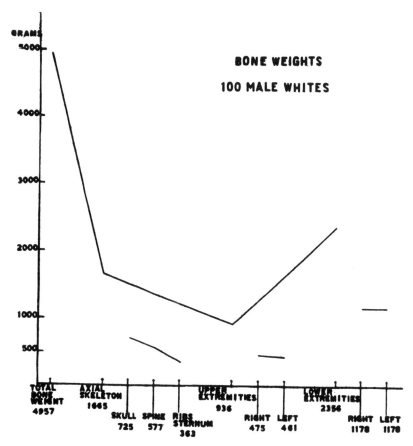

Fig. 53.   Distribution of total skeletal weight (figures below are mean weight in grams).

race; and (4) correlation with weight of entire skeleton or with other bones.   At best such data can only be corroborative, but it is all part of the total picture, so should be considered for whatever it may add.

For *entire skeleton* and for *axial skeleton*, on 100 adult male American whites Ingalls ('15) offers the following: (Table 75 and Figure 53).

In 1932, Ingalls made available data on the weight of the *foot bones* in the same sample.

In Table 76 the actual weights are given and in Table 77 weights

TABLE 76

THE WEIGHTS AND OTHER DATA LISTED IN THE TABLE BELOW ARE BASED ON 200 FEET, RIGHTS ONLY, FROM MALE WHITES*

	Mean in Grams	±	S.D.	±	C. of V.	±	Range Min.	Max.
1. Calcaneus	43.88	.46	9.72	.33	22.17	.78	20.7	73.8
2. Talus	28.77	.29	6.16	.21	21.43		14.4	44.6
3. Navicular	8.34	.09	1.88	.06	22.56		4.6	13.2
4. Cuneiform I	7.27	.08	1.71	.06	23.56		3.8	13.0
5. Cuneiform II	2.93	.03	.62	.02	21.30		1.7	4.6
6. Cuneiform III	3.90	.04	.93	.03	23.83		2.2	6.8
7. Cuboid	8.32	.10	2.16	.07	25.96	.93	4.3	14.3
8. Tarsus (nos. 1 to 7)	103.41	1.03	21.61	.73	20.90		51.8	158.2
9. Metatarsal I	12.38	.12	2.48	.08	20.07		7.2	19.9
10. Metatarsal II	6.47	.06	1.25	.04	19.26		4.0	10.4
11. Metatarsal III	5.65	.05	1.08	.04	19.18		3.4	10.0
12. Metatarsal IV	5.53	.05	1.14	.04	20.58		2.8	9.2
13. Metatarsal V	6.48	.06	1.26	.04	19.38		3.7	9.9
14. Metatarsus (nos. 9 to 13)	36.51	.31	6.42	.22	17.58	.61	22.8	56.4
15. Phalanges (Hallux)	5.72	.06	1.23	.04	21.43		3.2	9.7
16. Phalanges (II to V)	5.99						4.0	7.8
17. Phalanges (all)	11.71	.11	2.40	.08	20.53		7.2	17.5
18. Foot (nos. 8+14+17)	151.63						81.8	232.1

* From Ingalls, '32, Table 1.

TABLE 77

SAME MATERIAL AS TABLE 76: IN THE FIRST COLUMN THE WEIGHT IS REPRESENTED IN TERMS OF THE TOTAL FOOT WEIGHT; IN THE SECOND COLUMN IN TERMS OF THE SEGMENT OF THE FOOT TO WHICH THE BONE BELONGS*

	Per Cent	Per Cent
1. Calcaneus	28.95	42.45
2. Talus	18.98	27.83
3. Navicular	5.50	8.06
4. Cuneiform I	4.79	7.02
5. Cuneiform II	1.93	2.83
6. Cuneiform III	2.58	3.77
7. Cuboid	5.48	8.04
8. Tarsus (nos. 1 to 7)	68.21	100.00
9. Metatarsal I	8.16	33.91
10. Metatarsal II	4.27	17.72
11. Metatarsal III	3.72	15.47
12. Metatarsal IV	3.64	15.15
13. Metatarsal V	4.27	17.75
14. Metatarsus (nos. 9 to 13)	24.06	100.00
15. Phalanges (Hallux)	3.78	48.89
16. Phalanges (II to V)	3.95	51.11
17. Phalanges, all	7.73	100.00
18. Foot (no. 8+14+17)	100.00	—

* From Ingalls, '32, Table 2.

relative to total foot and relative to segments (tarsals, metatarsals, phalanges).

Bone weights in the foot are stable in the 19–30 and 31–40 years age groups. The foot bones share in the final (senile) loss of bone weight of the skeleton generally; this is more evident in the metatarsals and the phalanges than in the tarsals.

In 1935, Pyle reported on the left *hand bone* weights of 64 adult American whites. The data are given in Table 78.

Bone weights of the hand are, in order: metacarpals II, III, I, IV, prox. phalanx III, metacarpal V, prox. phalanx II, IV, capitate, prox. phalanx I, navicular, hamate, prox. phalanx V, mid. phalanx III, lunate, greater multangular, mid. phalanx IV, II, triquetral, lesser multangular, dist. phalanx I, mid. phalanx V, pisiform, dist. phalanx III, II, IV, V.

Carpal weight is the most variable. "There is some evidence that the bones which are heaviest at maturity acquire postnatal centers of ossification first." Metacarpal weights are less variable than phalangeal weights.

In 1954, Trotter* made a study of the weight of the skeleton based on 24 white American males, age 18–87 years. The long bones were weighed separately; the rest of the skeleton in groups of skull, vertebra, sacrum and coccyx, ribs, hand, foot. Matiegka's formula (based on skeletal rather than living measurements) was tested.† The middle one-half of each pair of femora was

---

* Trotter's description ('54, pp. 539–40) of the preparation of human skeletal material for study is as follows:

> Each cadaver was embalmed with either 10% formalin, or with a solution combining two parts of glycerine, two parts of 95% alcohol and one part of phenol crystals. Before dissection the bodies were stored for varying periods in 3% carbolic acid. Following removal of soft parts, the skeletons were prepared for the Collection by the Terry method. This involved immersion of the bones in hot water (96°–98°C.) for 72 hours or less after which the remaining soft parts were removed with either a hard bristle brush or a soft wire rotating brush. They were then laid on a tilted drain board and allowed to dry at room temperature. When thoroughly dry, the "greasy" skeletons were placed in a Leipzig degreaser and exposed to fumes from benzol for a period of approximately 17 hours. After removal from the degreaser they were allowed to stand for a day. The bones were then "sized" by dipping in a very thin solution of glue which contained 3% carbolic acid. Finally, they were dipped again in 10% formalin.

† It is based on stature and the max. transverse diameters of the lower end of humerus forearm, femur, and leg. The squared average of these four dimensions (o^2), times stature in cm. (L) = weight of skeleton (O), or $o^2 \times L = O$.

TABLE 78
WEIGHT OF THE LEFT CARPUS*

Carpal	Number	Mean Grams	Standard Deviation	Coefficient of Variability	Range Minimum	Maximum
Navicular	63	2.23 ± .04	0.53 ± .03	23.76 ± 1.52	1.27	3.56
Lunate	64	1.69 ± .03	0.39 ± .02	23.02 ± 1.44	0.91	2.54
Triquetral	64	1.18 ± .02	0.29 ± .02	24.24 ± 1.51	0.45	1.90
Greater Multangular	63	1.65 ± .03	0.40 ± .02	24.06 ± 1.52	0.94	2.75
Lesser Multangular	64	1.14 ± .02	0.28 ± .02	24.82 ± 1.58	0.62	2.00
Capitate	64	2.72 ± .05	0.64 ± .04	23.64 ± 1.51	1.15	4.60
Hamate	64	2.21 ± .04	0.48 ± .03	21.76 ± 1.40	1.23	3.55
Pisiform	61	0.61 ± .01	0.17 ± .01	27.37 ± 1.84	0.24	1.04
Total Carpals	57	13.56 ± .22	2.59 ± .16	19.02 ± 1.24	7.86	19.01
Metacarpal I	64	4.66 ± .07	0.87 ± .05	18.61 ± 1.17	3.00	6.97
Metacarpal II	64	7.12 ± .11	1.32 ± .08	18.51 ± 1.17	4.70	10.22
Metacarpal III	64	6.67 ± .11	1.26 ± .08	18.82 ± 1.17	4.40	9.50
Metacarpal IV	64	4.06 ± .07	0.78 ± .05	19.31 ± 1.17	2.47	5.70
Metacarpal V	64	3.47 ± .06	0.67 ± .04	19.37 ± 1.17	2.23	4.87
Total Metacarpals	57	25.99 ± .39	4.42 ± .28	17.01 ± 1.10	18.05	33.32
Proximal Phalanx I	51	2.27 ± .04	0.41 ± .03	18.06 ± 1.24	1.37	3.25
Proximal Phalanx II	51	3.22 ± .06	0.59 ± .04	18.26 ± 1.24	2.15	4.49
Proximal Phalanx III	51	4.02 ± .07	0.76 ± .05	18.93 ± 1.31	2.62	5.35
Proximal Phalanx IV	51	3.07 ± .05	0.57 ± .04	18.44 ± 1.24	1.89	4.19
Proximal Phalanx V	51	1.87 ± .03	0.35 ± .02	18.56 ± 1.31	1.07	2.69
Total Proximal Phalanges	51	14.42 ± .25	2.67 ± .18	18.38 ± 1.24	9.60	19.73
Middle Phalanx II	51	1.22 ± .02	0.26 ± .02	20.98 ± 1.46	0.72	1.72
Middle Phalanx III	51	1.82 ± .04	0.38 ± .03	21.04 ± 1.46	1.00	2.47
Middle Phalanx IV	51	1.47 ± .03	0.30 ± .02	20.41 ± 1.39	0.75	2.10
Middle Phalanx V	51	0.75 ± .02	0.16 ± .01	21.22 ± 1.46	0.37	1.15
Total Middle Phalanges	51	5.27 ± .01	1.07 ± .07	20.30 ± 1.39	3.11	7.42
Distal Phalanx I	51	0.88 ± .02	0.20 ± .01	22.15 ± 1.46	0.61	1.34
Distal Phalanx II	51	0.46 ± .01	0.12 ± .01	25.00 ± 1.77	0.27	0.64
Distal Phalanx III	51	0.50 ± .01	0.13 ± .01	25.20 ± 1.77	0.29	0.76
Distal Phalanx IV	51	0.40 ± .01	0.09 ± .01	22.83 ± 1.62	0.25	0.57
Distal Phalanx V	51	0.31 ± .003	0.03 ± .002	10.65 ± 0.74	0.18	0.45
Total Distal Phalanges	51	2.55 ± .24	0.53 ± .04	20.78 ± 1.46	1.71	3.58
Total Phalanges	51	22.32 ± .41	4.66 ± .31	20.88 ± 1.46	14.86	30.62
Total Carpus	48	61.38 ± .99	10.25 ± .71	16.70 ± 1.20	41.79	83.71

* From Pyle, '35, Table 1.   Reprinted from *Human Biology* by permission of the Wayne State University Press.

x-rayed and areas of compact bone determined with a planimeter. The sum of the areas of the compact bone of each pair was recorded in square cms.   Trotter's conclusions are as follows (pp. 549–50):

> The mean weight of the skeletons is 4459.9 gm. and the standard deviation 800.8 gm.   Stature is significantly correlated with skeleton weight but age and skeleton weight are not significantly correlated.   The correlation coefficient between the average weight of the femurs and the weight of the skeleton is .9591.   The standard error of estimate of skeleton weight, estimated from the average weight of the femurs is 231.71 gm.
>
> Matiegka's formula for estimating skeleton weight from stature and maximum transverse diameters of the distal ends of arm, forearm, thigh and leg was tested by substituting cadaver stature and the transverse diameters of the appropriate bones for the measurements of the living.   The correlation coefficient between the resultant estimated skeleton weights and the actual skeleton weights is .7007—practically the same as was found between cadaver stature and skeleton weight.
>
> Measurements of the femur tested for correlation with skeleton weight are length, area of a projection from an anterior view, and area of compact bone (as shown by x-ray) in the middle half of its length.   The last of these three variables provides the highest coefficient of correlation with skeleton weight.   The combination of stature, the area of compact bone in the middle half of the femur, and skeleton weight, has a multiple correlation coefficient of .8234 significant at the .001 level.   The standard error of estimate of skeleton weight determined from these two variables is 475.5 gm.
>
> Thus, of the independent variables which have been tested, and may be obtained from the living, the weight of the skeleton may be estimated with the least standard error of estimate from stature and the sum of the areas of compact bone in the middle half of the femurs (as shown in an x-ray, postero-anterior view).   The estimated weight will vary from the true weight in one-third of the cases by as much as, or more than, 475.5 gm. which is approximately 11% of the mean weight of this sample of White male skeletons in the Terry Collection.

The problem of skeletal weight in the living, based on measurements and weights of individual bones, was studied by Merz, Trotter, and Peterson ('56).   A series of 204 skeletons from the Terry Collection was used: American whites and Negroes, both

MEANS AND STANDARD DEVIATIONS (S.D.) OF THE VARIABLES ACCORDING TO RACE, SEX AND AGE*

Cases no.	Interval	X_1 Age (years) Mean	S.D.	X_2 Stature (cm) Mean	S.D.	X_3 Femur Length (cm) Mean	S.D.	X_4 Area Shaft (cm²) Mean	S.D.	X_5 Area Compact (cm²) Mean	S.D.	X_6 % Compact X_5/X_4 Mean	S.D.	X_8 Femur Weight (gm) Mean	S.D.	Y Skeleton Weight (gm) Mean	S.D.
							White Male										
4	18–29	21.5	4.4	172.0	12.3	46.2	3.1	60.4	12.4	26.8	7.1	44.2	6.3	364	100	4445	999
8	30–39	35.1	3.4	173.1	10.5	46.2	4.4	68.0	9.1	29.2	2.9	43.5	6.4	388	68	4245	624
9	40–49	44.9	3.0	173.0	7.0	46.2	2.0	70.9	5.6	32.1	3.2	45.6	8.1	435	70	4860	710
9	50–59	55.8	4.0	171.7	4.7	46.1	2.6	68.9	5.5	30.1	3.9	43.6	2.7	395	51	4369	569
9	60–69	66.2	2.3	172.1	4.9	46.3	1.7	71.0	5.1	31.3	4.1	44.0	3.8	415	70	4432	701
9	70–79	73.6	3.3	168.1	2.8	46.3	1.5	69.8	3.7	30.2	3.5	43.3	4.7	410	34	4575	349
8	80–87	82.9	2.5	168.9	7.5	46.0	2.4	69.3	7.5	27.0	3.0	39.1	3.9	358	46	3955	457
55	18–87	56.7	18.8	171.3	7.0	46.2	2.5	69.0	6.9	29.8	4.2	43.3	5.4	398	64	4417	646
							Negro Male										
8	18–29	24.1	4.3	174.9	7.0	48.6	3.2	70.2	9.4	29.7	3.3	42.5	2.6	448	71	4915	715
8	30–39	34.2	2.9	178.5	4.4	49.9	2.0	76.2	4.9	33.8	4.7	44.3	4.2	512	65	5621	675
8	40–49	45.7	2.8	170.6	8.4	47.6	4.0	70.2	10.8	31.3	3.6	44.9	3.6	439	94	4482	1009
8	50–59	56.2	2.3	171.4	5.7	48.0	2.1	73.1	7.3	34.2	5.1	46.7	4.1	451	81	4976	890
8	60–69	62.8	3.5	167.9	10.2	48.7	2.1	74.6	8.8	35.8	4.2	47.7	5.5	477	76	4988	480
8	70–79	73.6	3.5	172.8	10.4	48.7	3.5	76.0	11.5	31.5	3.0	42.3	7.4	477	126	5340	946
5	80–91	86.4	4.2	167.8	6.4	46.8	1.8	72.3	4.2	31.0	3.1	43.0	4.0	390	50	4611	832
54	18–91	52.8	19.6	172.2	8.2	48.4	2.8	73.2	8.6	32.5	4.2	44.6	4.9	460	86	5069	822
							White Female										
7	17–39	30.0	6.2	163.3	5.0	42.9	2.8	54.5	4.2	22.0	3.0	40.5	5.6	265	38	3197	543
4	40–49	46.5	1.7	161.2	7.8	42.8	2.8	58.9	10.3	20.8	7.1	34.7	6.6	264	105	3002	844
7	50–59	55.0	2.1	164.6	5.8	44.4	1.0	61.5	5.4	24.4	3.8	39.9	5.9	290	58	3320	507
8	60–69	65.0	2.9	158.1	7.4	42.2	2.4	56.4	3.0	18.7	4.0	33.2	7.5	231	31	2984	400
8	70–79	73.0	2.7	161.4	7.8	43.6	2.2	61.3	6.9	17.3	7.0	28.0	11.0	255	67	3022	709
5	80–89	86.4	3.4	153.6	8.3	42.5	2.2	61.9	6.0	11.2	3.7	18.0	4.9	192	51	2182	400
39	17–89	59.4	18.3	160.6	7.4	43.1	2.3	58.9	6.3	19.3	6.1	32.8	10.2	251	62	2989	630
							Negro Female										
12	16–29	22.2	3.9	161.6	8.4	43.5	1.9	55.2	5.0	22.8	2.5	41.4	4.8	316	46	3736	487
7	30–39	35.7	3.5	162.1	8.1	44.8	2.9	59.9	6.8	24.8	3.9	41.3	3.0	333	83	4030	790
8	40–49	44.5	2.6	160.4	6.9	46.0	2.3	62.9	6.0	26.4	5.4	42.0	7.8	346	61	3920	646
8	50–59	54.8	3.3	160.0	3.5	43.6	1.4	58.4	5.3	25.6	4.7	43.6	5.9	291	50	3388	443
6	60–69	63.8	2.2	158.8	5.6	43.1	1.5	60.9	5.5	23.4	3.4	38.5	5.3	325	74	3827	656
9	70–79	73.0	3.1	160.0	5.6	44.7	1.9	60.9	3.8	20.8	6.0	33.9	9.1	297	68	3373	634
5	80–91	83.8	4.5	158.4	7.5	44.9	3.2	63.7	6.7	22.8	1.7	36.1	4.4	289	51	3286	612
55	16–91	50.2	20.7	161.0	6.5	44.3	2.2	59.7	5.7	23.7	4.4	39.8	6.7	314	61	3659	628

* From Merz, Trotter, Peterson, '56, Table 2.

TABLE 80

REGRESSION EQUATIONS FOR ESTIMATION (E) OF SKELETON WEIGHT (GM.), WITH COEFFICIENTS OF CORRELATION (R OR R) AND STANDARD ERRORS OF ESTIMATE (GM)*

Independent Variables	Equations	r	R	Standard Error of Estimate (gm.)
	White Male			
Area compact	$E = 93.8X_5 + 1621.3$	.6091		517.1
	Negro Male			
Stature and area shaft	$E = 28.1X_2 + 42.6X_4 - 2884.8$		.6247	654.3
	White Female			
Area compact	$E = 73.2X_5 + 1578.7$	.7078		450.7
	Negro Female			
Age, area shaft, area compact	$E = -13.6X_1 + 60.8X_4 + 29.5X_5 + 13.1$		.6864	469.7

* Stature in this study was taken on cadavers. In applying this formula to the living, adjustment should be made by adding 2.5 cm to living stature. From Merz, Trotter, Peterson, '56, Table 7.

sexes (55 male W, 54 male N, 39 female W, 55 female N), age 16–29, and by decades to 80–91. The data used to determine Y, the weight of the skeleton are: X_1 age in years; X_2 cadaver stature in cms.; X_3 av. max. length of femurs in cms.; X_4 av. area of mid. $^1/_2$ of femur in a–p x-ray film in cms.^{2}; X_5 av. area of compact bone in mid. $^1/_2$ of femur in a–p x-ray film in cms.^{2}; X_6 av. area of compact bone in % av. area mid. $^1/_2$ of femur $(100X_5/X_4)$; X, av. weight of femurs in gms. These variables were presented in Table 79, according to race, sex, and age.

The regression formulae based on the data in Table 9 are presented in Table 80, as follows.

Trotter (56a) gives the following correlations with skeletal weight (SW):

Correlation	r
Stature and SW	.6909
Femur weight and SW	.9591
Femur length and SW	.5833
Femur cond. brdth. and SW	.5344
Area of femur and SW	.7159
Area compact bone femur and SW	.7634

There is no correlation with age.

The internal structure of the femur is more highly correlated with skeletal weight than any of its dimensions.

TABLE 81

(Weights of the entire skeleton and of its component parts, and weights of these parts expressed as percentages of total skeletal weight. Weights of the paired bones include weights of both right and left bones. Numbers in parentheses following coefficients of variation indicate the order of increasing size of these coefficients.)*

	Average Weight in Gm. and S.D.			Coefficient of Variation	Percentages of Skeletal Weight and S.D.	Coefficient of Variation
Skeleton	2882	±	365	12.66 (1)		
Skull	514	±	88	17.19 (6)	17.98 ± 2.99	16.64 (13)
Mandible	69.2	±	11.6	16.80 (5)	2.42 ± 0.41	17.08 (14)
Hyoid	1.13	±	0.49	43.61 (21)		
Vert. column	290	±	48.2	16.63 (4)	10.06 ± 1.03	10.23 (3)
Ribs (24)	185	±	37.2	20.09 (14)	6.42 ± 0.94	14.68 (11)
Sternum	13.5	±	3.96	29.32 (20)	0.47 ± 0.14	30.99 (17)
Clavicle	30.23	±	7.58	25.08 (18)	1.04 ± 0.20	18.90 (15)
Scapula	82.4	±	18.2	22.05 (16)	2.84 ± 0.42	14.86 (12)
Humerus	185	±	34.5	18.68 (10)	6.38 ± 0.66	10.29 (5)
Radius	63.1	±	12.7	20.16 (15)	2.18 ± 0.27	12.52 (7)
Ulna	76.8	±	14.8	19.20 (11)	2.66 ± 0.28	10.71 (6)
Hand	72.9	±	13.1	18.02 (8)	2.53 ± 0.36	14.33 (10)
Carpals, right	7.73	±	2.12	27.46 (19)	21.20 ± 3.95**	18.61
Os coxae	226	±	36.3	16.09 (3)	7.83 ± 0.68	8.73 (2)
Femur	510	±	77.5	15.19 (2)	17.67 ± 1.15	6.50 (1)
Patella	16.4	±	3.98	24.38 (17)	0.57 ± 0.12	20.34 (16)
Tibia	308	±	59.3	19.24 (12)	10.63 ± 1.09	10.27 (4)
Fibula	71.3	±	13.3	18.65 (9)	2.47 ± 0.31	12.56 (8)
Foot	167	±	29.4	17.60 (7)	5.79 ± 0.74	12.79 (9)
Tarsals, right	52.4	±	10.2	19.49 (13)	62.97 ± 2.28†	3.62

* From Lowrance and Latimer, '57, Table 1.
** Right carpals as percentage of entire right hand skeleton.
† Right tarsals as percentage of entire right foot skeleton.

For other racial/groups there are two studies on bone weights to be noted. Sitsen ('31) studied Javanese skeletons as follows (weights in gms.):

Stature Group	Pelvis Male	Scapula		Calvaria Male
		Male	Female	
Av. 150 cm.	287–472	87–140	59–78	528–697
Av. 160 "	296–488	93–149	63–84	563–744
Av. 170 "	314–518	99–158	67–90	598–790

Sitsen felt that bones in the lower 25–30% of the lower range of variation are atrophic. This, plus inherent variability, renders bone weight very doubtful in racial diagnosis.

Lowrance and Latimer ('57) offer data on 105 Asiatic skeletons, as in Table 81. (The exact provenience of these "Asiatic" skeletons is not known; all are adult; both sexes are represented.)

TABLE 82

PREDICTION EQUATIONS FOR ESTIMATING BONE ASSOCIATION*

(Dry weight in grams. Equations based on the right side only of paired bones)

White

Total skeletal weight =
8.841 Femur + 670.239 ± 278
10.823 (Tibia + Fibula) + 1036.579 ± 288
22.457 Humerus + 871.137 ± 327
32.817 (Radius + Ulna) + 800.010 ± 327
108.992 Clavicle + 1833.228 ± 420
16.197 Innominate + 1315.164 ± 241
3.739 Skull + 1760.950 ± 416

Femur weight =
.089 Total skeleton + 27.593 ± 28
1.121 (Tibia + Fibula) + 72.505 ± 26
1.965 Humerus + 109.678 ± 41
3.022 (Radius + Ulna) + 88.023 ± 39
9.120 Clavicle + 204.009 ± 48
1.470 Innominate + 139.354 ± 34
.240 Skull + 246.713 ± 54

Tibia + Fibula weight =
.071 Total skeleton − 5.292 ± 23
.733 Femur + .572 ± 21
1.650 Humerus + 49.532 ± 32
2.512 (Radius + Ulna) + 33.443 ± 30
7.415 Clavicle + 133.187 ± 39
1.100 Innominate + 98.584 ± 31
.201 Skull + 164.481 ± 43

Humerus weight =
.932 Total skeleton + 16.634 ± 12
.278 Femur + 38.482 ± 15
.352 (Tibia + Fibula) + 46.336 ± 15
1.250 (Radius + Ulna) + 19.021 ± 12
3.765 Clavicle + 67.482 ± 17
.515 Innominate + 57.576 ± 14
.089 Skull + 92.025 ± 20

Negro

Total skeletal weight =
8.988 Femur + 807.686 ± 251
9.652 (Tibia + Fibula) + 1468.833 ± 296
12.472 Humerus + 2529.405 ± 355
16.853 (Radius + Ulna) + 2576.237 ± 388
56.457 Clavicle + 3280.862 ± 385
12.678 Innominate + 2306.559 ± 274
No Significant correlation to Skull

Femur weight =
.076 Total skeleton + 70.915 ± 23
1.023 (Tibia + Fibula) + 89.930 ± 21
1.407 Humerus + 188.383 ± 28
1.988 (Radius + Ulna) + 183.385 ± 32
No significant correlation to Clavicle
1.123 Innominate + 218.453 ± 27
No significant correlation to Skull

Tibia + Fibula weight =
.058 Total skeleton + 56.488 ± 23
.726 Femur + 17.745 ± 18
1.118 Humerus + 138.634 ± 25
1.824 (Radius + Ulna) + 105.431 ± 25
No significant correlation to Clavicle
.785 Innominate + 181.783 ± 27
No significant correlation to Skull

Humerus weight =
.029 Total skeleton + 29.575 ± 17
.392 Femur + .078 ± 15
.439 (Tibia + Fibula) + 23.091 ± 16
1.237 (Radius + Ulna) + 17.367 ± 14
No significant correlation to Clavicle
.508 Innominate + 73.608 ± 17
No significant correlation to Skull

Radius + Ulna weight =
  .022 Total skeleton + 14.109 ± 8
  .197 Femur + 25.691 ± 10
  .250 (Tibia + Fibula) + 31.077 ± 9
  .580 Humerus + 18.262 ± 8
  2.768 Clavicle + 43.976 ± 11
  .341 Innominate + 43.694 ± 10
  .064 Skull + 63.254 ± 14

Clavicle weight =
  .005 Total skeleton + 1.969 ± 3
  .040 Femur + 6.348 ± 3
  .049 (Tibia + Fibula) + 7.881 ± 3

  .115 Humerus + 4.966 ± 3
  .184 (Radius + Ulna) + 2.937 ± 3
  .074 Innominate + 9.026 ± 3
  .017 Skull + 10.864 ± 3

Innominate weight =
  .052 Total skeleton − 38.985 ± 14
  .468 Femur − 7.774 ± 19
  .535 (Tibia + Fibula) + 22.849 ± 22
  1.174 Humerus + 5.053 ± 22
  1.665 (Radius + Ulna) + 6.630 ± 22

  5.442 Clavicle + 60.784 ± 27
  .160 Skull + 75.231 ± 29

Skull weight =
  .140 Total skeleton + 74.936 ± 81
  .896 Femur + 309.714 ± 103
  1.146 (Tibia + Fibula) + 331.875 ± 102

  2.368 Humerus + 315.520 ± 104
  3.640 (Radius + Ulna) + 289.313 ± 102

  14.865 Clavicle + 341.674 ± 101
  1.877 Innominate + 331.657 ± 98

Radius + Ulna weight =
  .015 Total skeleton + 52.265 ± 11
  .203 Femur + 33.718 ± 10
  .263 (Tibia + Fibula) + 34.257 ± 9
  .454 Humerus + 44.323 ± 9
  1.824 Clavicle + 77.057 ± 11
  No significant correlation to Innominate
  No significant correlation to Skull

Clavicle weight =
  .004 Total skeleton + 2.471 ± 3
  No significant correlation to Femur
  No significant correlation to (Tibia + Fibula)

  No significant correlation to Humerus
  .169 (Radius + Ulna) + 2.911 ± 3
  No significant correlation to Innominate
  No significant correlation to Skull

Innominate weight =
  .049 Total skeleton − 45.861 ± 17
  .514 Femur − 36.264 ± 18
  .506 (Tibia + Fibula) + 16.255 ± 22
  .834 Humerus + 42.324 ± 21
  No significant correlation to (Radius + Ulna)

  No significant correlation to Clavicle
  No significant correlation to Skull

Skull weight =
  No significant correlation to total skeleton
  No significant correlation to Femur
  No significant correlation to (Tibia + Fibula)

  No significant correlation to Humerus
  No significant correlation to (Radius + Ulna)

  No significant correlation to Clavicle
  No significant correlation to Innominate

* From Baker and Newman, '57, Appendix B.

The study of bone weights by Baker and Newman ('57) is specifically oriented to problems of skeletal identification. It is based on the skeletons of American and Negro male casualties in the Korean War (15 white killed in action, one Negro; 80 white POW'S, 19 Negro). The dry weights of total skeleton, skull, femur, tibia plus fibula, humerus, radius plus ulna, innominate, and clavicle were taken; the max. length of each long bone was measured; and the volume of clavicle and long bones was determined by the water displacement method. The statistical treatment of these data resulted in a number of equations and correlations.

The bone weights (gms.) fit into an equation for the prediction of living weights (in lbs.) as follows:

Whites
Living weight = .024 (Dry skeletal weight) + 50.593 ± 20.1
Living weight = .233 (Dry femur weight)   + 57.385 ± 22.2
Negroes
Living weight = .013 (Dry skeletal weight) + 85.406 ± 13.7
Living weight = .163 (Dry femur weight)   + 76.962 ± 13.3

Multiple correlation coefficients and regression equations of stature (in.) and weight (lbs.) to dry skeletal weight (gms.) were as follows:

	R	Regression
White	.642	Dry skeletal weight = 8.155 living weight + 91.736 stature − 3214.457 ± 462
Negro	.541	Dry skeletal weight = 5.545 living weight + 74.374 stature − 1273.608 ± 376

Multiple correlation coefficients and regression equations of stature (in.) and weight (lbs.) to dry femur weight (gms.) were as follows:

	R	Regression
White	.703	Right femur weight = .650 living weight + 12.314 stature − 530.073 ± 43.1
Negro	.706	Right femur weight = .405 living weight + 10.001 stature − 317.912 ± 29.2

Finally, in Table 82, Baker and Newman present for white and Negro American males prediction equations for estimating long bone associations (dry weight in gms., right side only of paired bones).

The general conclusions to be derived from this study are that it is possible to predict skeletal features from the living, and vice versa; moreover, in cases of multiple burial, skeletal components are correlated closely enough to permit bone weight to be used as a sorting-out factor, a process which is accurate enough to be acceptable as a standard procedure. Basically, there is no close correlation between bone weight and living weight except very broadly, i.e., a low bone weight betokens an individual below average body weight. The femur alone gives a better correlation. Bone weight intercorrelations are a bit lower in American Negroes than in American whites.

8. BONE DENSITY

The problem of differences in bone density (weight/volume) by race, sex, and age was studied by Broman, Trotter, and Peterson ('58) on 80 adult American white and American Negro skeletons. Bone weight was taken in a dry fat-free stage, and bone volume was measured by displacement of millet seed. Lumbar vertebrae and femur were used. The basic data are given in Table 83.

TABLE 83

MEANS AND STANDARD DEVIATIONS (S.D.) OF AGE (YRS.), WEIGHT (GM.), VOLUME (CM.³) AND DENSITY (WEIGHT/VOLUME) OF VERTEBRAE AND FEMURS ACCORDING TO RACE AND SEX*

Group	Age Mean	S.D.	Bones	Weight Mean	S.D.	Volume Mean	S.D.	Density Mean	S.D.
White male	64.0	12.8	Vertebrae	110.4	20.4	276.5	49.0	.408	.098
			Femurs	310.4	54.9	499.8	63.1	.628	.114
Negro male	59.6	13.9	Vertebrae	135.4	40.2	277.0	60.7	.483	.097
			Femurs	356.0	59.8	511.2	72.6	.700	.087
White female	67.2	17.1	Vertebrae	79.8	22.9	208.8	36.3	.380	.080
			Femurs	200.0	48.7	339.6	66.6	.598	.121
Negro female	60.3	19.8	Vertebrae	101.9	24.6	229.0	42.1	.458	.141
			Femurs	235.6	44.2	368.0	59.4	.652	.129

* From Broman, Trotter, Peterson, '58, Table 2.

The authors concluded as follows:

1. The mean density of the vertebrae is significantly less than that of the femurs in each of the four groups.

2. Although the mean densities of both vertebrae and femurs are less in Whites than in Negroes and less in females than in males only the difference between races is statistically significant.

3. There is a significant and parallel decrease in the densities of vertebrae and femurs with age in each group except for the Negro male group in which the slope for vertebrae is not significant.

4. The significance of the difference between races in the mean densities is reduced when a correction for differences in ages between the groups is made, and in the case of the femurs the difference is no longer significant.

Thus, on the basis of this study it is concluded that femurs are significantly more dense than lumbar vertebrae, that both are more dense in American Negroes than in American Whites but not more dense in males than females, that the density of both series of bones decreases significantly with age at approximately the same rate regardless of race or sex, and that after correction for age differences the difference between races is significant only for vertebare densities and not for femur densities.

In 1960, Williams and Samson studied bone density radiographically, using an electronic densitometer as a gauge. Their subjects were 16 adult white Americans, 16 East Indians of Pakistan. They found that bone density, as measured, was not related to race, sex, age, weight, or height. However, they did find a correlation with body size. The subjects were ranked on a percentile basis: 25% small, 50% medium, 75% large. Five tall, heavy subjects had an average or less bone density coefficient; six short, light subjects were above average; 21 subjects showed a bone density coefficient that tended to vary with weight.

9. BLOOD-TYPING FROM BONES

Candela ('36, '37, '40) and Boyd and Boyd ('37), among others, have developed techniques to determine blood types (usually in the ABO system) from bone. In recent years the reliability of such determinations has been seriously challenged by Thieme and Otten ('57) (see also Thieme, Otten, and Sutton, '56).

Thieme and Otten used 40 bone samples from individuals of known blood type; also, they used blood stains of known type after ageing and drying. The "inhibition test" was employed on the bones. This test depends on the reduction in titer of known antisera by the inhibiting action of specific antigens. The reduction in titer is detected by the differential agglutination of appropriate red cells added to the antisera.   The results are presented in Table 84.

The authors concluded that blood-type determination from bone gave extremely variable results, due to the influence of extraneous factors.   Bacterial action produces error, especially with elapsed time, in typing blood stains.   Moreover, there is a "large chance of error" in the inhibition test itself.

TABLE 84

ABO Blood Typing Results on Variously Treated and Aged Samples of Bones and Blood[1]*

Sample	Known Type	Number Tested	Typing Results[2]				Per Cent Wrong
			0	A	B	AB	
1. Human bone aged 2 years,	0	7	6	(1)	—	—	
buried in sandy soil	A	8	(5)	3	—	—	47
	B	3	(2)	—	1	—	
	AB	1	(1)	—	—	—	
1A. Whole blood stains on filter	0	6	6	—	—	—	
paper	A	6	6	6	—	—	0
a. Dried fresh, aged 9 months	B	4	—	—	4	—	
	AB	3	—	—	—	3	
b. Samples 3 weeks in open	0	6	4	(2)	—	—	
tubes, then dried on paper	A	6	(2)	4	—	—	37
	B	4	(1)	—	3	—	
	AB	3	(1)	(1)	—	1	
c. Samples 2 months in open	0	6	3	(3)	—	—	
tubes, then dried on paper	A	6	(3)	2	—	(1)	53
	B	4	(1)	—	3	—	
	AB	3	(2)	(1)	—	—	
d. Samples with 0.5 gm.	0	3	—	—	(2)	(1)	
polluted soil added, aged	A	3	(1)	—	(1)	(1)	100
in open tubes 2 weeks,	B	3	(3)	—	—	—	
then dried on paper							

* From Thieme and Otten, '57, Table 1.
Note: 1.   Numbers in parentheses are tests giving readings different from known type.   2.   No inhibition of anti-A or anti-B is recorded as 0.   Probably little or no specific blood group substance of any type remains.

10. BONE PATHOLOGY: AMPUTATIONS

Obviously, it is not within the scope of this book to do other than indicate the gross effects of amputation, i.e., atrophy (as noted in measurement), loss of weight, and change in internal structure (as seen radiographically).

Barber ('34) reported on 14 stump dissections involving arm or thigh.   In three cases (one double) he gave scapular and clavicular weights and lengths as follows:

No.	Scapula Weight Sound	Scapula Weight Amp.	Scapula Length Sound	Scapula Length Amp.	Clavicle Weight Sound	Clavicle Weight Amp.	Clavicle Length Sound	Clavicle Length Amp.
1531	90	106	177	178	34	32	154	153
730	63	31	163	148	23	11	147	119
1456*	54	40	153	153	20	13	151	141

* Both arms amputated. Measurements under Amp. are those of the side amputated at higher level.

In eight cases (two double) femur and pelvic dimensions are given as follows:

No.	Amputation of	Weight of Femur Sound	Weight of Femur Amp.	Weight of Os Innominatum Sound	Weight of Os Innominatum Amp.
1519	Left thigh			231	227
1995	Left leg	499	428	208	201
1800	Right leg	369	260	187.5	187
1991	Left thigh			185	157.5
1332	Left thigh			210	177
1686	Right thigh			245	221
1471	Left thigh, Right foot	470	357	231	203
1697	Both legs (Right higher)	468	459	235 (left)	228 (right)

The general effect of an amputation is to decrease weight and dimensions on the affected side. Such effect will depend, of course, upon site of amputation and upon the time factor,* i.e., elapsed time between operation and study of the bones. This has been demonstrated by Todd and Barber ('34). In amputation of upper arm scapular weight loss (as a % of the sound side) was 15% at "some months," and 43–52% at three years ($\pm$), after amputation. In amputation of leg or thigh femoral loss was about 7%, innominate loss 5–20%, in recent amputations, and 5–32% in femur, 2–32% in innominate, in "long standing" amputations. Figures 54 and 55 illustrate dimensional changes in left and right humeral amputations, respectively.

In amputations below the knee there are no decreases in dimensions, but femur and patella lose 13% of weight, innominate 7%, on the operated side. A few days after amputation rarefaction begins in all bones of the operated side; this increases rapidly for about 14 days; after this texture stabilizes. Figure 56 and 57 illustrate these textural changes in humeral amputations (Todd and

* Barber ('34) notes an age factor also, i.e., in children amputation of the humerus causes early closure of humeral epiphyses (head) and of acromial epiphysis (scapula).

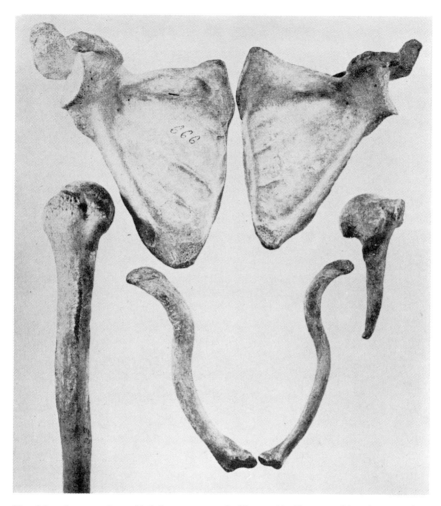

Fig. 54. Amputation of left humerus, male Negro 44–49 years old. Amputation between mid. and upper one-thirds of shaft. Shaft remnant more gracile due to atrophy; both clavicle and scapula show atrophy.

Barber, '34), affecting humeral stump, clavicle, and scapula; it is to be noted that osteoporotic changes are most marked near articular ends and at the sites of muscle attachments.*

* The effects of immobilization on normal bone (due to injury) have been noted by Conway and Stubenbord ('34). In the x-ray film bone density is decreased, cortex is thinned, medullary canal is apparently widened. These changes do not show up until three weeks post-immobilization.

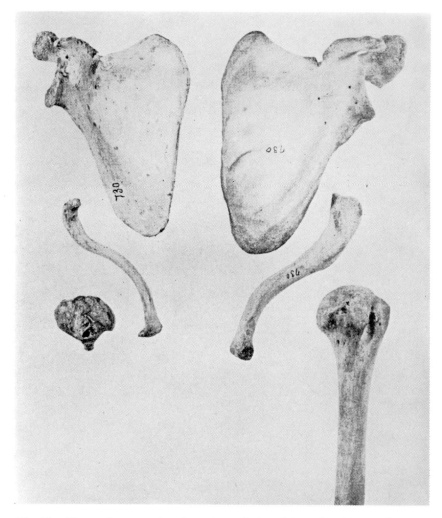

Fig. 55.   Humeral amputation through surgical neck in male white age 51 years.
Extreme atrophy with collapse of bony outlines and disorganization of joint surfaces of humeral head, scapula, and clavicle.

It is pertinent here to note that Jones ('10) warns against the
action of insects in simulating bone pathology.   In studying ancient
Nubian bones he noted (p. 264) that "syphilis has also been sup-
posed to have been not uncommon, but here . . . the damage caused
by beetles, gnawing the bones in the grave, was mistaken for the
effects of disease."

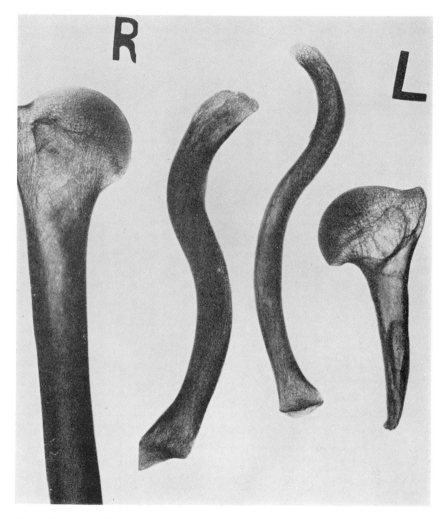

Fig. 56. X-ray film showing atrophic changes in humeral stump and clavicle. Left bones are smaller, thinner, demineralized.

Summarizing Statement

1. In the *skull* all major dimensions are reduced by 1–2% by drying. This is not enough to influence size and proportional interpretations. Endocranial volume, apart from pathology (micro- or macrocephaly) is of no import. There are no racial differences in the thickness of the vault bones, but they do get thinner with age.

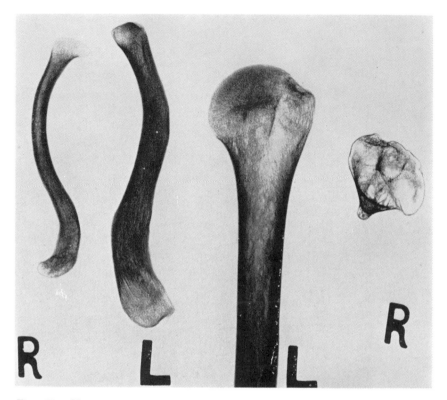

Fig. 57. X-ray film showing extreme atrophy of right humeral stump and
clavicle.

2.   In the *vertebral column* total length is reduced 2.7% by drying.
"Lipping" (osteophytosis) of the margins of the vertebral bodies
permits age estimates in lustra of 10 years.

3.   In the *sternum* there are no reliable sex differences.   For
estimation of age it may be used as corroborative.

4.   In the *ribs* all epiphyses are united by the 23rd year (the
bone is "adult" then).   Rib I tends to be longer in whites than in
Negroes.   There is no racial difference in length of rib XII.

5.   *Microscopy* of the bone is a potentially useful factor in evaluating age-changes, but at present standards are not available.
Individual variability seems to be extensive.

6.   *Bone weight* is variably correlated with total body weight.
The internal structure of bone (femur shaft) is more highly cor-

related with body weight. Bone weights have their greatest value in sorting out multiple burials.

7. *Bone density*, seen radiographically, decreases with age, but is not a reliable age indicator save in age-periods of a decade or two. It is strongly influenced by dietetic factors.

8. *Blood-typing* (ABO blood groups) from bones is not reliable.

9. In cases of *amputation* dimensional and textural changes are to be observed in the shoulder girdle (humeral amputation) and in the hip girdle (femoral amputation), on the side of amputation. These changes are atrophic. They may be useful in an individual case in establishing the possibility of non-amputation or amputation in fragmentary material.

REFERENCES

ALLBROOK, D. B.: Changes in lumbar vertebral body height with age. *AJPA* n.s., *14(1)*:35–39, 1956.

BAKER, P. T. and NEWMAN, R. W.: The use of bone weight for human identification. *AJPA* n.s., *15(4)*:601–618, 1957.

BARBER, C. G.: Ultimate anatomical modification in amputation stumps. *JBJS* o.s., 32, n.s., *16*:394–400, 1934.

BOYD, W. C. and BOYD, L. G.: Blood grouping in forensic medicine. *J. Immunol.*, *33*:159–172, 1937.

BROMAN, G. E., TROTTER, M. and PETERSON, R. R.: The density of selected bones of the human skeleton. *AJPA* n.s., *16(2)*:197–211, 1958.

CANDELA, P. B.: Blood group reactions in ancient human skeletons. *AJPA*, *21*: 429–432, 1936.

CANDELA, P. B.: Blood group determination upon Minn. and N.Y. skeletal material. *AJPA*, *23*:71–78, 1937.

CANDELA, P. B.: Reliability of blood tests on bones. *AJPA*, *27*:367–381, 1940.

CARVALHO, H. V. DE and BAILLOT, O.: Novas técnicas e novo processo de observacão microscopica dor ossos e sua applicacão medico-legal. *Arquivos de Medicina Legal e Identificão*, *3(7)*:37–41, 1933.

COBB, W. M.: The ossa suprasternalia in whites and American Negroes and the form of the superior border of the manubrium sterni. *JA*, *71(2)*:245–291, 1937.

CONWAY, F. M. and STUBENBORD, J. G.: The effects of immobilization on normal bone. *JBJS* o.s., *32*, n.s., *16*:298–302, 1934.

DESLYPERE, P. and H. BAERT: Assessment of age by the measurement of the Haversian canals of human bones: A critical study of the Balthazard and Lebrun method. *J. Forensic Med.*, *5(4)*:195–199, 1958.

DWIGHT, T.: The sternum as an index of sex and age. *JA*, *15(3)*:327–330, 1881.

DWIGHT, T.: The sternum as an index of sex, height, and age. *JA*, *24(4)*: 527–535, 1889/90.

FAZZARI, I.: Osservazioni sulla struttura radiologica dell' osso dell' anca nell' uomo. *Arch. Ital. di Anat. e di Embriol.*, *45*:413–439, 1941.

FRANCIS, C. C.: Growth of the human pituitary fossa. *HB, 20(1)*:1–20, 1948.

FRORIEP, A.: Uber die Bestimmung der Schädelkapazität, durch Messung oder durch Berechnung. *ZMA, 13*:347–74, 1910/11.

GIRDANY, B. R. and GOLDEN, R.: (See *Refs.*, Chap. II).

HAAS, L.: Einzelheiten aus der Röntgendiagnostik der Sella türcica. *Fortschr. auf dem Gebiet der Röntgenstr.*, *50(1)*:465–468; *50(2)*:468–469, 1934.

HAAS, L.: The size of the sella turcica by age and sex. *Am. J. Roentgenol. Rad. Ther.*, *Nucl. Med.*, *72*:754–761, 1954.

HANSEN, G.: Die Altersbestimmung am proximalen Humerus und Femurende in Rahmen der Identifizierung menschlicher Skelettreste. *Wissenchaft. Zeitschr. Hunboldt Univ.* Berlin, *Math.-natür-wissenchaft, 1(1)*:1–73, 1953/54.

HINTZSCHE, E.: Zur Morphologie und Anthropologie des menschlichen Brustbeins. *Anth. Anz., 1(4)*:192–199, 1924.

INGALLS, N. W.: Observations on bone weights. *AJA, 48(1)*:45–98, 1915.

INGALLS, N. W.: Observations on bone weights. II. The bones of the foot. *AJA, 50(3)*:435–450, 1932.

JONES, F. WOOD: 1910 (see *Refs.*, Chap. III).

KADANOFF, D.: Über die Beziehung zwischen der Grösse der Sella turcica und der Schädelgrösse. *Anat. Anzeig., 87*:321–333, 1939.

LANIER, R. R., JR.: Length of first, twelfth, and accessory ribs in American whites and Negroes; their relationship to certain vertebral variations. *AJPA n.s., 2(2)*:137–146, 1944.

LOWRANCE, E. W. and LATIMER, H. B.: Weights and linear measurements of 105 human skeletons from Asia. *AJA, 101*:445–459, 1957.

LUTKEN, P.: Investigation into the position of the nutrient foramina and the direction of the vessel canals in the shafts of the humerus and femur in Man. *Acta Anat., 9*:57–68, 1950.

MCKERN, T. W. and STEWART, T. D.: 1957 (see *Refs.*, Chap. II).

MERZ, A. L., TROTTER, M. and PETERSON, R. R.: Estimation of skeletal weight in the living. *AJPA n.s., 14(4)*:589–609, 1956.

MICHELSON, N.: The calcification of the first costal cartilage among whites and Negroes. *HB, 6*:543–557, 1934.

OLIVIER, G. and PINEAU, H.: Determination du sexe par les poids des os. *Bull. et Mem. de la Soc. d' Anth. de Paris*, T. 9, Ser. 10, pp. 328–339, Masson, Paris, 1957.

PRUETT, B. S.: Hypophyseal fossa in Man. *AJPA, 11*:205–222, 1927.

PYLE, S. I.: Bone weight in human carpus. *HB, 7(1)*:108–118, 1935.

PYLE, S. I.: Observation on the size and position of the nutrient foramen in the radius. *HB, 11*:369–378, 1939.

ROYSTER, L. T. and MORIARTY, M. E.: Study of size of sella turcica in white and colored males and females between 8–9 years as measured by flat x-ray films. *AJPA, 14*:451–459, 1930.

SISTEN, A. E.: Zur Bedeutung des Gewichtes bei der Anthropologischen Untersuchung des Skelettes. *Anth. Anzeig. 8(1)*:82–88, 1931.

STEWART, T. D.: The rate of development of vertebral osteoarthritis in American whites and its significance in skeletal age identification. *The Leech, 28(3,4,5)*: 144–151, 1958.

STEWART, T. D.: Metamorphosis of joints of the sternum in relation to age changes in other bones. *AJPA, n.s., 12(4)*:519–535, 1954.

STIEVE, H. and HINTZSCHE, E.: Über die Form des menschlichen Brüstbeins. *ZMA, 23*:361–410, 1923/25.

THIEME, F. P., OTTEN, C. M. and SUTTON, H. E.: A blood typing of human skull fragments from the Pleistocene. *AJPA n.s., 14(3)*:437–443, 1956.

THIEME, F. P., and OTTEN, C. M.: The unreliability of blood typing aged bone. *AJPA n.s., 15(3)*:387–398, 1957.

TIRELLI, V.: Considerazioni di medicina legale sulla ossa umane. *Arch. de Antropol., Crim. Psich. e Med. Legale., 31(ser. 4)*:80–94, 1910.

TODD, T. W.: Thickness of the male white cranium. *Anat. Rec., 27(5)*:245–256, 1924.

TODD, T. W.: The nature of mummification and maceration illustrated by the male White Skull. *JA, 59(2)*:180–187, 1925.

TODD, T. W.: The nature of mummification and maceration. II. Female white and Negro skulls. *JA, 60(3)*:309–328, 1926.

TODD, T. W. and PYLE, S. I.: Effects of maceration and drying upon the vertebral column. *AJPA, 12(2)*:303–319, 1928.

TODD, T. W. and BARBER, C. G.: The extent of skeletal change after amputation. *JBJS, o.s., 32, n.s., 16*:53–64, 1934.

TODD, T. W. and KUENZEL, W.: The estimation of cranial capacity. AJPA, *8(3)*: 251–259, 1925.

TROTTER, M.: Synostosis between manubrium and body of sternum in whites and Negroes. *AJPA, 18(4)*:439–442, 1933/34.

TROTTER, M.: A preliminary study of estimation of weight of the skeleton. *AJPA n.s., 12(4)*:537–551, 1954.

TROTTER, M.: Variable factors in skeleton weight. *HB, 28*:146–153, 1956.

TROTTER, M.: Variable factors in skeleton weight, (pp. 36–43 in Brozek, *op. cit.* 1956 a.).

TURKEWITSCH, B. G.: Alters-und Geschlechtseigenschaften des anatomische Baues des menschlichen knochernen Labyrinthes. *Anat. Anzeig., 70*:225–234, 1930.

VALLOIS, H. V.: Le poids comme caractére sexuel des os longs. *L' Anth., 61*: 45–69, 1957.

WASHBUBN, S. L.: The relation of the temporal muscle to the form of the skull. *Anat. Rec., 99(3)*:239–248, 1947.

WEISL, H.: The articular surfaces of the sacro-iliac joint and their relation to the movements of the sacrum. *Acta Anat., 22(1)*1:–14, 1954.

WILLIAM, G.: The identification of persons by X-ray examination of bone trabeculation. *Police College Mag., 3*:135–47, 1954.

WILLIAMS, D. C. and SAMSON, A.: Bone density of E. Indian and American students. *J. Am. Dietetic Assoc., 36(5)*:462–466, 1960.

IX

From Skull to Head: Restoration of
Physiognomic Details

1. THE PROBLEM

A skull may tell of age, of sex, of race, and thus in part contribute to *cranial* identification. But it may do more: it may provide a further individualization, for it may give clues as to *cephalic* identification. This is to say that the dead skull is, in a sense, the matrix of the living head; it is the bony core of the fleshy head and face in life. Upon the cranial framework (which is really subjacent to all soft tissues) we may build bit by bit, until details of physiognomy take shape, and a reasonably acceptable facsimile of a living human head emerges.

This is a tricky thing to achieve, for the skull doesn't give all the clues it should. We recognize a person by so many little details, so many subtle nuances, that it is hard to recapture precise individuality. Only a rather gross likeness may be achieved. (See Suk, '35.) Furthermore, the average identification specialist is not gifted in the necessary direction wherein art must supplement science. I refer to the creation of a bust (head and neck) in modelling clay, built upon the nuclear skull. A competent sculptor, working under my direction, using data supplied by me, has been my answer.

There are three main aspects to the skull-to-head problem, which we shall consider: (1) comparison of the skull with portraits of the presumed deceased; (2) comparison of the skull with photographs of the presumed deceased; (3) actual restoration of a head from the skull. There is available another method which will be discussed in Chapter X, i.e., reconstruction based on x-ray films of the skull. We shall now consider portraits, photographs, and plastic restoration.

2. THE RELATION OF THE SKULL TO PORTRAITS

Actually this is often more or less an exercise in historic authenticity. Anatomists and physical anthropologists who had access to skulls of famous persons pondered the relation between the skulls

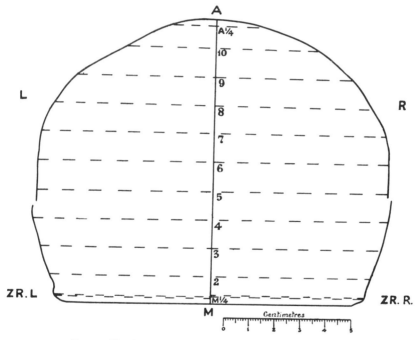

George Buchanan's Skull, Transverse Contour.

Fig. 58. George Buchanan's skull: transverse contour.

and the portraits of the persons. Were the portraits "true to life," so to speak? Did they faithfully depict the cephalo-facial proportions and relationships of the deceased? Did the artist "cheat" a bit here and there to flatter the subject? In a sense these are academic questions, but in a broader sense the skull-portrait prob-lem is a forerunner of the skull-photograph, the skull-bust, and the skull-roentgenography problems.

TABLE 85

Comparison of the Cranial Measurements of George Buchanan with those of Other Skulls*

Cranial Character	Average London Poor 17th Century ♂s.	Skull of George Buchanan	Skull of Sir Thomas Browne	Skull of Jeremy Bentham	Deviation of Buchanan skull Century ♂s. Difference S.D.
Capacity	1481	1360(??)	1509	1475	− .93
Length (Flowers)	186.1	171.3	190.0	183.5	− 2.75
Length (Maximum)	188.8	174.0	194.6	186.0	− 2.29
Breadth (Parietal)	142.4	140.0	143.7	147.0	− .41
Breadth (Minimum frontal)	96.8	98.8	87.4	99.0	+ .34
Height (Basio-vertical)	130.4	130.6(?)	122.0	—	+ .04
Height (Basio-bregmatic)	129.7	129.9(?)	121.9	132.0	+ .04
Height (Auricular)	110.0	111.0	102.6	116.0	.00
Skull Base	100.1	100.9(?)	102.7	102.0	+ .18
Arc, Transverse (Apex)	309.0	304.0	297.0	325.0(?)	− .39
Arc, Sagittal	378.8	355.4	380.0	365.0(?)	− 1.65
Arc, (Nasion to Bregma)	129.3	119.5	129.0	130.0(?)	− 1.51
Arc, (Bregma to Lambda)	128.1	124.0	123.0	120.0(?)	− .51
Arc (Lambda to Opisthion)	120.6	111.9(?Reconst.)	128.0	115.0(??)	− 1.11
Chord (Lambda to Opisthion)	97.3	91.3(?Reconst.)	99.8	97.1(?)	− 1.17
Horizontal Circumference	530.0	503.0	549.0	540.0(?)	− 1.70
Alveolar Point to Nasal Spine	19.2	21.5	21.7(?)	22.0(??)	+ .82
Facial Height	70.5	69.6	73.1(?)	73.0(?)	− .20
Facial Breadth	91.4	92.5(?)	90.9	97.0(??)	+ .18
Bizygomatic Breadth	131.0	130.0	132.3	127.0(?)	− .21
Nasal Height, R.	51.8	51.0	52.2	52.8	− .28
Nasal Height, L.	51.7	51.7	52.2	52.8	.00
Nasal Breadth	24.6	25.6(?)	22.6	26.7	+ .40
Dacryal Subtense	12.8	12.0	12.8	11.9(?)	− .45
Dacryal Chord	22.2	22.2	20.9	22.2(?)	.00
Dacryal Arc	36.1	32.0	32.7	33.0(?)	− 1.15
Simotic Subtense	4.6	4.5	5.0	4.3	− .09

Simotic Chord	9.2	10.4	8.7	9.5	+.63
Breadth, R. Orbit	42.3	45.8	43.7	45.2(?)	+2.24
Breadth, L. Orbit	42.4	44.8	42.8	46.0(?)	+1.62
Height, R. Orbit	34.3	35.9	36.3	36.0(?)	+.68
Height, L. Orbit	34.3	36.8	36.7	36.0(?)	+1.09
Palate Height	11.1	10.5	16.5	12.0(?)	−.42
Palate Breadth	39.3	36.8	37.5(??)	35.0(?)	−.82
Palate Length to base of Spine	46.0	38.7(??)	49.0(??)	47.0(?)	−2.75
Profile Length	94.4	89.5(?)	98.3(?)	89.0(?)	−.92
Length, Foramen Magnum	36.8	32.6(Reconst.??)	34.6	36.2(?)	−1.40
Breadth, Foramen Magnum	30.6		30.1	31.0(?)	
Profile Angle	85°.9	87°.8	84°.7(?)	93°.0(?)	+.60
Angle at Nasion	64°.2	60°.5(?)	65°.4	58°.0	−1.01
Angle at Basion	42°.5	42°.3(?)	42°.7(?)	44°.5	−.05
Angle at Alveolar Point	73°.3	77°.2(?)	71°.9(?)	77°.5	+1.07
1st Cephalic Index (100 B/L)	75.4	80.5	73.8	79.0	+1.47
2nd Cephalic Index (100 H/L)	69.3	75.1(?)	62.7	70.9	+1.80
3rd Cephalic Index (100 B/H)	109.1	107.2(?)	117.8	111.4	−.40
Compound Cephalic Index (100(B-H)/L)	6.7	5.4(?)	11.2	8.1	−.36
Facial Index	77.1	75.2(?)	80.4	75.3(?)	−.30
Nasal Index, R.	47.5	50.2	43.3	50.6	+.63
Nasal Index, L.	47.5	49.5	43.3	50.6	+.46
Foraminal Index	83.4	—	85.7	85.6	—
Dacryal Index	58.1	54.1	61.2	53.6(?)	+.43
Simotic Index	50.7	43.3	57.5	45.3(?)	+.57
1st Palate Index (Breadth/Length)	85.4	95.1(??)	76.5(??)	74.5	+1.75
2nd Palate Index (Height/Breadth)	28.5	28.5	33.7(??)	34.3(?)	.00
Occipital Index	58.0	58.3(?)	55.8	61.3	+.11
Orbital Index, R.	81.0	78.4	83.1	79.6(?)	−.43
Orbital Index, L.	80.9	82.1	85.7	78.3(?)	+.23
External Orbital Width	98.1	98.5	98.0	100.4(?)	+.10

* From Pearson, '26.

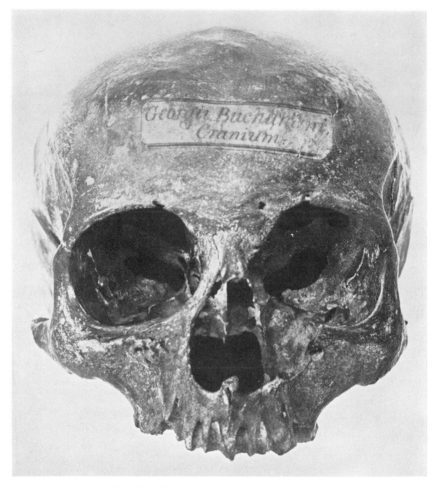

Fig. 59.   Buchanan's skull: norma facialis.

This is a very fascinating subject and it would be easy to be carried away with it.   It has all the elements of careful historical research, precise craniometric study, and acceptable scientific deduction.   Many famous persons have been thus "brought to life": Schiller and Kant (Welcker, 1883, 1888); Raphael (Welcker, 1884); Bach (His, 1895).   In the hands of the Biometric School of London University the finest studies have been prepared: Sir Thomas Browne (Tildesley, '23); Robert the Bruce (Pearson, '24); George Buchanan and Jeremy Bentham (Pearson, '26); St.

Magnus and St. Rognvald (Reid, '26); Lord Darnley (Pearson, '28); Cromwell (Pearson and Morant, '34: portraits, busts, and death masks).*

Of all of the foregoing I shall discuss in detail only one, the '26 study of George Buchanan by Pearson.

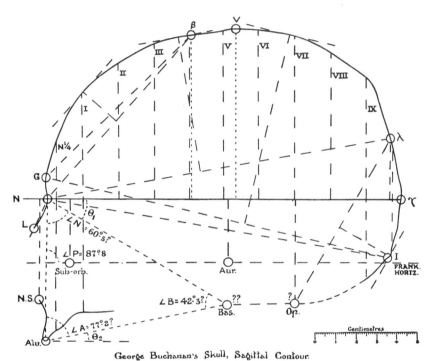

George Buchanan's Skull, Sagittal Contour.

Fig. 60. Buchanan's skull: sagittal contour.

The first step is the careful and precise measurement of the skull (col. 2 of Table 85), its comparison with other historic skulls (cols. 3 and 4 Table 85), and a sample of the contemporaneous 17th century population (cols. 1 and 5 of Table 85).

If anything Buchanan tended to have an absolutely smaller skull compared to that of the average 17th century person.

* These I have studied in detail. There are others, mentioned in Appendix II of Glaister and Brash ('37). Wilde ('59) discusses a French skeleton of the 15th century, using family records of reference to pathology (paralysis) and to general bodily traits. Hug ('59/'60) similarly describes a Swiss skeleton dated Ca. 1676, relating skull to painting.

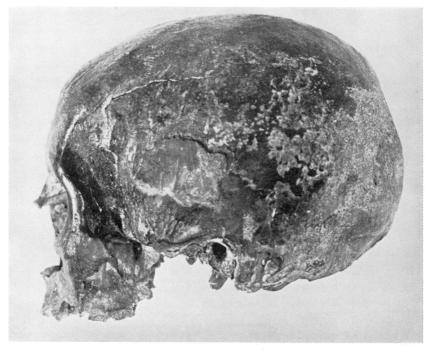

Fig. 61. Buchanan's skull: norma lateralis (left profile).

The next step is the preparation of contoural cranial drawings based on the measurements. These may be three in number:

1) A *transverse* contour, as in Figure 58, and a photograph of the skull/in facial view (norma facialis), as in Figure 59.

2) A *sagittal* contour, as in Figure 60, and a photograph of the skull in left lateral view (norma lateralis), as in Figure 61.

3) A *horizontal* contour, as in Figure 62, and a photograph of the skull from above (norma verticalis), as in Figure 63.

The general impression is that of a skull with a broad, low vault; with a rather receding forehead and a rounded occiput; and with a short oval outline as seen from above.

The next, and final step, is to see how these cranial contours fit into or with known portraits. And here a major problem arises. The contoural cranial drawings are full face, full lateral, full vertical, each at right angles to the other. Portraits are rarely so carefully oriented. As a rule a facial view is seen slightly from

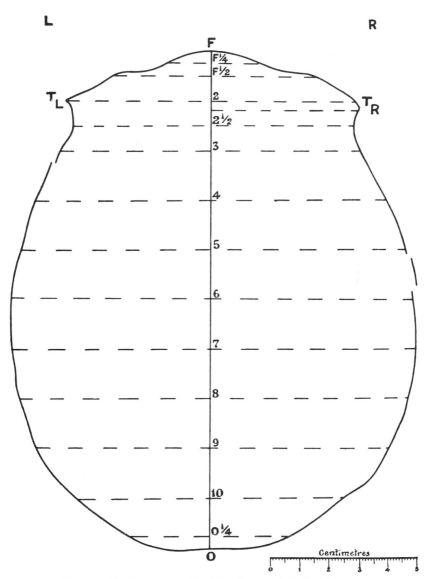

George Buchanan's Skull, Horizontal Contour.

Fig. 62. Buchanan's skull: horizontal contour.

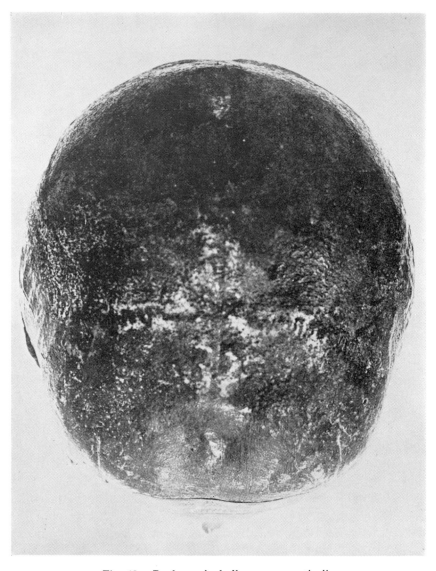

Fig. 63.   Buchanan's skull: norma verticalis.

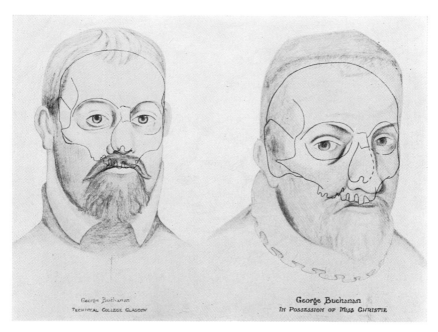

Fig. 64a-b. Facial skull tracing fit to Glasgow and Christie portraits of George Buchanan.

either the left or the right side (left or right "three-quarters view"). Therefore a *precise matching* is defeated at the start.

The matching of transverse contour with portrait, as done by Pearson, is seen in Figures 64–66, which I have chosen from Pearson's total series. Figures 64a-b give the portrait much too high a vault, as does Figure 65b and Figure 66a. Figure 65a is not too bad in the vault, but misses on breadth. Figure 66b gives the best fit of all, in vault height, in cranial breadth, in facial width, and in upper facial height.

As far as I'm concerned the skull-portrait approach is a fascinating exercise in historicity, but little else. Portraitists too often aim at a flattering or idealistic likeness rather than a trait-for-trait veracity.

3. THE RELATION OF THE SKULL TO PHOTOGRAPHS

The difficulty here is apt to be the same as in portraiture, viz., that of orientation. The usual photograph is almost always a

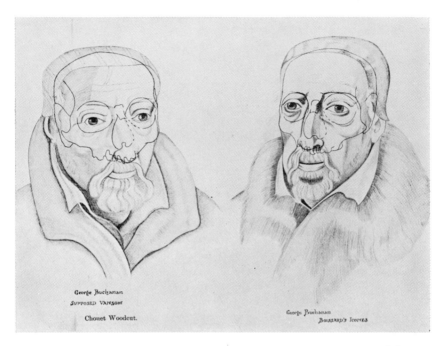

Fig. 65a-b.   Facial skull tracings fit to Chonet and Boissard portraits of George Buchanan.

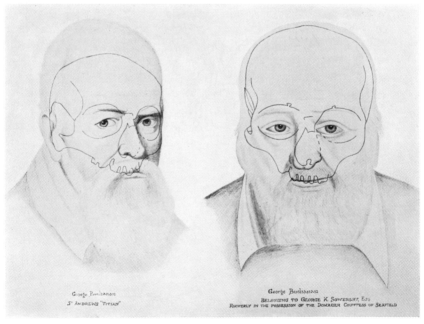

Fig. 66a-b.   Facial skull tracings fit to St. Andrews and Sowersby portraits of George Buchanan.

254

deviated one, i.e., neither facial nor lateral views are in true transverse or sagittal planes.

Lander ('17/'18) reported on the examination of a skeleton of known age, sex, and race, for which a photograph was available (see Figure 67), and concluded solely on the basis of visual inspection, "it seems improbable that anyone examining the skull would postulate a type of face similar to that seen in the photograph." In their discussion of Cromwell's skull Pearson and Morant ('34) refer to a study by Derry who photographed the head and skull of

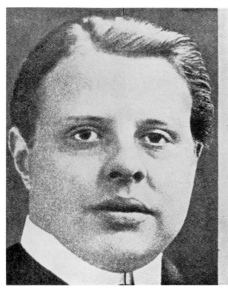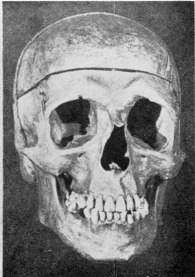

Fig. 67. Portrait and skull.

an executed Egyptian criminal. Allowing for the fact that head and skull were photographed in slightly different positions the fit is pretty good. Prinsloo ('53) used photographs of the presumed victim, related them to tracings of the skull, and achieved a satisfactory comparison.

The most successful use of skull-photograph comparison is that of Glaister and Brash ('37) in the famous "Buck Ruxton Case." I shall discuss here only the evidence for the skull attributed to Mrs. Ruxton. (Mary Rogerson's skull was similarly studied). In this case there were two skulls, listed as No. 1 and as No. 2.

Both were female. It was assumed that one was that of Mrs. Ruxton, the other that of the housemaid Mary Rogerson.

In Figures 68–69, skulls #1 and #2 are superimposed in a view that is acceptably frontal or facial, on "Portrait A" of Mrs. Ruxton; 68 does not fit, 69 does. In Figures 70-71, skulls #1 and #2 are superimposed, in a lateral view, on "Portrait B" of Mrs. Ruxton; 70 does not fit, 71 does. It is evident that Skull No. 2 is that of Mrs. Ruxton.

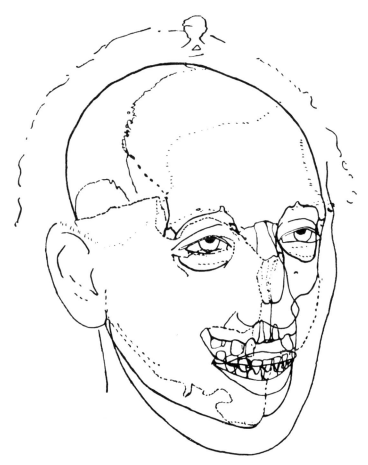

Fig. 68.   Outline of Skull No. 1 in "Photograph A" position, superimposed on outline of Mrs. Ruxton's "Portrait A." They do not correspond.

As a test of the validity of the method and the soundness of the deduction Glaister and Brash photographed a cadaver head and its resultant skull in the same position as Mrs. Ruxton's "Portrait A." This is shown in Figure 72. The skull was traced in two views, comparable to "Portrait A" and "Portrait B," and the tracings superimposed upon outlines of the cadaver head. The fit is undeniably a good one (Figures 73–74).

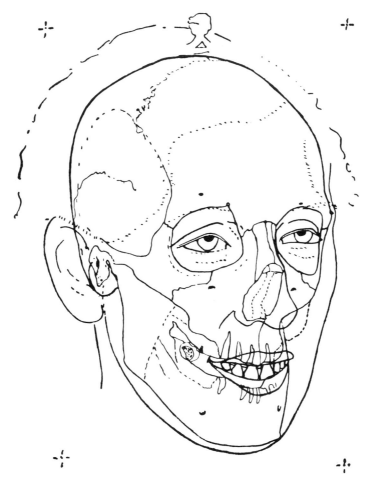

Fig. 69. Outline of Skull No. 2 in "Photograph A" position, superimposed on outline of Mrs. Ruxton's "Portrait A." They appear to correspond well. The crosses are registration marks on outlines to enable more precise superimposition.

I recommend a skull-photograph comparison whenever possible. Allowances can be made for a degree of non-comparability in *head positioning* in the photographs, as relates to the far more precisely oriented *cranial tracings*. Important corroborative and possibly conclusive evidence may thus be established.

4. THE RESTORATION OF THE HEAD FROM THE SKULL

The data upon which this work is based are from the careful measurement of the tissue thicknesses of the cadaver head and face.

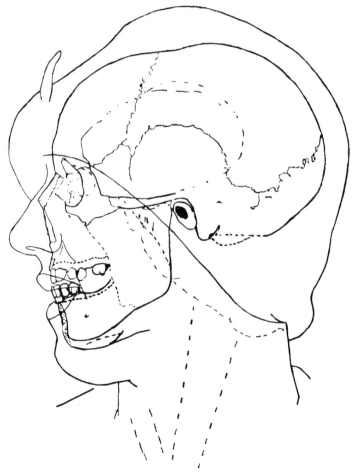

Fig. 70.   Outline of Skull No. 1 in "Photograph B" position superimposed on outlines of Mrs. Ruxton's "Portrait B."   The facial outlines do not correspond.

The basic work is that of His (1895; see Stewart, '54). He used a thin, sharp needle bearing a small piece of rubber. This was pushed into the flesh, at right angles to the bone, at a number of sites, until the point of the needle struck bone. As the needle penetrated the piece of rubber was displaced upwards from the point. The distance from point to piece of rubber was then recorded, in mm., as the thickness of the tissue at that site.

In Figure 75 the sites chosen by His are shown, numbered.

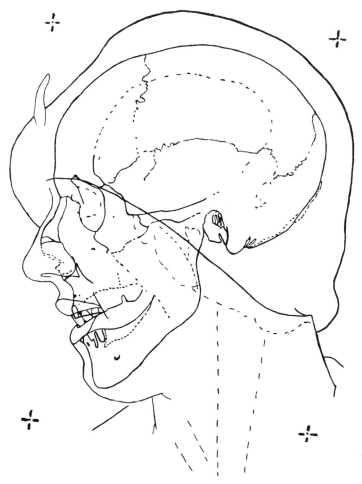

Fig. 71. Outline of Skull No. 2 in "Photograph B" position superimposed on outline of Mrs. Ruxton's "Portrait B." The outlines correspond well.

In Table 86 the corresponding thicknesses are shown (Figure 75 and Table 86 are from Stewart, '54).

In 1898, Kollmann and Büchly extended the work of His, also on cadavera. Four descriptive categories of bodily condition were set up: thin (T); very thin (VT); well nourished; (WN); very well nourished (VWN). Tissue thicknesses were averaged accordingly. In Table 87 average male (VT and WN) and average female (T and WN) tissue thicknesses are given, together with max.-min. variation for both sexes.

In Figures 76 and 77 the measuring points, identified by the abbreviations in Table 87, are shown in frontal (facial) and lateral views.

In Table 88 Kollmann and Büchly compare their results with those of His and pool the data to give mean values, plus max.-min. range, for 45 *male* cadavera (all moderately well nourished).

In Table 89 Kollmann and Büchly compare their results with

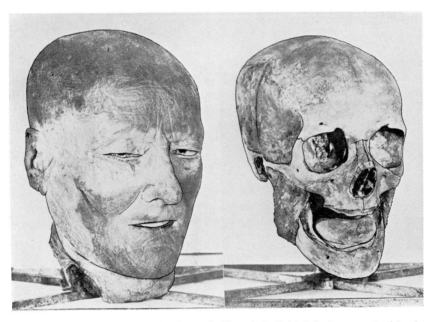

Fig. 72. Head of anatomical subject (left) and skull (right) photographed in the same position as the head of Mrs. Ruxton in her "Portrait A" (subject is female, age 84; salient details emphasized via inking).

TABLE 86

ANALYSIS OF TISSUE DEPTHS AT 15 POINTS OVER FACE AS DETERMINED ON CADAVERS*

Point of Measurement	Death After Wasting Illness (9 Males) mm.	Suicides (Sound)				Range (37) mm.
			Males		Females 18–52 Yr. (4) mm.	
		All (28) mm.	17–40 Yr. (16) mm.	50–72 Yr. (8) mm.		
A. Midline measurements:						
1. Hairline	3.4	4.08	4.03	4.1	4.16	2.5– 5.0
2. Glabella	3.9	5.17	4.91	5.3	4.75	3.0– 6.0
3. Nasion	4.8	5.45	5.50	5.6	5.0	3.0– 7.0
4. Nasal bridge	3.0	3.29	3.25	3.5	3.0	2.0– 3.5
5. Root of upper lip	10.8	11.25	11.38	11.6	9.75	8.0–14.0
6. Philtrum of upper lip	8.16	9.37	9.53	9.5	8.26	6.5–12.0
7. Mentolabial furrow	8.5	10.0	9.62	10.9	9.75	7.0–14.0
8. Chin eminence	8.5	11.05	10.66	12.2	10.75	8.0–15.0
9. Under chin where mandible has minimum depth	4.1	6.16	5.97	6.4	6.5	2.5– 8.0
B. Side face:						
10. Center of eyebrow	4.6	5.80	5.69	6.1	5.5	4.0– 8.0
11. Middle of lower border or orbit	3.75	4.90	4.56	5.6	5.25	4.0– 6.5
12. Mandibular border, in front of masseter	4.75	8.37	7.90	9.4	8.1	3.5–12.0
13. Over zygomatic arch	3.8	6.05	5.75	6.4	6.75	2.5– 9.0
14. Ascending ramus, at center of masseter	13.0	17.55	18.0	18.1	17.0	10.0–22.0
15. Gonial angle	8.0	12.08	12.12	12.3	11.5	5.5–16.0

* From Stewart, '54, Table XXV, after His (1895).

those of His and pool the data to give mean values, plus max.-min. range, for 8 *female* cadavera (all moderately well nourished).

The studies by His and by Kollmann and Büchly are so basic that all other work since then has involved either testing or the availability of similar data on other groups.   Czekanowski ('07) and von

TABLE 87

FACIAL TISSUE THICKNESSES IN MALES AND FEMALES (WHITE)*

Measuring Points (with Abbr. Used by K. and B.)		Averages				Range of Variation			
		Male		Female		Male		Female	
		VT	WN	T	WN	Max.	Min.	Max.	Min.
St. 1	Upper forehead	—	3.07	1.86	3.02	4.0	2.0	4.2	2.0
St. 2	Lower forehead	3.0	4.29	2.93	3.90	5.8	3.0	5.4	3.2
NW	Nasal root	3.1	4.31	3.53	4.10	6.0	3.0	4.7	2.5
NR	Mid nasal bone	2.5	3.13	2.1	2.57	5.0	2.1	4.0	2.0
NS	Tip of nasal bone	2.1	2.12	1.46	2.07	3.0	1.3	3.0	1.6
OW	Root of upper lip	14.7	11.65	7.1	10.1	14.7	8.3	11.0	8.0
LG	Philtrum	11.0	9.46	6.2	8.1	13.0	6.1	10.0	7.0
LF	Mental sulcus	8.8	9.84	7.2	10.95	13.5	8.0	14.1	7.8
KW	Chin prominence	5.7	9.02	4.96	9.37	13.0	5.0	12.1	7.7
K3	Under the chin	5.1	5.98	3.66	5.86	9.0	3.0	9.4	3.8
ABr	Mid eyebrow	3.8	5.41	4.1	5.15	6.8	2.0	5.5	4.6
UA	Mid infraorbital	2.1	3.51	3.76	3.65	6.1	2.1	4.4	3.0
UK	Front of Masseter	5.0	7.76	3.6	6.16	12.0	2.3	8.5	4.7
JB	Root of zygomatic arch	5.8	7.42	6.6	7.1	11.0	3.9	9.8	4.8
JB1	Highest point of zygomatic arch	3.0	4.33	2.76	5.32	7.8	1.8	8.0	3.1
WB	Highest point on malar	3.2	6.62	4.2	7.73	10.9	3.2	9.5	6.7
MS	Mid of Masseter	—	17.01	11.5	14.83	24.5	6.3	19.0	12.0
KW	Jaw angle	4.5	8.72	3.75	7.56	15.1	3.0	10.2	4.7
NL	From root of nose to alar margin	57.0	52.0	50.66	46.75	63.0	41.0	50.0	44.0
NB	Nasal breadth at alae	33.0	35.65	31.33	34.75	43.0	29.0	38.0	32.0
NT	Nasal depth from tip to root of lip	28.0	24.75	27.0	22.50	29.0	20.0	24.0	19.0
HO	Height of upper lip	19.0	21.55	19.0	20.50	27.0	18.0	23.0	19.0
RK	Oral cleft to chin prominence	35.0	33.45	29.0	25.50	42.0	28.0	30.0	25.0

* From Kollmann and Büchly, 1898.   Table 2.

Eggeling ('13) are good critique sources.   Ziedler ('19/'21) presents data on the facial soft parts of the Negro.   Harslem-Riemschneider ('21/'22) reports on the facial musculature and tissues of 14 Papuans and Melanesians.   Stadtmüller ('23/'25) combines the foregoing racial data in a comparative tabulation and adds information on a male from Java. Suzuki ('48) gives useful information on the thickness of the soft parts of the Japanese face (good, medium, and poor nourishment states).

The use of tissue thicknesses is primarily designed for a plastic reconstruction, i.e., the modelling of a bust. However, the data can be used in another manner, which is easier and quicker, though not so complete a restoration. In Figures 78–80 I show this (Krog-

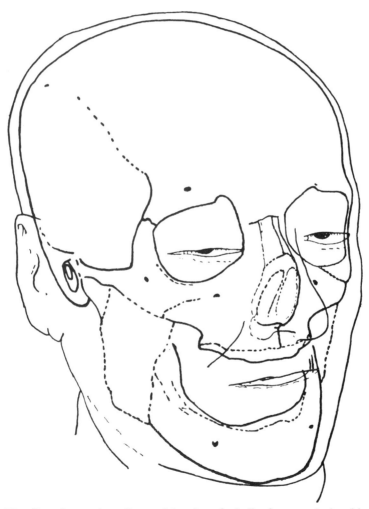

Fig. 73. Superimposed outlines of head and skull of anatomical subject in "Photograph A" position (compare with Fig. 69).

man, '43, Pt. II).   In Figure 78 is shown the facial view of the skull of a male Negro, age 65 years.   In Figure 79 small blocks of clay, to average tissue thickness of a moderately well-nourished white male (as in Table 88), have been placed at 15 sites.   In Figure 80 one-half of the face is sketched in, with physiognomic details added (drawing by John Adams).   Virchow ('14) has done much the same in his "half skull-half mask" approach.

TABLE 88

AVERAGE AND RANGE OF FACIAL TISSUE THICKNESSES IN 45 MALE WHITE CADAVERA*

Measuring Points (with Abbrev. Used by K. and B.)		Averages			Range of Both Studies	
		His (24)	Kollmann-Büchly (21)	Combined 45	Maximum —	Minimum —
St. 1	Upper forehead	4.06	3.07	3.56	5.0	2.0
St. 2	Lower forehead	5.10	4.29	4.69	6.0	3.0
NW	Nasal root	5.55	4.31	4.93	7.0	3.0
NR	Mid nasal bone	3.37	3.13	3.25	5.0	2.1
NS	Tip of nasal bone	—	2.12	2.12	3.0	1.3
OW	Root of upper lip	11.49	11.65	11.57	14.7	8.3
LG	Philtrum	9.51	9.46	9.48	13.0	6.1
LF	Mental sulcus	10.26	9.84	10.05	14.0	8.0
KW	Chin prominence	11.43	9.02	10.22	15.0	5.0
K3	Under the chin	6.18	5.98	6.08	9.0	3.0
ABr	Mid eyebrow	5.89	5.41	5.65	8.0	2.0
UA	Mid infraorbital	5.08	3.51	4.29	6.1	2.1
UK	Front of Masseter	8.65	7.76	8.20	12.0	2.3
JB	Root of zygomatic arch	6.07	7.42	6.74	11.0	3.9
JB1	Highest point of zygomatic arch	—	4.33	4.33	7.8	1.8
WB	Highest point on malar	—	6.62	6.62	10.9	3.2
MS	Mid of Masseter	18.05	17.01	17.53	24.5	6.3
KW	Jaw angle	12.21	8.72	10.46	16.0	3.0
NL	From root of nose to alar margin	—	52.0	52.0	63.0	41.0
NB	Nasal breadth at alae	—	35.65	35.65	43.0	29.0
NT	Nasal depth from tip to root of lip	22.63	24.75	23.69	29.0	20.0
HO	Height of upper lip	22.12	21.55	21.83	27.0	18.0
RK	Oral cleft to chin prominence	49.12	33.45	41.28	57.0	28.0

* From Kollmann and Büchly, 1898.   Table 4.

The more detailed plastic reconstruction, modelled in clay, is shown in Figure 81, in a step-by-step study by Stewart ('54) (see also Krogman, McGregor, Frost, '48).

The skull-head plastic reconstruction method has never been thoroughly tested.   In Kupffer and Hagen (1881) it was found that Kant's skull dimensions varied from the cast dimensions, ranging from −4 mm. (cast smaller) in orbital height to +24 mm. (cast larger) in horizontal circumference. In 1946, I took measurements on a cadaver head (American Negro male, ca. 40 years), on the

TABLE 89

AVERAGE AND RANGE OF FACIAL TISSUE THICKNESSES IN 8 FEMALE WHITE CADAVERA*

Measuring Points (with Abbrev. Used by K. and B.)		Averages			Range of Both Studies	
		His (4)	Kollmann-Büchly (4)	Combined 8	*Maximum* —	*Minimum* —
St. 1	Upper forehead	4.16	3.02	3.59	4.5	2.0
St. 2	Lower forehead	4.75	3.90	4.32	5.5	3.2
NW	Nasal root	5.0	4.10	4.55	5.5	2.5
NR	Mid nasal bone	3.0	2.57	2.78	4.0	2.0
NS	Tip of nose	—	2.07	2.07	3.0	1.6
OW	Root of upper lip	9.75	10.1	9.92	11.0	8.0
LG	Philtrum	8.26	8.1	8.18	10.0	6.0
LF	Mental sulcus	9.75	10.95	10.35	14.1	7.5
KW	Chin prominence	10.75	9.37	10.06	13.0	7.7
K3	Under the chin	6.5	5.86	6.18	9.4	3.8
ABr	Mid eyebrow	5.5	5.15	5.32	7.0	4.6
UA	Mid infraorbital	5.25	3.65	4.45	6.0	3.0
UK	Front of Masseter	8.1	6.16	7.13	8.5	4.7
JB	Root of zygomatic arch	6.75	7.1	6.92	9.8	4.8
JB1	Highest point on zygomatic arch	—	5.32	5.32	8.0	3.1
WB	Highest point on malar	—	7.73	7.73	9.5	6.7
MS	Mid of Masseter	17.0	14.83	15.91	19.0	12.0
KW	Jaw angle	11.5	7.56	9.53	12.0	4.7
NL	Nasal root to alar margin	—	46.75	46.75	50.0	44.0
NB	Nasal breadth at alae	—	34.75	34.75	38.0	32.0
NT	Nasal depth from tip to root of lip	21.5	22.50	22.0	24.0	19.0
HO	Height of upper lip	21.0	20.50	20.75	23.0	19.0
RK	Oral cleft to chin prominence	43.25	25.50	34.37	43.25	25.0

* From Kollmann and Büchly, 1898. Table 3.

cleaned skull, and on the plastic reconstruction.* The only serious errors that resulted were in bipalpebral breadth which we underestimated on the bust (−13 mm.), and bigonial breadth, which we overestimated on the bust (+10.5 mm.).† *All the midline features* were within ±4 mm., though skewed to the minus side (bust smaller than head). Arising from the results of this

* I was assisted by Miss Mary Jane McCue, a sculptress. I told her no more than I would were the skull an unknown identified by me; I gave her tissue data from Kollman and Büchly on male whites. From time to time I checked the progress of the restoration.

† Bipalpebral breadth measures the distance between the outer corners of the eyes. Bigonial breadth is across the jaw angles.

test I venture to put down here a few useful "rules of thumb."
(See Krogman, McGregor, Frost, '48.)

1. Relation of eyeball to bony orbit.

The apex of the cornea, when viewed from norma frontalis, is at
the juncture of two lines, one drawn from the medial edge of the
orbit (maxillofrontale) to the lateral margin of the orbit (ectoconchion); and the other line bisecting the orbit between the superior
and inferior margins.

The outer point of the cornea is approximately tangent to a
centrally located line drawn from the superior and inferior margins
of the orbit.

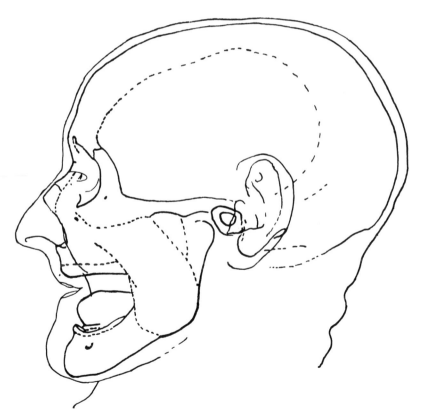

Fig. 74.   Superimposed outlines of head and skull of anatomical subject in the
"Photograph B" position (compare with Fig. 71).

2. Nose tip. (Modified more or less by racial type, and contours of underlying bony structure.)

The width of the bony nasal aperture, in Caucasoids, is about three-fifths of the total nasal width as measured across the wings.

The projection of the nose is (from subnasale to pronasale) is approximately three times the length of the nasal spine (as measured from the lower margin of the nasal opening to the tip of the spine). The nasal spine is, however, rarely completely preserved.

3. Location of ear.

The most lateral part of the cartilaginous portion of the ear-tube is 5 mm. above, 2.6 mm. behind, and 9.6 mm. lateral, to the most lateral part of the bony portion of the ear-tube. (Montagu, '38.)

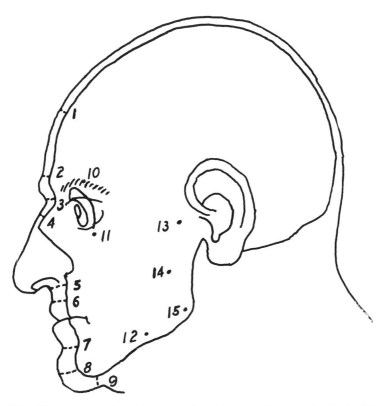

Fig. 75. Diagram showing sites where the tissue depths given in Table 86 were measured.

4. Width of mouth.

The width of the mouth is approximately the same as inter-pupillary distance; or, alternatively, the distance between two lines radiating out from the junction of the canine and first premolar on each side.

5. Length of ear.

The ear length (from top to bottom) is often roughly equal to nose length. (Ear size and proportion are extremely variable.)

A relevant aspect of the skull-head restoration problem is the theme of tissue restoration in mummification. Gillman ('33/'34) restored a Bantu arm, forearm, and part of the wrist, that had been naturally dessicated for some 150–200 years. He first cites Ruffer's work on Egyptian mummies: alcohol 100 parts; 5% sodium car-

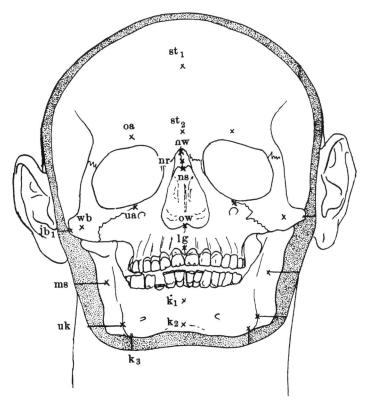

Fig. 76. Diagram of a frontal view of a human skull, showing the points used by Kollmann and Büchly.

bonate sol. 60 parts. After a variable time, depending on "the bulk and nature of the tissue," the solution is replaced by 30% alcohol, and "more alcohol is added day by day."

Gillman put the Bantu arm in a solution of 1 gm. sodium hydroxide in 100 cc. of 33% alcohol. By the 14th day the part was deemed sufficiently restored and the softening process was completed. The arm was then washed in running water for 12 hours, then transferred to 10% formalin for a week. It was finally hardened in 90% alcohol. Gillman states that "the natural ridges that

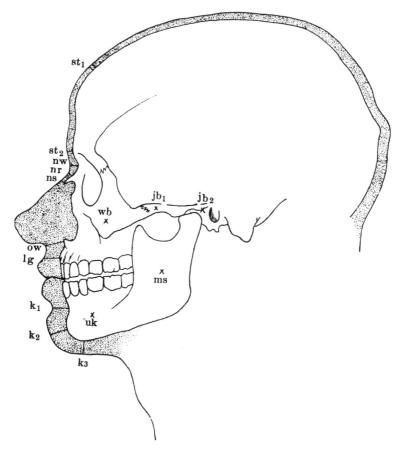

Fig. 77. Diagram of a lateral view of a human skull showing the points used by Kollmann and Büchly.

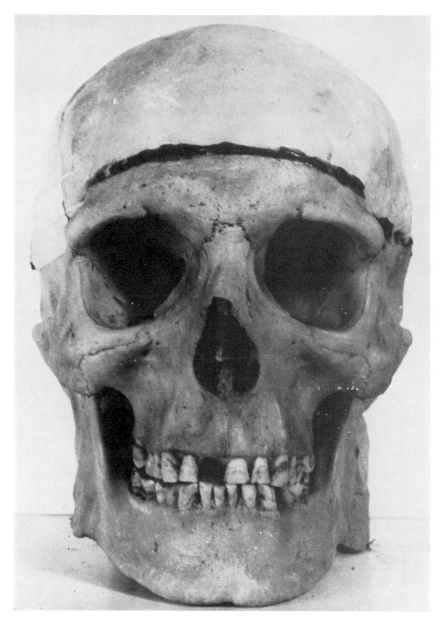

Fig. 78.   Facial view of skull of male Negro, age 65 years (autopsied).

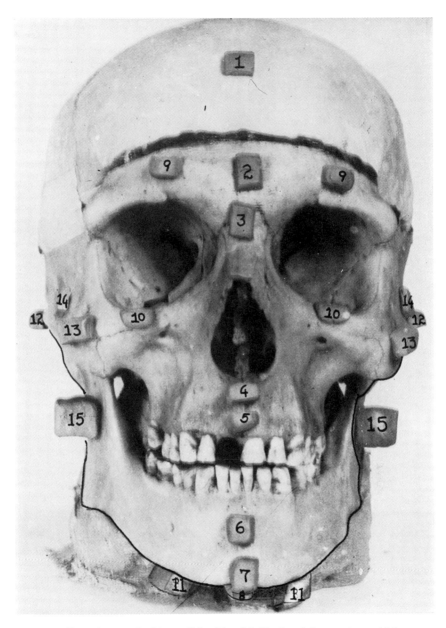

Fig. 79. Facial view of subject of Fig. 78, with blocks of clay to tissue thickness at selected sites.

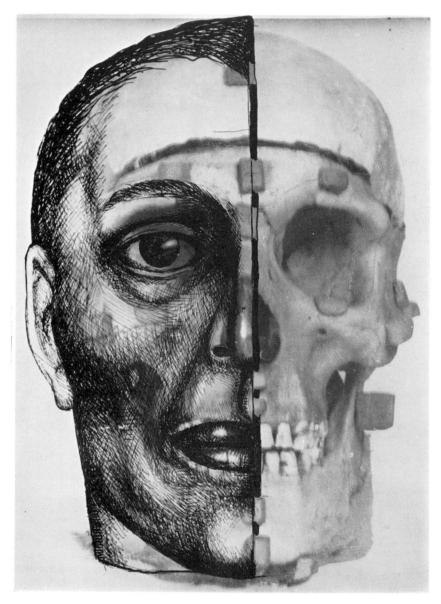

Fig. 80.   Facial view of subject of Figs. 78–79, with soft tissues drawn in on the right half.

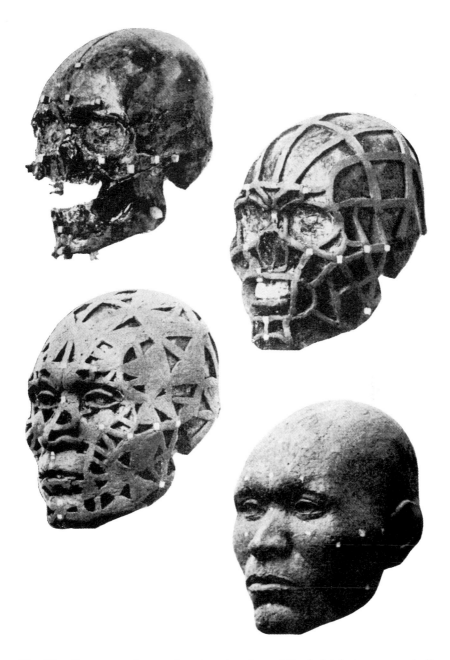

Fig. 81. Four stages in a sculptor's restoration of the facial features on a skull. Note that the lower jaw has been firmly attached to the skull, the missing teeth restored, and blocks proportional to the tissue depth attached at designated points. By connecting the blocks with strips of clay, the surface was built up and ultimately the features were modeled in. Further stages beyond those shown would include the addition of hair and neck.

occur in the skin can be restored"; if so, this might permit finger and palm prints.

Montagu ('35) tested Gillman's method on a mummified Egyptian foot. He used 40 gms. of sodium hydroxide in 4000 cc. of 30% alcohol. The foot was soaked for 49 hours, washed in water for 35 hours. It was "much damaged." Montagu suggests a "weaker solution."

Summarizing Statement

1. The comparison of skull to portrait is mainly an interesting historic exercise. It is a useful technique to emphasize the variability and individuality of such a procedure.

2. The comparison of skull to photograph is more useful, and may serve to establish identity. If photographs depart (as they usually do) from a full facial, or a full lateral, view, corrections can be made so that skull tracings (facial and lateral) can be fairly accurately superimposed on the photographs.

3. The use of schedules of tissue thicknesses to model a head from the skull is a useful procedure. Certainly eyes, nose, mouth, ears, can be reconstructed as part of a physiognomic restoration. But it must be pointed out that details of coloration, of expression, of eyebrows, etc., and of the whole subtle complex of "living appearance" can hardly be re-created. The best one may say is that this sort of restoration is a possible added factor in individualization of skeletal remains.

REFERENCES

CZEKANOWSKI, J.: Untersuchungen über das Verhältnis der Kopfmasse zu den Schädelmassen. *Arch f. Anth.*, NF 6:42–89, 1907.

EGGELING, H. VON: Die Leistungsfähigkeit physiognomischer Rekonstruktionsversuche auf Grundlage des Schädels. *Arch f. Anth.*, N.F., *12*:44–47, 1913.

GILLMAN, J.: Restoration of mummified tissues. *AJPA*, *18*:363–369, 1933/34.

GLAISTER, J. and BRASH, J. C.: *The Medico-legal Aspects of the Buck Ruxton Case.* E. and S. Livingston, Edinburgh, 1937.

HALL, M.: Über Gesichtsbildung. *MAGW*, *28*:57–100, 1898.

HARSLEM-RIEMSCHNEIDER, L.: Die Gesichtsmuskulatur von 14 Papua und Melanesieren. *ZMA*, *22*:1–44, 1921–22.

HIS, W.: Anatomische Forschungen ueber Johann Sebastian Bach's Gebeine und Antlitz nebst Bemerkungen ueber dessen Bilder. *Abhandl. Math.-phys. Classe d. Köng. Sächs. Gesells. d. Wissensch.*, *22*(whole ser. 37):379–420, 1895.

HODGKINSON, L. A.: The endocranial equivalent of the Frankfurt Plane and the exocranial position of the interior auditory meatus. *JA*, *65*:96–107, 1930/31.

HUG, E.: Das fragliche Skelett des Ülrich von Hütten. *Bull. d. Schweiz. Gesellsch. f. Anth. u. Ethnol.*, *36*:34–46, 1959/60.

KOLLMANN, J. and BÜCHLY, W.: Die Persistenz der Rassen und die Reconstruction der Physiognomie prähistorischer Schädel. *Arch. f. Anth.*, *25*:329–359, 1898.

KROGMAN, W. M.: 1939 (see *Refs.*, Chap. II).

KROGMAN, W. M.: Role of the physical anthropologist in the identification of human skeletal remains. *FBI Law Enforce. Bull.*, Pt. I., *12(4)*:17–40, 1943. Pt. II, *12(5)*:12–28, 1943.

KROGMAN, W. M. (with McCUE, MARY JANE): The reconstruction of the living head from the skull. *FBI Law Enforce. Bull.*, 8 pp. (reprint), July, 1946.

KROGMAN, W. M., McGREGOR, J. and FROST, B.: A problem in human skeletal remains. *FBI Law Enforce. Bull.*, 6 pp., (reprint), June, 1948.

KUPFFER, C. and HAGEN, F. B.: Der schädel Immanuel Kants. *Arch. f. Anth.* *13*:359–410, 1881.

LANDER, K. F.: The examination of a skeleton of known age, race, and sex. *J.A.*, *52(Ser.3,V.18)*:282–291, 1917/18.

MONTAGU, M. F. A.: Restoration of an Egyptian mummified foot. *AJPA*, *20(1)*: 95–103, 1935.

PEARSON, K.: The skull of Robert the Bruce, King of Scotland 1274–1329. *Biom.*, *16*:253–272, 1924.

PEARSON, K.: On the skull and portraits of George Buchanan. *Biom.*, *18*:233–256, 1926.

PEARSON, K.: The skull and portraits of Henry Stewart, Lord Darnley, and their bearing on the tragedy of Mary, Queen of Scots. *Biom.*, *20*:1–104, 1928.

PEARSON, K. and MORANT, G. M.: The Wilkinson head of Oliver Cromwell and its relationship to busts, masks, and painted portraits. *Biom.*, *26*:269–378, 1934.

PRINSLOO, I.: The identification of skeletal remains. *J. Forensic Med.*, *1(1)*:11–17, 1953.

REID, R. W.: Remains of St. Magnus and St. Rognvald, entombed in Saint Magnus Cathedral, Kirkwall, Orkney. *Biom.*, *18*:118–150, 1926.

SIMPSON, K.: Rex v. Dobkin: the Baptist church cellar murder. *Medico-Legal and Criminol Rev.*, *11*:132–145, 1943.

SIMPSON, K.: Rex vs. George Haigh: the acid-bath murder. *Medico-Legal and Criminol Rev.*, *18*:38–47, 1950.

STADTMÜLLER, F.: Zur Beurteilung der plastischen Rekonstruktions methode der Physiognomie auf dem Schädel. *ZMA*, *22*:337–372, 1921/22; also *23*:301–314, 1923/25.

STEWART, T. D.: 1954 (see *Refs.*, Chap. II).

SUK, V.: Fallacies of anthropological identifications and reconstructions. A critique based on anatomical dissections. *Publ. Fac. Sci. Univ. Masaryk*, Prague, *207*:1–18, 1935.

SUZUKI, K.: On the thickness of the soft parts of the Japanese face. *J. Anth. Soc. Nippon*, *60*:7–11, 1948.

TILDESLEY, M. L.: Sir Thomas Browne: His skull, portraits, and ancestry *Biom.*, *15*:1–76, 1923.

VIRCHOW, H.: Die Anthropologische Untersuchung der Nase. *ZE*, *44*:289–337, 1912.

VIRCHOW, H.: Halb Schädel halb Maske, *ZE*, *46*:180–186; 504–507, 1914.

WELCKER, H.: Schiller's Schädel und Todtenmaske, nebst Mittheilungen über Schadel und Todtenmaske Kants. Braunschweig. 1883.

WELCKER, H.: Der Schädel Rafael's und der Rafaelporträts. *Arch f. Anth. 15*: 417–440, 1884.

WELCKER, H.: Zur Kritik des Schillerschädels. *Arch. f. Anth.*, *17*:19–60, 1888.

WILDE, A. G.: De Etude de l'identification d' un squelette du XV eme siecle. *Compt. Rend. Assoc. Anat.*, *45(104)*:789–799, 1959.

WILDER, H. H.: The restoration of dried tissue, with special reference to human remains. *Am. Anth.*, *6(1)*:1–13, 1904.

WILDER, H. H.: The physiognomy of the Indians of Southern New England. *Am. Anth.*, *14(3)*:415–436, 1912.

WILDER, H. H. and WENTWORTH, B.: 1918, (see *Refs.*, Chap. I).

ZIEDLER, H. F. B.: Beiträge zur Anthropologie der Gesichtsweichteilen der Neger. *ZMA*, *21*:153–184, 1919/21.

X

The Use of Radiography in Skeletal Identification

1. GENERAL CONSIDERATIONS

As a rule the use of radiography to identify skeletal details presupposes at least two sets of x-ray films, i.e., a before-and-after set. This assumes that certain bonea are found and x-rayed; tentative identification is made; x-ray films taken during the life of the presumed individual are then secured and comparison made on a bone-by-bone or trait-by-trait basis. More rarely radiography may be used in a given instance quite apart from comparison. Cornwell ('56) reviews the use of radiography of skeletal material where previous x-ray films are available. Morgan and Harris ('53) suggest the use of radiography of charred masses to ascertain if human bones are contained therein. In such a case a burned mass showed "the characteristic pattern of the burned skull after explosion of the cranium and the characteristic retraction of the scalp." They add, though this is not germane to our present discussion, that x-ray films are also useful in "the finding, location, and as an aid to removal of, foreign bodies such as bullets, shotgun pellets, knife blades, ice picks, and various other types of opaque lethal foreign bodies."

2. RADIOGRAPHY OF THE SKULL

In 1921, Schüller pointed out that the *frontal sinuses*, seen radiographically, were useful in identification. In 1931, Dr. Thomas A. Poole (cited by Cornwell, '56, and by Mayer, '35) stated that the frontal sinuses of no two persons were alike. The frontal sinuses appear as extensions from the nasal cavity in the second year of life. They grow slowly until puberty, at which time they increase rapidly, growing until about the 20th year. The frontal sinuses are larger in males than in females, and in females the scalloped upper archings, while smaller, are more numerous. In about 5% of adults no frontal sinuses may be observed radiographically; in 1%, either right or left, it may be absent unilaterally (although

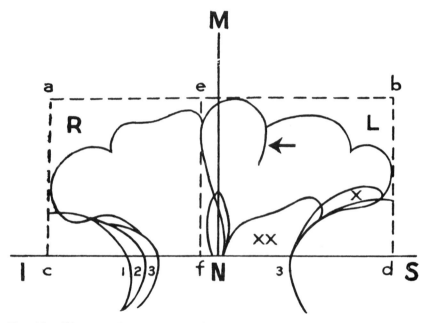

Fig. 82. Diagram of x-ray picture (forehead-nose position) of frontal sinuses.

often the "absence" is due to an extremely deviant septum). In senility the walls of the frontal sinuses become thinner, and the sinuses appear as larger. Occasionally, in old age, a continuity with the diploë develops, extending from supraorbital region to the vertex of the vault. In acute or chronic inflammations, in some endocrine dysplasias, and in other conditions (trauma, osteites of various kinds) which may occur in the lifetime of an individual, changes may be manifested in the frontal sinuses that will afford unmistakable criteria of comparison.

Schüller ('43) orients the head (skull) in the "forehead-nose posi-

tion," i.e., forehead and nose are in contact with the x-ray cas-
sette; the central axis of the x-ray tube is oriented to the supra-
orbital margins. Especial attention is paid to the line of the frontal
spetum, the upper borders of the sinus, partial septa, and supraorbital cells. In Figure 82 the tracing of an x-ray film of a frontal
sinus is shown. Schüller's comments and his method of measurement are given as below (p. 556):

> The following are the bony details to be observed in the plate:
> the line of the frontal septum; the upper border of the frontal sinus;
> partial septa; supraorbital cells. In the skull [shown in Figure 1] the
> line of the septum deviates from the mid-line towards the right side;
> the upper border is scalloped with two arcades on the right and
> three on the left frontal sinus; one partial septum is present
> (marked by an arrow) between the medial and the two lateral
> arcades of the left frontal sinus; two cells are seen in the lower half
> of the left frontal area, the lateral cell, marked by one cross, repre-
> senting a supraorbital extension, the medial cell, marked by two
> crosses, representing a *bulla frontalis* of the ethmoid.
>
> In order to measure the diameters of the frontal sinuses I use a
> simple construction—namely, a vertical line corresponding to the
> median sagittal section of the forehead (MN), a horizontal line (IS)
> corresponding to the projection of the *jugum (planum) sphenoidale*,
> one rectangle (R + L) framing the upper border and the two lat-
> eral borders of both combined frontal sinuses (*abdc*) and another
> rectangle (L) framing the larger sinus (*ebdf*).
>
> The line MN can be determined readily in the great majority
> of cases, because the dense line of the frontal crest is generally easily
> seen in the x-ray picture corresponding to the attachment of the
> *falx cerebri* on the inner surface of the vertical plate. Sometimes
> the outlines of a narrow groove are visible; this is the anterior part
> of the longitudinal sinus. A persistent frontal suture may indicate
> the midline, or the rim of the *crista galli* facilitates its recognition.
> Finally, the position of characteristic shadows representing ossifica-
> tions along the *falx cerebri* or calcifications of the pineal body may
> serve the same purpose.
>
> The line IS is drawn perpendicularly to the mid-line. It repre-
> sents the level of the *jugum (planum) sphenoidale*, which forms the roof
> of the body of the sphenoid bone on the floor of the anterior cranial
> fossa, just behind the *lamina cribrosa*. This line of the *jugum sphe-
> noidale* lies in the same horizontal level as the bottom of the frontal

sinus in the majority of cases, as it is seen in profile pictures of the anterior cranial fossa. In the standard forehead-nose view, the projection of the *jugum sphenoidale* is always visible as a straight or slightly curved outline, which crosses the projection of the medial border and/or the medial wall of the orbit (1, 2, 3 in Figure 82). The line IS, joining these points perpendicular to MN, indicates the level of the floor of the frontal sinuses. The horizontal line IS forms the base for the construction of the rectangular frames of the two combined frontal sinuses (R + L) and the larger left sinus (L); a horizontal line is drawn through the highest point of the left frontal sinus, and three vertical lines are drawn, two along the most lateral points of the left and the right sinus, and one along the right border of the left sinus. The exact measurements are taken of the width (*ab*) of the rectangular frame for both combined sinuses, the width (*eb*) of the rectangle for the left sinus and the height (*ef*) of the rectangle for the left sinus. These three measurements, combined with the description of the frontal septa, of the arches of the upper border of the frontal sinuses and of the separate cells in the supraorbital region, should allow one to identify the frontal sinus of each individual skull. It is obvious that the three measurements are sufficient as fundamentals for the classification of large numbers of cases and may be used as the basis of a filing system for the x-ray pictures.

Culbert and Law ('27) and Law ('34) present a case-history of identification via "sinus-prints" (so to speak); plus certain details of the *mastoid process*. In this case there were found 13 points of "identity" in the frontal sinuses and seven in the right mastoid (there had been a left mastoidectomy).

The sphenoid bone and its component parts has been suggested by Voluter, in his V-Test (see Ravina, '60) as possessing great value in identification. The area of the sella turcica is especially important by virtue of its centrally-protected nature, i.e., it is often the last area of the skull to be affected by various erosive or destructive processes. The V-Test considers the following variables: the form and volume of the sella turcica; the angle formed by the basal plane (the clivus) and the anterior cranial base (this is the "Sattlewinkel" or "sellar angle" of established craniometry); the details of the osseous structure and the pneumatization of the sella; size and shape of the sphenoidal sinus. All of these factors, in varying degrees, and in varying combinations, are, says Voluter, as variable as are fingerprints. The procedure is one of *matching*, i.e., comparison of x-ray films of the presumed victim with those taken ante-mortem.

The use of radiography to calculate endocranial dimensions, to derive an encephalic index, and to estimate endocranial volume, has been discussed by Mollison ('25/'26), Neuert ('31) and Haas ('52). On the x-ray film, in lateral view, Neuert following Welcker, located the most foreward point on the forehead (excluding the supraorbital ridges) and the most posterior point on the occiput to give *length;* the anterior point of the foramen magnum and the highest point on the vault contour to give *total height;* the roof of the external auditory meatus and the highest point on the vault contour to give *auricular height;* in the a-p view he located, right and left, the point marking maximum transverse breadth of the head.

The following corrections are then to be made:

Dimension	Very Thin Scalp	Av. Scalp	Very Thick Scalp
From L subtract	5 mm.	10 mm.	15
From B subtract (not over M. temp)	6 "	10 "	13
From B subtract (over M. temporalis)	12 "	to	30
From AH subtract (L = length, B = breadth, AH = auricular height)	4 "	6 "	8

In total skull-head calculations to be used in the estimation of endocranial dimensions allowance must be made for both tissue and bone. There is considerable difference of opinion here as is seen from the following tabulation (compiled by Krogman, 37) of corrections (in mm.):

Author	Length	Breadth	Height
Merkel	10–12	5–6	5–6
Langerhans	10	—	—
Weeks	11.1	—	5.9
Gladstone			
Male	7.25	7.4	3.79
Female	7.12	6.98	3.50
Anderson	9	9	7
Ley and Joyce	8	10	5
Parsons	9.7	11.4	8
Todd	11.4	13.6	9.5
Wood Jones	6	7	5
Lee	11	11	11

A general average of 10 mm. for length, 10 mm. for breadth, and 8 mm. for height is acceptable.

For horizontal circumference corrections are as follows:

Scalp	Male	Female
Thin	14 mm.	20 mm.
Av.	21 "	28 "
Thick	28 "	35 "

The calculation of endocranial volume ("brain volume") has been given variously by earlier physical anthropologists. Manouvrier used the formula L × B × AH/2, with the result to be divided by a constant varying with age and sex:

Age	Male	Female
Birth–5 years	1.05	1.05
5–10 "	1.06	1.06
10–15 "	1.07	1.07
16–20 "	1.10	1.08
20–25 "	1.15	1.10
25–X "	1.20	1.15

Froriep used $(L - 1)/2 \times (B - b)/2 \times (H - h)/2 \times 4$, on the skull, where 1 = frontal and occipital thickness, b = parietal thickness, R and L, b = vault thickness.

Lee and Pearson present the formulae most frequently used to calculate endocranial volume from measurements of the head:

$$\text{Male} = 0.000337 \, (L\text{-}11) \, (B\text{-}11) \, (AH\text{-}11) + 406.01 \text{ cc.}$$
$$\text{Female} = 0.000400 \, (L\text{-}11) \, (B\text{-}11) \, (AH\text{-}11) + 206.60 \text{ cc.}$$

Haas, on lateral and a-p x-ray films of the head, measured max. length, height from foramen magnum to vertex, max. breadth at squamous suture and came up with a module (L + B + H) 3 and an index B/L × 100. He figures on a *16% magnification*.

In 1953, Thörne and Thyberg suggested the feasibility of using "mass miniature radiography of the cranium" as a technique in identification. Two sets of films (lateral and p-a) were taken at 1 m. distance, twice (one month apart) of 100 children and adults. Tracings, using dimensions, indices, and angles, were made of the x-ray films. The first and second sets of films, in each individual case, were compared for matching. "It was possible to perform such an identification in all cases without difficulty."

Sassouni ('57, '58, '59; see also Krogman and Sassouni, '57) has made a major contribution in this area. He x-rayed 498 young adult American males (white and Negro) in left lateral and postero-anterior views in the Broadbent-Bolton Roentgenographic Cephalometer. Two sets of such records were secured, the first to be considered an ante-mortem (AM) series, the second a post-mortem (PM) series. The procedure is given by Sassouni ('59, pp. 4–6) as follows:

On the postero-anterior film twenty-four measurements were taken from thirty subjects (Fig. 83). The range of variation and the standard deviation were calculated for each measurement. The films of the AM and PM series were measured by two different persons and the total range of error assessed for each measurement. The ratio between standard deviation and error was calculated and only those in which the ratio S.D/E. was greater than two were retained. Two diameters were eliminated because of duplication. Thus, the selected measurements from the postero-anterior film are: bigonial breadth, mastoid to apex height, bimaxillary breadth, bizygomatic breadth, maximum cranial breadth, sinus breadth, incision height, and total facial height.

From the lateral film (Fig. 84) a similar study was done. The ratio between standard deviation and range of error was calculated for the twenty-four lateral measurements. Eight measurements with a ratio S.D/E. greater than two were selected (after eliminating overlapping measurements). These are: cranial height 8 cm. posterior, 4 cm. posterior, above, and 4 cm. anterior to sella· cranial length along nasion-sella line, 4 cm. above, and 8 cm. above; total facial height nasion-menton.

The coefficient of correlation "r" was calculated between these sixteen measurements (8 postero-anterior and 8 lateral) taken from ninety subjects. The communalities (h) of each measurement were calculated (Thurstone, '47). The index of selectivity

$$S = \frac{S.D.}{E.} - h\left[\frac{S.D.}{E.} - 1\right],$$

was calculated for each measurement and the smallest eliminated. Then, the communalities and the new indices of selectivity were calculated again; the smallest S was eliminated and so on, until only five measurements were left.

The five measurements which proved to be critical are:

> Length of cranium, 4 cm. above the Na-S line
> Total facial height (Na-Me)
> Sinus breadth
> Bigonial breadth (Go-Go)
> Bizygomatic breadth (Zy-Zy)

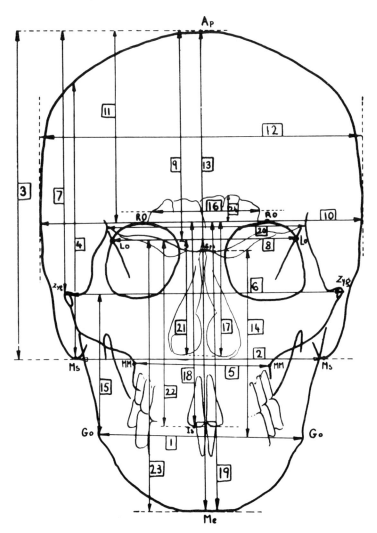

Fig. 83. Frontal view, showing 24 measurements taken on x-ray film. The eight basic measurements are: 1, 3, 5, 6, 12, 16, 18, 19.

The first dimension is from the lateral film, the other four from the p-a film. Accordingly, to save time and money, the lateral film was discarded. Hence, the p-a view, with its eight frontal measurements, becomes the critical x-ray film.

Sassouni concludes as follows ('59, p. 7)

> A test of identification was conducted. The eight measurements were taken on 500 AM films and through proper coding were put on a Univac tape. One hundred films were selected at random from the 500 PM films. The same eight distances were measured and, one by one, tests of identification tried on a Univac machine. In seventy-four tests out of 100, one answer, the right one, was ob-

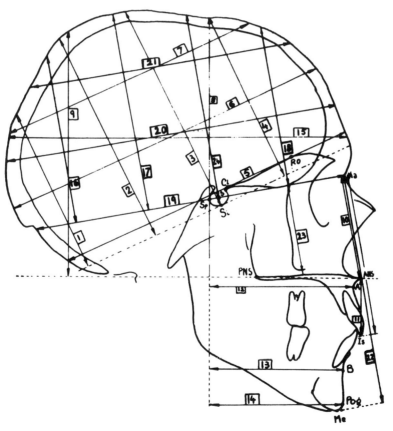

Fig. 84. Lateral view, showing 24 measurements taken on x-ray film. The eight basic measurements are: 16, 17, 18, 19, 20, 21, 22, 24.

tained. The remaining twenty-six contained some error of measurement either on the AM or the PM series. A cross-checking method was developed in order to locate and to neutralize the error. Twenty-three out of 26 were thus identified. This brings the total to 97% identification. The three remaining films could either be identified by further cross-checking or by leaving them until all are identified and by direct comparison of the remaining films. It can be stated, therefore, that 100% identification is achieved through the method proposed here.

According to the index of selectivity and the number of measurements, the actual and theoretical selection was estimated. With twenty measurements and with an index of selectivity of three each, one individual can be identified out of three and one-half billion subjects.

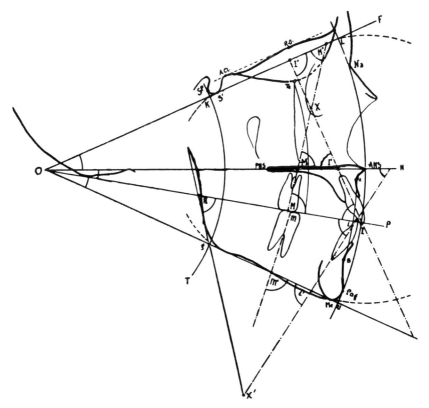

Fig. 85.   Analysis of lateral x-ray film to show planes and arcs.

Lateral cephalometric x-ray films may be used for identification in yet another way. Sassouni ('55) has developed an "analysis" of individuality employing four basic *planes* of reference (see Fig. 85, Sassouni, '57) a cranial base plane (OS'F) a platal plane, (ANS-PNS-O) an occlusal (dental) plane (PMO), and a mandibular (base) plane (Me-G-O); two basic arcs, with point 0 as center: anterior (L-Na-ANS-I-Pog), and posterior (S^P-g). The lateral film may be correlated with the p-a x-ray film as in Fig. 86 (Sassouni, '57).

A concrete problem may be considered. Let us suppose that a skull is found sans maxillary teeth and mandible. How could an entire face be reconstructed? First of all the part found is x-rayed, in lateral and p-a views, in the Broadbent-Bolton apparatus. Then the tracing is made of the films, in both views, according to the Sassouni "Analysis." Assuming that the maxillo-mandibular dentition, and the maxillo-mandibular relationships bear an acceptable relationship to upper face and skull, the occlusal and mandibular planes can be drawn in so as to meet at O; similarly, the anterior and posterior arcs can be drawn in. Hence, the mandible can be drawn in its presumedly vertical and a-p relationships. This procedure is shown in Fig. 87 (Sassouni, '57). How well it worked is seen in Fig. 88 (Sassouni, '57).

Obviously this method is not 100% fool-proof. It assumes a "normal," well-proportioned face, i.e., all planes meet at or near *O*, and the anterior and posterior arcs delimit an orthognathous (straight) face in good occlusion. The restoration is admittedly hypothetical. However, I feel that it gives a reasonably acceptable facsimile of cranio-facial proportions that is a useful adjunct in identification work. At least it is one more design in the entire mosaic; at best it is another good check-method for comparison with portarits, photographs, etc.

3. RADIOGRAPHY OF OTHER BONES

Greulich ('60a,'60b) has developed criteria of identification in x-ray films of *wrist* and *hand*, studying traits in distal radius, distal ulna, carpals, metacarpals, and phalanges. He maintains that traits of individuality are established in these bones in late adolescence and remain "relatively unchanged" until well into the 30's.

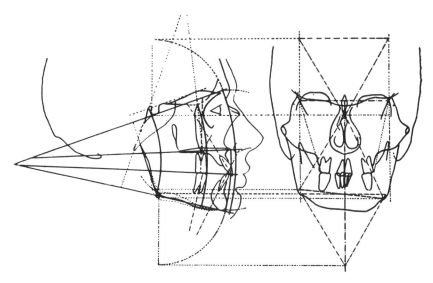

Fig. 86. Tracings of lateral and frontal x-ray films, oriented to demonstrate three-dimensional correlation.

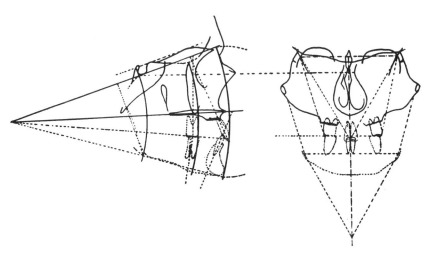

Fig. 87. Reconstruction of cranio-facial relationships in hypothetical case where maxillary dentition and entire mandible are missing.

So individual are these bony traits that Greulich was able, via x-ray films of wrist and hand, to differentiate between identical twins. For a single individual it was quite easy to pair right and left hands from among a series of such wrist-hand x-ray films. American whites, American Indians (Apaches), and Japanese-Americans, were studied, with the result that apparent "racial differences" were noted. In Figures 89–91, from Greulich ('60b), details of wrist, carpals, metacarpals, and phalanges are shown.

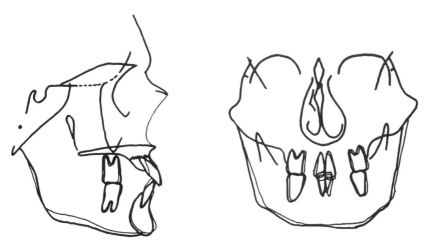

Fig. 88. The actual case shown in Fig. 87. The original maxillo-mandibular tracing is in heavy lines, the reconstruction in thin lines. The difference between the two is the error involved.

In 1959, Schranz reported on age-changes* in the *humerus*, seen both grossly and radiographically. He gives an age sequence as follows:

15–16 years: metaphysis (growing end of shaft) still cartilaginous.
17–18 years: incipient union; diaphyseal internal structure still ogival.
19–20 years: union nearly complete; internal structure of epiphysis is radial, of diaphysis ogival.

* In another Chapter we have already referred to the use of the x-ray film in demonstrating age-changes in the *pubic symphysis* and in the *scapula*.

21–22 years: union complete, with few traces of cartilage still on external surface; internal structures as in 19–20 years.

23–25 years: development of metaphysis complete; internal structure of epiphysis no longer quite radial, of diaphysis still ogival; medullary cavity is far from the surgical neck.

26–30 years: radial nature of internal structure of epiphysis is fading; that of diaphysis still ogival; medullary cavity not to surgical neck yet.

31–40 years: internal structure of epiphysis no longer radial: that of diaphysis more columniform; most superior part of medullary cavity is near surgical neck.

41–50 years: columniform structure of diaphysis is discontinuous; cone of medullary cavity is up to surgical neck; between the cone and the epiphyseal line lacunae may occur.

51–60 years: pea-sized lacunae show on the major tubercle.

61–70 years: outer surface of the bone is rough; cortex is thin; diaphyseal internal structure is irregular; medullary cavity is up to epiphyseal line; bean-sized lacunae occur in major tubercle; the head shows transparency.

75+ years: external surface of the bone is rough; major tubercle has lost its prominence; cortex is thin; little spongy tissue remains in the medullary cavity; epiphysis (head) very fragile, with increasing transparency.

In all this the female has an age-priority of two years at puberty, five years at maturity, and seven to 10 years in the senium. The femur, Schranz says, does not show such distinctive age-changes as does the humerus.

In Figures 92–95 age-stages of 21–22, 31–40, 61–74, 75+ years, respectively, are shown.

4. THE USE OF RADIOGRAPHY IN MASS DISASTER (FIRE)

The identification of all but three of the 119 victims (41 male, 78 female) of the "Noronic" disaster (Sept. 19, 1949) is a classic illustration of the use of radiography (in conjunction with other data) to establish individuality in extensively burned bodies (Brown, '50; Singleton, '51; Brown, Delaney, Robinson, '52).

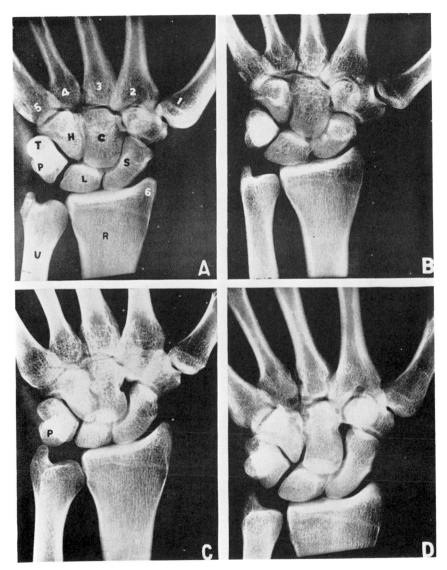

Fig. 89. X-ray film of wrist area: 1–5 = metacarpals I–V; 6 = styloid proc. of radius; 7 = styloid proc. of ulna; shown are capitate (C), hamate (H), triquetrum (T), pisiform (P), lunate (L), scaphoid (navicular) (S); R = radius; U = ulna.

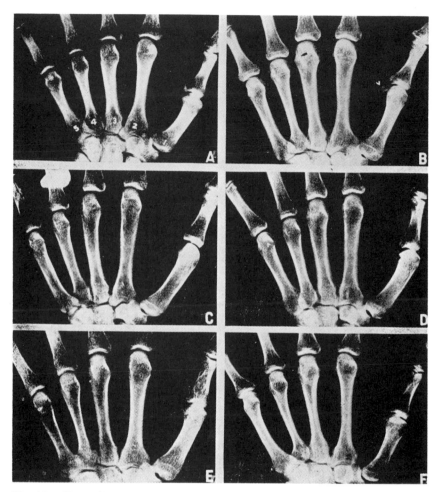

Fig. 90.   X-ray film of wrist area: 1–5 = metacarpals I–V; black arrow in B at head of metacarpal III points to diagnostic white line; the white "V" in B points to a regular sesamoid bone, a diagnostic feature.   The Λ at head of metacarpal V in D points to an occasional sesamoid bone.

In general a-p x-ray films of trunk sections were taken; a-p and lateral of head and of extremities (whenever these parts were available).   In 35 cases pre-mortem files of x-ray films were available for comparison.*   The films taken of the burned bodies were, of course, comparable only up to a point, i.e., missing portions,

* Of these 35, identification was made in 24, was inconclusive in five, and failed in six.

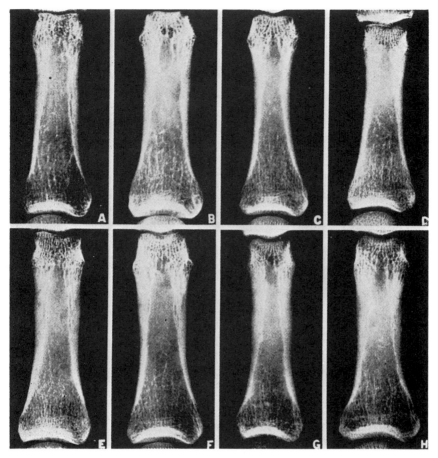

Fig. 91. X-ray films of phalanx 1, finger III, in eight young males, showing individual differences in form and internal structure.

distortion and bending, were limiting factors. Singleton reports that old fractures or infections "played very little part"; congenital bone anomalies were more useful; the most useful method was a trait-comparison, of which he says: "In most cases . . . identification consisted of an accurate matching of normal bony landmarks, particularly margins of joints. The conformation of the bony structures of an individual is a permanent characteristic of that individual, and is not subject to change by plastic operations. . ." Areas which yielded positive identification are as follows: skull,

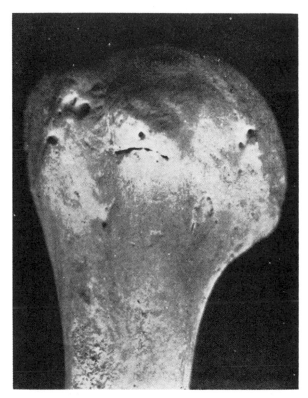

Fig. 92.   Proximal end of macerated humerus, male, age 21 years; remnant of
closure seen near major tubercle.

four traits; cervical vertebrae, two traits; thoracic vertebrae and thorax, 13 traits; lumbar vertebrae and pelvis, nine traits; foot and ankle, one trait.   In Figure 96 is shown a bony trait analysis in a specific case.

In an over-all summary Brown *et al.*, observe (p. 17): "The most important evidence for the identification was contributed by the recognition of property and valuables in 32 cases, by dental studies in 25, by roentgenogram comparison in 19, by pathology and medical histories in 16, and by fingerprints in six cases."

Summarizing Statement

1.   There is no doubt that radiography is an extremely important adjunct in skeletal identification.   It assumes, basically, that *com-*

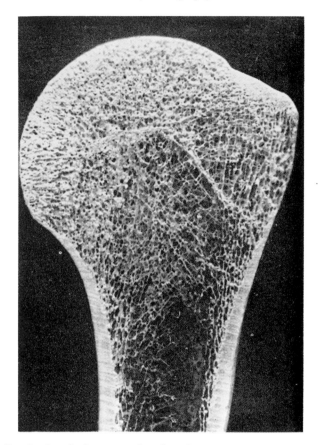

Fig. 93. Proximal end of macerated and sectioned humerus, male, age 35 years; internal structure of epiphysis no longer characteristic; that of diaphysis is columniform; cone of medullary cavity near surgical neck.

parison is possible, i.e., that there are two sets of x-ray films, an ante-mortem set, and a post-mortem set. The procedure is then one of a detail-by-detail check.

2. In the skull the frontal sinuses, the sphenoidal complex, and the mastoid area offer the best criteria of individuality.

3. The use of radiography to calculate cranial capacity, or the use of any skull-to-head correction for the same purpose, is not much more than an exercise which is only very grossly corroborative.

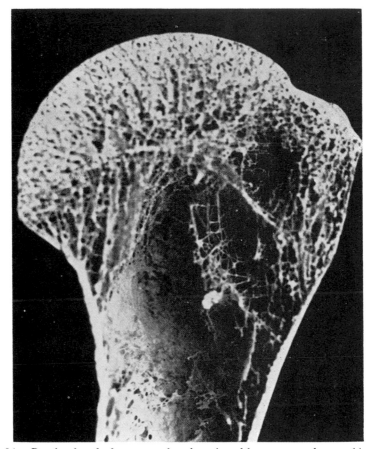

Fig. 94.   Proximal end of macerated and sectioned humerus, male, age 64 years; medullary cavity has reached metaphysis; note independent cavity in major tubercle.

4. The use of roentgenographic cephalometry on a mass basis has been validated as a positive tool in identification by Sassouni. His is the only study wherein variables have been statistically "weighed" for the individuality of complete independence. If his method were put to use en masse, as in the Armed Forces, identification of remains (where skull is available) would become a certainty.

5. Use of roentgenographic cephalometry, based on canons of proportion, can be extended to fragmentary cranial material, permitting reconstruction of the entire cranio-facial complex.

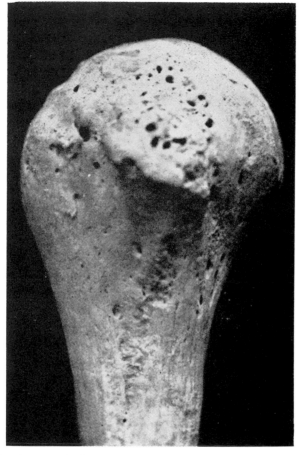

Fig 95. Proximal end of macerated humerus, female, age 97 years; major tubercle atrophied and not prominent.

6. In skeletal parts other than the skull it has been demonstrated by Greulich that radiography of the carpal bones shows individual details; Schranz has demonstrated, via radiography, certain age-changes in the humerus.

7. In assessing use of radiography in skull and in other areas I unhesitatingly choose the skull: (1) it or its parts are more frequently present; (2) the study of the traits of individuality in the skull is on an infinitely greater basis of standardization; (3) other

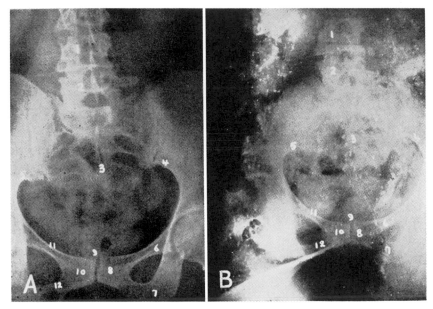

Fig. 96.   Comparison of x-ray films of Mrs. F. L. (A) and victim E-14 (B).
Details are so similar that identity was established.

skeletal parts, notably carpals, are frequently very incomplete or
are missing.

8. The use of radiography in mass disaster identification is of
first-rank importance, as so ably demonstrated in the "Noronic"
fire.

REFERENCES

BROWN, T. C.:   Medical identification in the Noronic Disaster. *Finger Print. and Ident. Mag., 6(32)*:3–14, 1950.

BROWN, T. C., DELANEY, R. J. and ROBINSON, W. L.:   Medical Identification in the "Noronic" Disaster. *JAMA, 148*:621–627, 1952.

CORNWELL, W. S.:   Radiography and photography in problems of identification: a review. *Med. Radiog. and Photog., 32(1)*:1, 34–35, 1956.

CULBERT, W. L. and LAW, F. M.:   Identification by comparison with roentgenograms of nasal accessory sinuses and mastoid processes. *JAMA, 88*:1634–1636, 1927.

GREULICH, W. W.:   Value of x-ray films of hand and wrist in human identification. *Science, 131*:155–156, 1960a.

GREULICH, W. W.:   Skeletal features visible on the roentgenogram of hand and wrist which can be used for establishing individual identification. *Am. J. Roentgenol. Rad. Therapy and Nuclear Med., 83(4)*:756–764, 1960b.

HAAS, L.: Roentgenological skull measurements and their diagnostic applications. *Am. J. Roentgenol., 67*:197–209, 1952.

KROGMAN, W. M.: Cranial types from Alishar Hüyük and their relation to other racial types, ancient and modern, of Europe and Western Asia. (In H. H. von der Osten, "The Alishar Hüyük, Seasons of 1930–32," Pt. III, Oriental Institute Publ., Vol. 30, pp. 213–293. 1937.)

KROGMAN, W. M. and SASSOUNI, V.: A Syllabus of *Roentgenographic Cephalometry* Growth Center, U. of Pa., Phila., 1957.

LAW, F. M.: Roentgenograms as a means of identification. *Am. J. Surg., 26*: 195–98, 1934.

MAYER, J.: Identification by sinus prints. *Virginia M. Monthly, 62*:517–519, 1935.

MOLLISON, TH.: Über die Kopfform des Mikrokephalen Mesek. *ZMA, 25*:109–128, 1925/26.

MORGAN, T. A. and HARRIS, M. C.: The use of X-rays as an aid to medico-legal identification. *J. Forensic Med., 1(1)*:28–38, 1953.

NEUERT, W. I. A.: Zur Bestimmung des Schädelinhaltes am Lebenden mit Hilfe von Röntgenbildern. *ZMA, 29*:261–287, 1931.

RAVINA, A.: L'identification des corps pare le V-Test. *Le Presse Médicale, 68*: 178, 1960.

SASSOUNI, V.: A roentgenographic cephalometric analysis of cephalofacio-dental relationships. *Am. J. Orthod., 47(7)*:477–510, 1955.

SASSOUNI, V.: Palatoprint, physioprint, and roentgenographic cephalometry as new methods in human identification (Preliminary report). *J. Forensic Sci., 2(4)*:429–443, 1957.

SASSOUNI, V.: Physical individuality and the problem of identification. *Temple Law Quart., 31(4)*:12 pp., reprint, 1958.

SASSOUNI, V.: Cephalometric identification: a proposed method of identification of war-dead by means of roentgenographic cephalometry. *J. Forensic Sci., 4(1)* 10 pp., reprint, 1959.

SASSOUNI, V.: Identification of war dead by means of roentgenographic cephalometry. Tech. Rep. EP-125, HQ, Q. M. Research and Engineering Command, Natick, Mass., 1960.

SCHRANZ, D.: Age determinations from the internal structure of the humerus. *AJPA n.s., 17(4)*:273–278, 1959.

SCHÜLLER, A.: Das Röntgengram der Stirnhohle: Ein Hilfsmittel für die Identitätsbestimmung von Schädeln. *Monatschr. f. Ohrenh., 55*:1617–1620, 1921.

SCHÜLLER, A.: Note on the identification of skulls by X-ray pictures of the frontal sinuses. *Med. J. Australia, 1*:554–556, 1943.

SINGLETON, A. C.: The roentgenological identification of victims of the "Noronic" disaster. *Am. J. Roentgenol., 66*:375–384, 1951.

THÖRNE, H. and THYBERG, H.: Identification of children (or adults) by mass miniature radiography of the cranium. *Acta Odontol. Scand., 11(2)*:129–140, 1953.

Thurstone, L. L.: *Multiple Factor Analysis.* U. of Chicago Press, 1947.

Appendix I

Osteology of the Human Skeleton

In this *Appendix* I propose to present information more by pictures than by description. Therefore, from the number of anatomical and radiological textbooks available, I have chosen the two which in my opinion tell the most via useful and reasonably simple illustrations. These are Hamilton's *Textbook of Human Anatomy* ('57) and Etter's *Atlas of Roentgen Anatomy of the Skull* ('55).

There are 206 bones in the adult human skelton, i.e., one in which all epiphyses or other centers of bone growth have united with diaphyses or with other bony structural elements.

In the *skull* we may note bones as follows (nos. in parentheses refer to total nos. right and left):

1. Cranium (8)
    frontal (1)
    parietal (2)
    occipital (1)
    temporal (2)
    sphenoid (1)
    ethmoid (1)
2. Face (14)
    nasal (2)
    vomer (1)
    inferior nasal concha (2)
    lacrimal (2)
    zygoma (2)
    palatine (2)
    maxilla (2)
    mandible (1)
3. Ear ossicles (6)
    malleus (2)
    incus (2)
    stapes (2)
4. Hyoid (1)
    Skull total = 29

In the *vertebral column* the bones are as follows:

1. Cervical vertebrae (7)
2. Thoracic vertebrae (12)
3. Lumbar vertebrae (5)
4. Sacrum (1, representing five fused sacral vertebrae).
5. Coccyx (1, representing three to five fused coccygeal vertebrae)

Vertebral total = 26

In the *thoracic* cage the bones are as follows:

1. Ribs (24)
2. Sternum (1, representing manubrium plus body, the latter of which represents the fusion of four elements).

Total thoracic cage = 25

In the *arm* the bones are as follows:

1. Shoulder girdle (4)
   scapula (2)
   clavicle (2)
2. Upper arm (2)
   humerus (2)
3. Forearm (4)
   radius (2)
   ulna (2)
4. Hand (54)
   carpals (16)
   navicular or scaphoid (2)
   lunate (2)
   triquetral (2)
   pisiform (2)
   multangulum major or trapezium (2)
   multangulum minor or trapezoid (2)
   capitate (2)
   hamate (2)
   metacarpals (10)
   phalanges (28)

Total arm = 64

In the *leg* the bones are as follows:

1. Pelvis (2, each pelvic bone representing the union of three bones, ilium, ischium, pubis)
2. Thigh and knee (4)
   femur (2)
   patella (2)
3. Leg (4)
   tibia (2)
   fibula (2)
4. Foot (52)
   tarsals (14)
   talus (2)
   calcaneus (2)
   cuboid (2)
   navicular (2)
   cuneiform I (2)
   cuneiform II (2)
   cuneiform III (2)
   metatarsals (10)
   phalanges (28)

Total leg = 62

A recapitulation is as follows:

Skull	29
Vertebral column	26
Thoracic cage	25
Arm	64
Leg	62
Total	206

To illustrate the *skull* I have chosen four pictures from Etter, showing both photographic and radiographic views.   In Figure 97 the frontal or facial view is shown, and in Figure 98 the postero-anterior x-ray view is shown.   In like manner Figure 99 and Figure 100 give lateral views and lateral x-ray views, respectively.

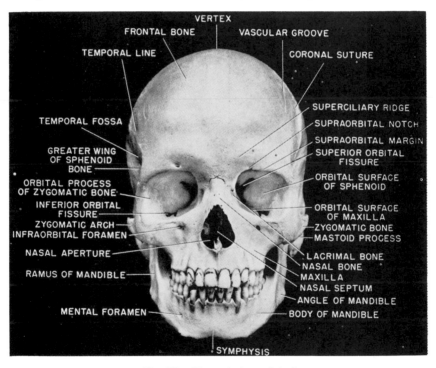

Fig. 97.   Frontal view of skull

Figure 97 should be carefully studied not only for its bones, sutures, (see Chapter III) and other structures, but also because it will serve to illustrate some of the bony landmarks used in measuring *breadths* of skull and face, and *heights* of facial structures.   Figure

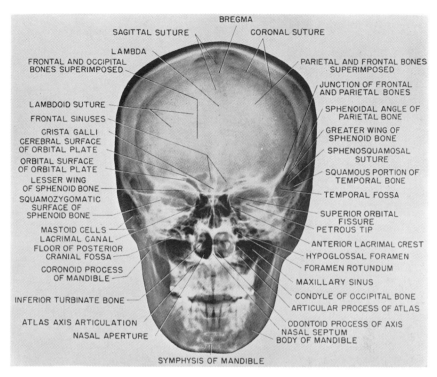

Fig. 98. Frontal x-ray view of skull (this is a postero-anterior film).

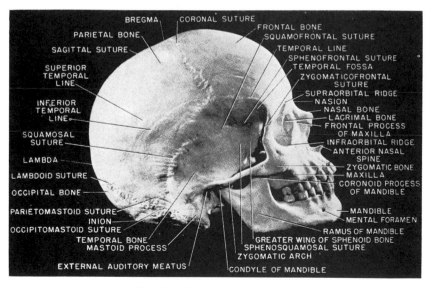

Fig. 99. Lateral view of skull.

303

98 is especially important for the demonstration of frontal and sphenoidal sinuses and other structures mentioned in Chapter X.

Figure 99 is important for its osteological detail and for its significance for measuring cranial *heights* and *lengths;* as well as for
cranio-facial *depths.* Figure 100 is basic for the roentgenographic
cephalometry referred to in Chapters IX-X.

The infra-cranial skeleton will be discussed via eight illustrations
from Hamilton. Figures 101 and 102 show anterior and posterior
views of the right shoulder girdle (clavicle, scapula, humerus).

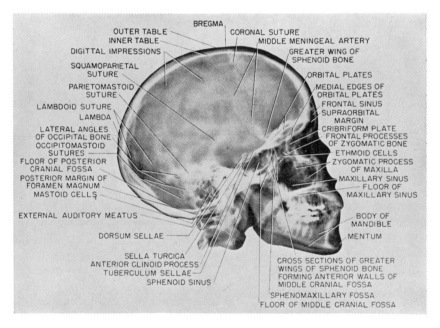

Fig. 100.   Lateral x-ray view of skull.

In the scapula (shoulder-blade) note that the concave sub-
scapular fossa faces forward, while the convex supraspinous and
infraspinous fossae, separated by the spine, face backward. The
glenoid fossa, for articulation with the humerus, faces outward or
laterally. These traits serve to differentiate *right* and *left* scapulae.

In the humerus the head faces inward or medially, as does also
the medial epicondyle. In the posterior view the olecranon fossa
(for the olecranon process of the ulna) is seen to be on the back of the

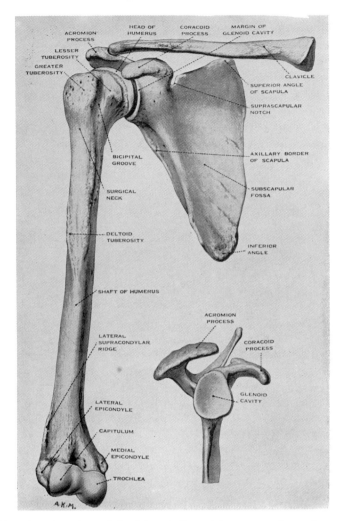

Fig. 101.   Anterior view of shoulder girdle and humerus.   Inset shows position
of glenoid cavity.

humerus.   If the bone is held vertically with head and medial
epicondyle turned to the mid-line of the body, and with the concave
olecranon fossa posteriorly or behind, *right* and *left* humeri can be
differentiated.

In Figures 103–104 anterior and posterior views of the right
radius and ulna are shown.   The radius is on the thumb or outer

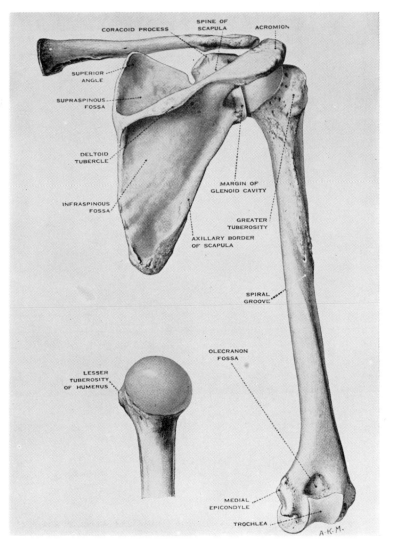

Fig. 102.   Posterior view of shoulder girdle and humerus.   Inset shows head of
humerus.

side of the forearm, the ulna on the little finger or inner side.   The
head of the radius and the olecranon process of the ulna are at the
upper ends of the respective bones.   In the radius, held with head
end up, the lower end has a styloid process which is laterally placed;
the anterior surface of the lower end is concave, the posterior sur-

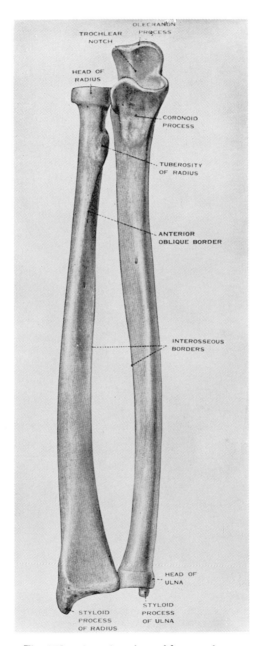

Fig. 103. Anterior view of forearm bones.

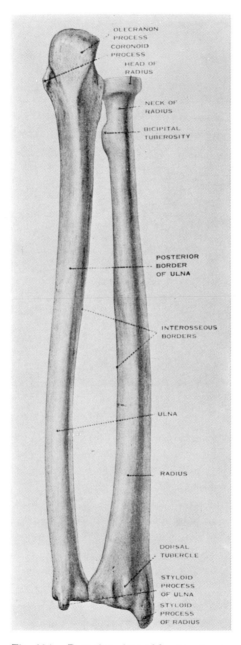

Fig. 104.   Posterior view of forearm bones.

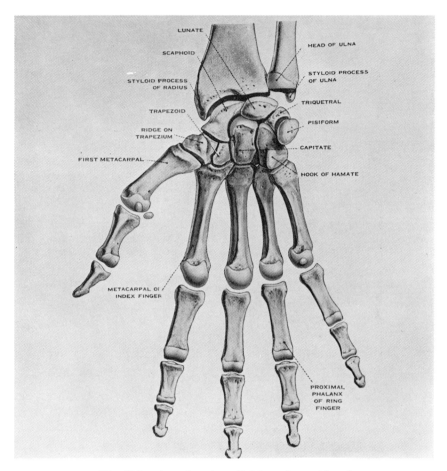

Fig. 105.   Anterior view of right wrist and hand.

face is convex.   These details serve to differentiate *right* and *left* radii.   In the ulna, held with olecranon process up, the concave semilunar part of the olecranon is anterior; at the lower end the styloid process is medially placed.   These details should serve to differentiate *right* and *left* ulnae.

In Figures 105 and 106 anterior and posterior views of wrist and hand are shown.   I shall not here go into details of *right* and *left*, for these are relatively very minute and specialized.

In Figure 107 are shown anterior and posterior views of the right femur (thigh-bone) and right patella (knee-cap).   In the femur the

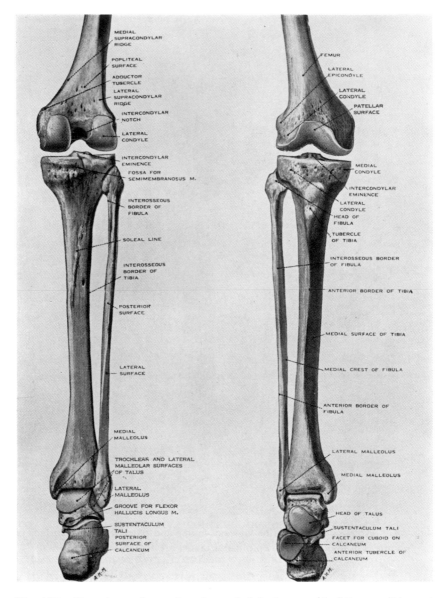

Fig. 108. Posterior and anterior views of right lower end of femur, tibia and fibula, talus and calcaneus.

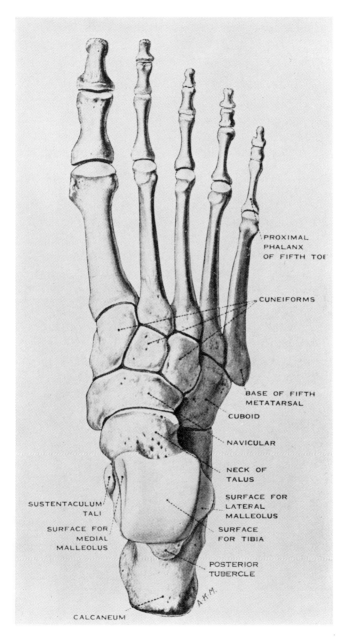

Fig. 109.   Dorsal or upper view of bones of foot.

face of the tibia is concave and more flattened. These details should serve to differentiate *right* and *left* tibiae. The fibula has an upper head and a lower lateral malleolus. Upper and lower ends of the fibula are harder to define than in other long bones: upper end is a bit larger and more blunt; lower end is a bit smaller and is rhomboid in shape and more pointed; at the lower end, laterally and almost posterior in position, there is a well-defined groove for a muscle tendon. If the bone is held in its long axis, with head upward, malleolus down and laterally faced, groove postero-lateral in position, it ought to be possible to differentiate *right* and *left* fibulae.

In Figure 109 is shown a view of the foot skeleton seen from above. The big toe is medial or inner, the little toe lateral or outer. Cuneiforms I-III are numbered medial to lateral, i.e., beginning on the big toe side. As for the hand I shall not go into details, *right* and *left*, of the foot bones.

I have emphasized *right* and *left* in this brief discussion not because a right-left differentiation is important for ageing, sexing, stature reconstruction, etc., but because to know right from left is useful in sorting out mass collections or lots of bones. If, for example, there are three tibiae, all left, then three individuals *must* be represented.

It remains but to repeat what I said in Chapter I, Introduction. This *Appendix* is merely for a quick reference, a once-over-lightly. It may serve for a general skeletal orientation, but it cannot substitute for either the careful and critical use of a textbook on human bones or, preferably, referral to a qualified specialist in skeletal identification.

REFERENCES

ETTER, L. E.: *Atlas of Roentgen Anatomy of the Skull.* Thomas, Springfield, 1955.

HAMILTON, W. J. (ed.): *Textbook of Human Anatomy.* Macmillan, New York and London, 1957.

(In Etter's book there is a Section on "The Radiographic Anatomy of the Temporal Bone" by J. B. Farrior, and a Section on "The Roentgen Anatomy of the Skull in the Newborn Infant" by S. G. Henderson and L. E. Sherman.)

Appendix II

Definitions of Selected Osteologic End-Points and Measurements

Here I shall rely upon *Appendix I* in the sense that bony landmarks (the end-points of measurement) will refer to bones already pictured and discussed. I shall also define the most frequently taken measurements on skull and long bones. The texts most useful here are Comas ('60), Martin-Saller ('56–'61), and Montagu ('60). I wish to make it completely clear that I am selecting *only* the more common skeletal end-points and measurements. Taken by and large, I shall include in *Appendix II* practically all of the craniometric or osteometric data mentioned in the text of this book.

THE SKULL

Of all the skeletal parts the skull has classically been the object of measurement and description (See Chapter VII). Largely upon this structure have been reared systems of racial, sexual, and age classification.

In Figure 110 (Comas, '60) is shown a facial view of the skull. Of all the points shown thereon I wish to define the following:

I In the mid-line, unpaired.

> Gn or gnathion: the point where the curvature of the anterior surface of the mandible becomes confluent with the base; this is the "lowest" point on the chin.
> Id or infradentale: the highest point or tip on the bony septum between the two lower central incisors.
> Pr or prosthion (also supradentale or upper alveolar point): the lowest point or tip on the bony septum between the two upper central incisors.
> Sn or subnasale: the level of the lower margin of right and left nasal apertures, projected to the midline.
> N or nasion: junction of internasal suture with nasofrontal suture.
> B or bregma: junction of sagittal and coronal sutures.

315

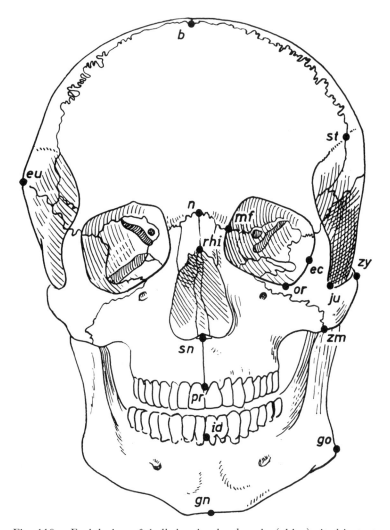

Fig. 110.   Facial view of skull showing landmarks (abbr.) cited in text.

II   Lateral points (paired).

Eu or euryon: points marking maximum biparietal breadth of the skull.
Zy or zygion: points marking maximum bizygomatic breadth of the face.
Mf or maxillofrontale: where the prolongation of the anterior lacrimal crest
    crosses the maxillo-frontal suture.
Or or orbitale: the lowest point on the lower margin of the orbit.
Ec or ectoconchion: the point on the lateral margin of the orbit marking the
    greatest breadth, measured either from maxillofrontale or from dacryon.

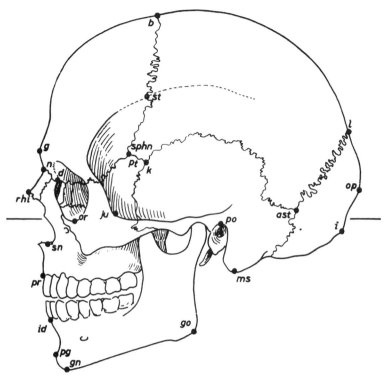

Fig. 111.   Lateral view (left) of skull showing landmarks (abbr.) cited in text.

In Figure 111 from Comas ('60) is presented a left lateral view of the skull, showing additional points.

I   In the mid-line, unpaired.

Pg or pogonion: the most forward projecting point on the mandible.

G or glabella: the most forward projecting point on the forehead (frontal bone).

L or lambda: intersection of sagittal and lambdoid sutures.

Op or opisthocranion: point marking maximum skull length, measured from glabella.

Ap or apex (not shown): point on sagittal contour of skull located by projection of a vertical to the Frankfort Horizontal (which see), erected at porion (see below).

II   Lateral points, paired.

Po or porion: most lateral point on the roof of the external auditory meatus (bony ear-hole).

Go or gonion: the most prominent point on the curve marking the transition between the body and the ascending ramus of the mandible. Gonion may also be located by bisecting the angle formed by the intersection of lines tangent to the lower border of the body and the posterior border of the ascending ramus.

D (dac) or dacryon: point marking junction of sutures between lacrimal, maxillary, and frontal bones.

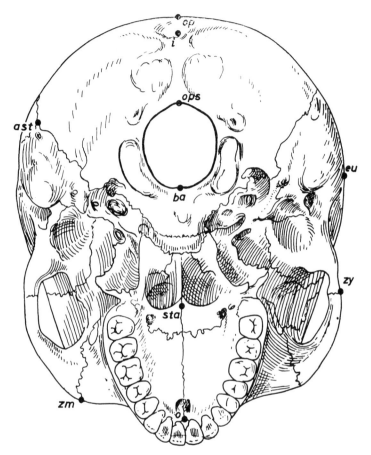

Fig. 112.   Basilar view of skull showing landmarks (abbr.) cited in text.

In Figure 112 (Comas, '60) is shown a basilar view of the skull. Additional points here are as follows:

I   In the mid-line, unpaired.

   Ops or opisthion: most posterior point on the posterior margin of the foramen magnum.

   Ba or basion: most anterior point on the anterior margin of the foramen magnum.

   Sta or staphylion: where a line tangent to the most anterior border of the posterior margins of the palatine bones crosses the midline.

   O or orale: where a line tangent to the lingual (palatal) margins of the alveoli (sockets) of the upper central incisors crosses the midline.

II   Lateral points, paired

   Enmo or endomolare (not shown):   the most lingual or palatal margins of the alveoli of the permanent upper second molars.

Two of the foregoing points, porion and orbitale, are basic to the construction of a universally accepted reference plane: *The Frankfort Horizontal* (or FH). This plane is established when right and left poria and left orbitale are in the same horizontal plane. This plane is internationally recognized as determining a standard plane of reference for craniometry. The phrase "measured in the FH" is one guarantee of a standardized measuring technique.

A number of cranio-facial *dimensions* are based on the points above defined.

I On the skull
      Max. length = gl-op
      Max. breadth = eu-eu
      Total height = ba-br
      Auricular height = po-ap
      Cranial base length = ba-n
      Basi-alveolar length = ba-pr

II On the face
      Total face height = n-gn
      Upper face height = n-pr
      Total face breadth = zy-zy
      Orbit
          breadth = mf-ec or d-ec
          height = max. height at right angles to breadth, measured from orbitale
      Nasal aperture
          height = n-sn
          breadth = max. breadth at right angles to height
      Palate
          length = sta-o
          breadth = enmo-enmo

The foregoing dimensions may be expressed as *indices*, the more common of which are as follows:

Length-breadth or cranial (eu-eu/gl-op ×100)	
dolichocranic or long skull	X– 74.9%
mesocranic or mid skull	75– 79.9%
brachycranic or broad, short skull	80– X%
Length-total height (ba-br/gl-op ×100)	
chamaecranic or low skull	X– 69.9%
orthocranic or mid skull	70– 74.9%
hypsicranic or high skull	75– X%
Breadth-total height (ba-br/eu-eu ×100)	
tapeinocranic or low, broad skull	X– 91.9%
metriocranic or mid skull	92– 97.9%
acrocranic or high, narrow skull	98– X%
Length-auricular height (po-ap/gl-op ×100)	
chamaecranic or low skull	X– 57.9%
orthocranic or mid skull	58– 62.9%
hypsicranic or high skull	63– X%
Breadth-auricular height (po-ap/eu-eu ×100)	
tapeinocranic or low, broad skull	X– 79.9%
metriocranic or mid skull	80– 85.9%
acrocranic or high, narrow skull	86– X%

Total facial index (n-gn/zy-zy ×100)
    euryprosopic or broad face   X– 84.9%
    mesoprosopic or mid face   85– 89.9%
    leptoprosopic or narrow face   90– X%
Upper facial index (n-pr/zy-zy ×100)
    euryen or broad upper face   X– 49.9%
    mesen or mid upper face   50– 54.9%
    lepten or narrow upper face   55– X%
Orbital (h/mf-ec ×100)
    chamaeconch or low orbit   X– 75.9%
    mesoconch or mid orbit   76– 84.9%
    hypsiconch or high orbit   85– X%
Orbital (h/d-ec ×100)
    chamaeconch or low orbit   X– 82.9%
    mesoconch or mid orbit   83– 88.9%
    hypsiconch or high orbit   89– X%
Nasal (b/n-sn ×100)
    leptorrhine or narrow nose   X– 46.9%
    mesorrhine or mid nose   47– 50.9%
    chamaerrhine or wide nose   51– X%
Palatal (sta-o/enmo-enmo ×100)
    dolichouranic or long narrow palate   X– 79.9%
    mesouranic or mid palate   80– 84.9%
    brachyuranic or short, broad palate   85– X%
Gnathic (ba-n/ba-pr ×100)
    orthognathic or straight profile   X– 97.9%
    mesognathic or mid profile   98–102.9%
    prognathic or protrusive profile   103– X%

THE LONG BONES

For the infra-cranial skeleton I shall consider only certain long-bones: humerus; radius; ulna; femur; and tibia. As an over-all summary I'd say two linear dimensions and two or three transverse or sagittal diameters are all that need concern us here.

As a rule each long bone has a *Maximum morphological length,* measuring total length from one end to the other, parallel to the long axis of the bone. However, there is also a *Physiological length* (also called oblique length or bicondylar length) which is the functional length of the long bone. Figure 113 (Comas, '60) illustrates what I mean.

In the Figure the physiological length is shown as dimension number 1. It is measured this way: on an osteometric board the femoral condyles are both placed tangent to a base-line; this "slants" the bone, so to speak, to one side; the length taken is projected from the base-line to the top of the femoral head. Now, assume that the distance between condyles and head is measured parallel to the axis of the shaft and at right angles to the base-line;

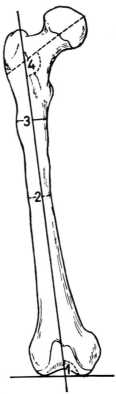

Fig. 113. The measurement of the physiological length of the femur (1), the transverse diameter at mid-level (2), the sub-trochanteric level (3), and the collo-diaphyseal angle (4).

this would give total morphological length which is, as a rule, from five to ten millimeters longer than the physiological length.

Now, let me consider each of the five bones above mentioned, in turn.

Humerus
 1. Max. morphological length = total distance from head to furthest point on lower end, measured parallel to the shaft.
 2. Physiological length = lower end parallel to base-line, with total distance then taken to top of head.
 3. Bicondylar breadth: distance between medial and lateral epicondyles.

Ulna
 1. Max. morphological length = total length from top of olecranon process to tip of styloid, measured parallel to the shaft.
 2. Physiological length = from lip of coronoid process of semilunar notch to lower articular surface, excluding the styloid process.

Radius

1. Max. morphological length = total length from top margin of head to tip of styloid process, measured parallel to the shaft.
2. Physiological length = from depth of depression (fovea) on top of head to lower articular surface, excluding the styloid process.

Femur

1 and 2. Max. morphological and physiological lengths have been discussed above.

The shaft of the femur is so shaped that it varies at mid-level and at subtrochanteric level. Hence, several transverse and sagittal diameters are useful.

3. Mid transverse diameter = max. transverse diameter of shaft at mid-level, at right angles to long axis of the shaft.
4. Mid sagittal diameter = max. sagittal diameter of shaft at mid-level, at right angles to the foregoing.
5. Subtrochanteric transverse diameter = max. transverse diameter of shaft, just below the lesser trochanter, at right angles to the long axis of the shaft.
6. Subtrochanteric sagittal diameter = max. sagittal diameter of shaft, just below the lesser trochanter, at right angles to the foregoing.
7. Bicondylar breadth = max. transverse diameter across the condylar end of the femur, at right angles to the long axis of the shaft.
8. Collo-diaphyseal angle = angle formed by the intersection of a line representing the long axis of the shaft and a line representing the axis of the neck and head. The angle may be expressed as in number 4 of Figure 113, or the reciprocal of the angle may be given.

The subtrochanteric diameters may be employed in a ratio, subtroch. sag. diam./ subtroch. trans. diam. X100 to give the *Platymeric Index* with values as follows:

platymeric or flattened	X–84.9%
eurymeric or moderate	85–99.9%
stenomeric or rounded	100–X%

Tibia

1. Max. morphological length = total length from intercondylar eminences to tip of the medial malleolus, measured parallel to the shaft.
2. Physiological length = from the depression on the top of the medial half of the condylar surface to the lower articular surface near the medial malleolus, but excluding it.

The tibia is also a bone with variable shaft diameters. Hence, two diameters are taken at the level of the nutrient foramen, which can be seen in Figure 108, on the posterior aspect of the tibia, about a third of the way down from the upper end.

3. Transverse cnemic diameter = max. transverse diameter, at level of the nutrient foramen, at right angles to the long axis of the shaft.
4. Sagittal cnemic diameter = max. sagittal diameter, at level of the nutrient foramen, at right angles to the foregoing.

These two tibial diameters may be expressed as a *Platycnemic Index:* trans. cnemic diam./sag. cnemic diam. X 100, with values as follows:

platycnemic or very flat	X–62.9%
mesocnemic or mod. flat	63–69.9%
eurycnemic or broad	70–X%

This concludes this brief *Appendix*. For further details and/or additional end-points and measurements the following list of books may be consulted.

REFERENCES

COMAS, J.: *Manual of Physical Anthropology*. Thomas, Springfield, 1960.

MARTIN, R. and SALLER, K.: *Lehrbuch der Anthropologie* (ed. 3). Gustav Fischer, Stuttgart. In 1956–61 to date there have appeared 11 Lieferungen.

MONTAGU, M. F. A.: *An Introduction to Physical Anthropology* (ed. 3), Thomas, Springfield, 1960.

MONTAGU, M. F. A.: *A Handbook of Anthropometry*. Thomas, Springfield, 1960.

Author Index

Subject Index

A

ABO blood groups, in bone, 235
Adoption, racial problems in, 3
Age-changes, in humerus, seen via X-ray film, 289, 290
Aino, long bones of (*see* Long bones)
Alvar, used on bones, 12, 13
American Indian, 204
American Negro, 62, 156, 158, 162, 164, 165, 168, 181, 182, 184
American white, 156, 158, 162, 164, 165, 168, 181, 182, 184
Amputation, effect on bone (*see* Bone, atrophy of)
Arm, bones of, 301
Arrested growth (*see* "Scars")
"Asians," skeleton of (*see* Skeleton)

B

Bach, skull of, 248
Bear, paw skeleton of, 4
Bentham, Jeremy, skull and portrait of, 248
Birth centers, in skeleton, 19, 20, 59, 60
Blood groups, in bones, 234, 235
Bone (bones)
  atrophy of, in amputation, 235, 236, 237
  blood-type, determined in, 234, 235
  changes in, due to immobilization, 237
  density of
    determined electronically in Pakistan skeletons, 234
    race differences, 233, 234
  growth of
    arm (*see* Arm)
    leg (*see* Leg)
    skull (*see* Skull)

thorax (*see* Thorax)
vertebral column (*see* Vertebral column)
non-human, 4
preservation of
  in situ and in uncovering, 10, 11, 12, 13, 21
weight of
  axial skeleton, 222
  entire skeleton, 222
  foot, 222, 223, 224
  left hand, 224
  (*see also under* Skeletal weight)
Brachial index (*see* Index)
Broadbent-Bolton Roentgenographic Cephalometer, 283
Browne, Sir Thomas, skull and portrait of, 248
Buchanan, George, skull and portrait of, 248, 249, 250, 253
"Buck Ruxton Case," 255ff.

C

Calcification of costal cartilage, 220
Carpal bones, in x-ray film, used for identification, 287, 288
Cartilage, bone preformed in, 18
Cephalic dimensions derived from cranial dimensions on x-ray film, used in identification, 281
Chinese, long bones of (*see* Long bones)
Circumstances, types of, in skeletal identification (*see* Types of cases)
Clavicle, epiphyses of, 51, 52
Collections, skeletal
  Chicago Natural History Museum, 5
  French, by Rollet (Paris), 5
  Hunterian, London, 5, 8